Pediatric
Gastroenterology

Advanced Textbook Series

- *Pediatric Endocrinology,* Wellington Hung, M.D., Gilbert P. August, M.D., and Allen M. Glasgow, M.D.

- *Pediatric Gastroenterology,* edited by Mervin Silverberg, M.D.

IN PREPARATION:

- *Pediatric Cardiology,* Courtney L. Anthony, M.D. and Rica G. Arnon, M.D.

- *Sexual Development and Disorders in Childhood and Adolescence,* edited by Raymond M. Russo, M.D.

An Advanced Textbook

Pediatric Gastroenterology

Edited by

Mervin Silverberg, M.D.
Professor of Pediatrics
Cornell University Medical College
New York, New York
Director, Department of Pediatrics
North Shore University Hospital
Manhasset, New York

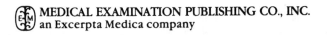

MEDICAL EXAMINATION PUBLISHING CO., INC.
an Excerpta Medica company

Advanced textbook of pediatric gastroenterology.

    Bibliography: p.
    Includes index.
    1. Pediatric gastroenterology. I. Silverberg,
Mervin. (DNLM: 1. Gastrointestinal diseases--
In infancy and childhood. WS 310. C744)
RJ446. C66 1982   618. 92'33   82-8307
ISBN 0-87488-657-0

Printed in the United States of America

notice

The editor and authors and the publisher of this book have
made every effort to ensure that all therapeutic modalities
that are recommended are in accordance with accepted
standards at the time of publication.

The drugs specified within this book may not have specific
approval by the Food and Drug Administration in regard to
the indications and dosages that are recommended by the
editor and authors. The manufacturer's package insert is
the best source of current prescribing information.

To my wife, Gittel, and my children
Shonni, John, Lori, Robbin, Jodi, and Jordanna
with affection and gratitude

Contents

viii   Contents.

Contributors

HARVEY AIGES, M.D., Assistant Professor, Department of Pediatrics, Cornell University Medical College; Senior Assistant Attending, Department of Pediatrics, North Shore University Hospital, New York

EUGENE ARONOW, M.D., Clinical Instructor, Department of Medicine, Cornell University Medical College; Senior Assistant Attending, Department of Medicine, North Shore University Hospital, New York

FREDRIC DAUM, M.D., Associate Professor of Clinical Pediatrics, Cornell University Medical College; Chief, Division of Pediatric Gastroenterology, Department of Pediatrics, North Shore University Hospital, New York

ELLEN KAHN, M.D., Assistant Professor of Pathology, Cornell University Medical College; Attending, Department of Laboratories, North Shore University Hospital, New York

FIMA LIFSHITZ, M.D., Professor of Pediatrics, Cornell University Medical College; Chief, Division of Endocrinology, Metabolism, and Nutrition; Physician-in-Charge, Pediatric Research; Associate Director, Department of Pediatrics, North Shore University Hospital, New York

ARNOLD SCHUSSHEIM, M.D., Assistant Attending, Department of Pediatrics, North Shore University Hospital, New York

DAVID SCHWARTZ, M.D., Senior Assistant Attending, Department of Surgery, North Shore University Hospital, New York

MERVIN SILVERBERG, M.D., Professor of Pediatrics, Cornell University Medical College; Director, Department of Pediatrics, North Shore University Hospital, New York

SAUL TEICHBERG, Ph.D., Assistant Professor, Department of Pediatrics, Cornell University Medical College; Chief, Electron Microscopy Laboratory, Departments of Pediatrics and Laboratories, North Shore University Hospital, New York

RAUL A. WAPNIR, Ph.D., M.P.H., Professor of Biochemistry in Pediatrics, Cornell University Medical College; Head, Pediatric Research Laboratory, Department of Pediatrics, North Shore University Hospital, New York

ASSOCIATE CONTRIBUTORS

MOSHE BERANT, M.D., Associate Professor of Pediatrics, Technion - Faculty of Medicine, Director of Pediatrics B, Rambam Medical Center, Haifa, Israel

ULYSSES FAGUNDES-NETO, M.D., Assistant Professor of Pediatrics, Escola Paulista de Medicina; Chief, Division of Pediatric Gastroenterology, Sao Paulo, Brazil

Foreword

One compelling sign of the fact that pediatric gastroenterology has indeed come of age is the appearance of the Advanced Textbook of Pediatric Gastroenterology, which Mervin Silverberg and his colleagues at North Shore University Hospital, a teaching center of Cornell University Medical College, have compiled. Its range of density reflects this group's interests and accomplishments in the physiologic and nutritional approach to disorders of the gut in infants and children. At a time when new journals devoted to this subspecialty appear almost monthly, it is good to have a vantage point from which to view and measure the impending deluge of new laboratory and clinical research reports. In the Advanced Textbook we have what this experienced and pioneer collaborative enterprise knows, thinks, believes, and advises.

The editor has addressed his compilation to pediatricians, foremost, of course, surgeons, practitioners, and medical students. Practitioners of adult gastroenterology will have to read and consult this volume to see just how "little people" differ from "big people." There is much we have to learn from the study of the growing gut, occupied as we have been with the developed gut and more recently the aging gut. One does not need to be much of a fortune teller to predict that this book will take an active place in all serious libraries of gastroenterology.

Henry D. Janowitz, M.D.
Clinical Professor of Medicine;
Head, Division of Gastroenterology
Mt. Sinai School of Medicine

Preface

In the spring of 1973, I attended the second National Digestive Disease Conference in Airlie House, Virginia, sponsored by the National Institute of Health, Arthritis, Metabolism, and Digestive Diseases. The most outstanding deficiency among the vast array of gastroenterological talent and presentations was the virtual absence of any reference to the problems and diseases in patients under the age of 18. This neglect epitomized the myopic view of many adult gastroenterologists, even at that late date.

The previous year, Dr. **Lawrence Gartner** and I had organized the first society dedicated to pediatric gastroenterology, The Pediatric Gut Club. The organization is now called the North American Society for Pediatric Gastroenterology and has over 150 active members. From these apparently humble beginnings, the field of pediatric gastroenterology has now become a potent force in the clinical and research activities of societies and funding agencies throughout North America. The volume of scientific articles and papers in this specialty during the past decade is very impressive and testifies to the tremendous progress we have made.

These rapid developments and the myriad of unanswered questions they raise leave room for new and fresh approaches to the field. The present textbook emerges from the numerous discussions and often heated arguments generated in one of the largest pediatric gastroenterological centers in the country at North Shore University Hospital. It is a team effort, with contributions by clinicians, biochemists, physiologists, and morphologists, both inside and outside our department. Diversification and variety is subtly introduced by the many different teachers and colleagues each of us has previously encountered. The emphasis in most chapters is true to the basic goals of the book; i.e., the elucidation of etiology, pathogenesis, diagnosis, differential diagnosis, and management. Overlap between chapters is inevitable, but it is hoped that this heterogeneity will add to both completeness and controversy.

The contributors have tried to be as clear and concise as possible. However, a good deal more information is left to motivated readers through the use of the exhaustive bibliography and a good local library.

My apologies go to the few readers who are more involved with and are desirous of new and updated writings in hepatology. We excluded the liver in the interests of keeping the volume modest in size and to qualify as a text exclusively on the gastrointestinal tract and pancreas. The three recently published excellent textbooks on liver disease in children also played a role in our decision.

The book is designed for prospective readers among pediatricians, surgeons, general practitioners, allied medical specialists, and medical students. Hopefully, gastroenterologists will also find new concepts in diagnosis and management, as well as recent research developments, to make this book of value to them. Additionally, the lucid organization of the text is basic enough to be of value to paramedical personnel, such as nurses and basic scientists, from many related biological fields.

I am especially indebted to the department secretarial staff who bore the burden of repeated revisions, modifications, and literature searches in addition to carrying on their extensive daily duties. Particular thanks are due to Evelyn McDonald, who was responsible for the major part of the work on the manuscript, as well as her associates, Louise Gabriel and Linda Thomas.

MORPHOLOGY OF THE GASTROINTESTINAL TRACT

Ellen Kahn, M. D.

GENERAL CHARACTERISTICS

The pharynx, esophagus, stomach, small and large intestines share a certain number of histological characteristics which will be described together. Special attention will be given to identifying patterns characteristic for each of the segments (1-6).

The wall of the gastrointestinal tract is composed of four layers, the mucosa or mucous membrane, submucosa, muscularis or muscularis externa, and adventitia or serosa (Fig. 1).

The mucosa is the innermost layer formed by epithelial elements, lamina propria, and muscularis mucosa.

The epithelium varies in the different segments and will be described in more detail. It assumes a squamous stratified, or glandular pattern, depending on its function—protective or secretory. Admixed with and supporting the epithelium is a layer of reticular connective tissue—the lamina propria—containing elastic, reticulum and collagen fibers, lymphocytes, plasma cells, and eosinophilic granulocytes, as well as lymphatic and blood capillaries. Separating the lamina propria from the submucosa is the muscularis mucosa. It is made up of two thin layers of smooth muscle, an inner circular and an outer longitudinal, connected by elastic fibers and extending to the basement membrane of the epithelium.

The submucosa, situated between the muscularis mucosa and the muscularis externa, is a fibrous connective tissue layer containing blood and lymphatic vessels and a nerve fiber plexus, the submucosal or Meissner plexus, with nonmyelinated, postganglionic sympathetic fibers, and parasympathetic ganglion cells.

The muscularis externa, mainly responsible for contractability, is made up of two large layers of smooth muscle, an inner circular coat and an outer longitudinal one; a helicoidal pattern has been noted in both. A prominent nerve fiber plexus—myenteric or Auerbach plexus—is found between these layers, with preganglionic parasympathetic and postganglionic sympathetic fibers terminating in parasympathetic ganglion cells, and postganglionic parasympathetic fibers terminating in smooth muscle.

The adventitia is the outermost layer of connective tissue which, when covered by a single layer of mesothelial cells, is called serosa.

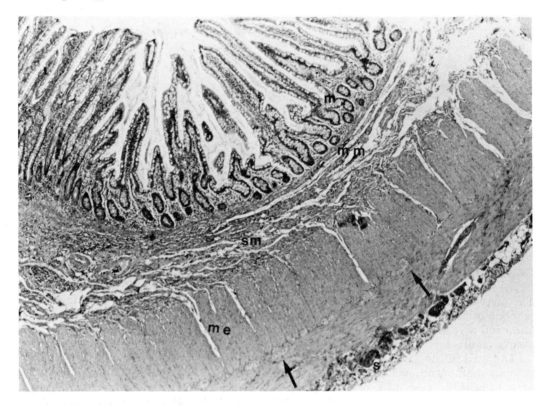

FIGURE 1 General architecture of the gastrointestinal tract: (m) mucosa; (mm) muscularis mucosa; (sm) submucosa; (me) muscularis externa; (s) serosa; (mp) myenteric plexus; arrow. Hematoxylin-eosin stain. Original magnification x 39.

NEUROENDOCRINE CELLS

Specialized cells are found throughout the gastrointestinal tract and because of their association with specific endocrine functions they are called enteroendocrine or neuroendocrine cells.

Initially, these were divided into two groups depending on their ability to reduce silver nitrate: argentaffin cells, containing granules able to reduce silver nitrate, and argyrophilic cells with granules that reduce silver nitrate only in the presence of a chemical reducer. Argentaffin cells may be stained by bichromate salts as well, and also are called enterochromaffin cells.

With the development of different methods of study, specifically electron microscopy and immunofluorescence, new cell types were defined and their function and distribution characterized, including extragastrointestinal sites. These cells, also known as halo cells, have a basal position in relation to the remaining epithelial cells, are oval or triangular, pale with dark-stained granules or agranular (7). Seven types were defined following the Wiesbaden, 1969 nomenclature based on electron microscopic characteristics: A, D, EC, ECL, G, S, and L cells (8).

The A cells secrete enteroglucagon; EC (enterochromaffin cells) are responsible for serotonin production; ECL (enterochromaffinlike cells) store biogenic amines;

G cells secrete gastrin; the S cells, secretin. The function of the D and L cells initially was not established; later, D cells were linked to the production of growth hormone release inhibiting hormone GH-RIH, somatostatin (9). This hormone seems to inhibit the release of secretory granules of the parietal and of the entero-endocrine cells of the gastrointestinal tract.

With the creation of the APUD concept (10), new cell types are defined. APUD stands for amine (amino acids) precursor, uptake, and decarboxylation, and en-compasses a group of cells characterized by a possible common embryonic neural crest origin and common cytochemical and electron microscopic features. The cy-tochemical properties are quite specific for the APUD cells, and consist of the con-tent or uptake of fluorogenic amines (catecholamine, 5-hydroxytryptamine, etc.), the capability to take up amino precursors, such as 5-hydroxytryptophan and dihy-drophenylalanine, and the presence of amino acid decarboxylase. Other cytochemi-cal features, such as metachromasia, content of nonspecific esterase and/or choli-nesterase, and alpha-glycerophosphate dehydrogenase, are less specific.

Ultrastructurally, the neuroendocrine cells share the general morphology of peptide-secreting cells (Fig. 2). More important for their characterization are the membrane-bound granules with variable electrodense cores, surrounded by a pale halo, averaging 100-250 nm. These can be demonstrated by light microscopy with the Grimelius stain, as dark granules, or more specifically by immunofluores-cence, and with the immunoperoxidase method (13). Electron microscopy and im-munocytochemistry resulted in identification of additional cell types and better char-acterization of others already described. These include gastric D1 cells, secreting gastrin inhibitory polypeptide-GIP; intestinal EC cells, motilin-producing; D cells, associated with enterogastrone; ECL cells, responsible for fundin secretion; duo-denal S cells, secretin producing (11); intestinal EG (L cells), originating entero-glucagon (12); and VIP (vasoactive intestinal peptide) H cells. Two types of EC cells were defined (13): the EC1 cells, producing a substance P (peptidelike), and the EC2 cells, secreting motilin. An ECN cell also was recognized as being re-sponsible for an as yet noncharacterized peptide. EC cells also produce melatonine, a substance close to 5-hydrotryptamine.

It is apparent that neuroendocrine cells may store more than one biogenic amine and some of these polypeptides also have been demonstrated in CNS cells (13). Thus the distribution of the neuroendocrine cells in the gastrointestinal tract is now clearly defined, but many problems remain to be resolved such as specific staining characteristics and embryonic origin. Additionally, about 5-20% of these cells are still unclassified (7).

PHARYNX

The general structure was mentioned previously (see Fig. 1). The epithelium of the mucosa is of a nonkeratinizing stratified squamous type, except in the naso-pharynx where it is a pseudostratified columnar ciliated epithelium. It is associated with few glands, and with lymphoid subepithelial nodules corresponding to the pharyngeal tonsil.

Striated muscle forms the muscularis. The adventitial outer layer is fibrous.

ESOPHAGUS

The esophagus obeys the general plan as outlined previously for the gastrointestinal tract.

The esophageal mucosa is covered by thick nonkeratinizing squamous stratified epithelium (Fig. 3) with a few melanoblasts. This epithelium terminates abruptly

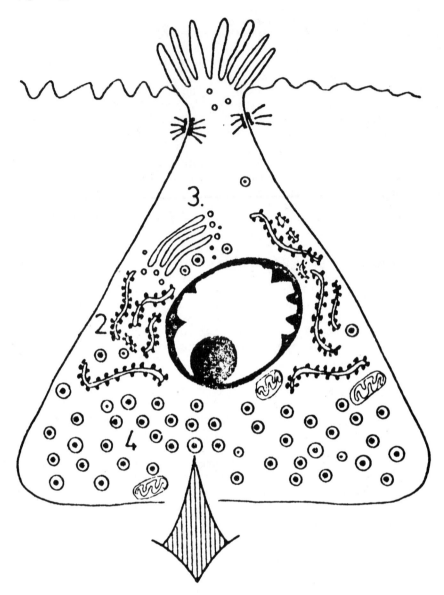

FIGURE 2   Schematic drawing of the principal features of a neuroendocrine cell:
(1) microvilli; (2) rough endoplasmic reticulum; (3) Golgi complex; (4) secretory
granules. (From Ref. 13. Reprinted with permission.)

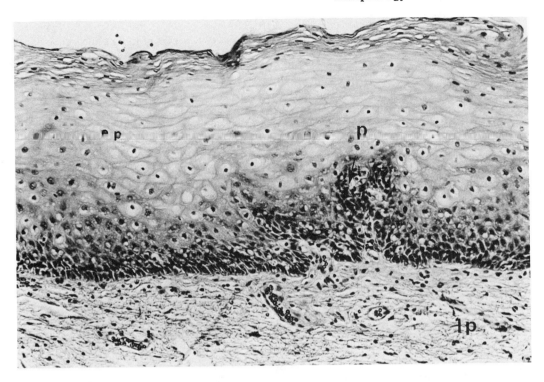

FIGURE 3   Esophageal mucosa. Note the nonkeratinizing squamous stratified epithelium (ep) in the upper half: (lp) lamina propria; (p) papilla; Hematoxylin-eosin stain. Original magnification x 150.

1.5 cm above the distal end of the esophagus, appearing grossly as a gray-pink irregular line. Fingerlike projections of the lamina propria, the papillae, extend halfway up into the surface epithelium and are responsible for the corrugated appearance of the distal esophagus.

Two types of glands are encountered in the esophagus: cardiac and esophageal. The cardiac glands are found in the lamina propria—in the distal and proximal portion of the esophagus—with characteristics, as the name indicates, of those of the cardia (see stomach). The esophageal and cardiac glands are both mucous-secreting, the former situated in the submucosa and predominant in the upper half of the organ.

The muscularis is made up of striated muscle only in the upper third. These are mixed with smooth muscle in the middle third of the esophagus, whereas in the lower third, smooth muscle fibers are the only elements. Only the myenteric plexus is present.

The outer layer is the adventitia with two types of nerves: argyrophilic, controlling coordination of swallowing, and nonargyrophilic, with motor functions.

STOMACH

In addition to the previously noted general architecture, the stomach has the following characteristics:

The <u>mucous membrane</u> varies in the different segments of the stomach, i.e., the cardia, fundus (the portion of the stomach above a horizontal line that passes through the cardia), body pyloric antrum and canal. The body occupies most of the proximal two-thirds and the antrum, the distal third of the organ (Fig. 4). Transitional mucosa between cardia and fundus on the one hand, and body and pyloric mucosa on the other, have a mixed pattern (4), i.e., it contains both cardiac and fundic glands in the former and body and pyloric glands in the latter.

One of the gross characteristics of the gastric mucosa are the folds or <u>rugae</u>. These disappear with distention of the organ and are more prominent in the <u>body</u> than in the antrum. Another gross characteristic of the gastric mucosa are the <u>foveolae</u> or pits noted on the mucosal surface. These are depressions of the surface epithelium into which tubular glands open—about four in each. Surrounded by small amounts of fibrous connective tissue, the pits constitute the superficial layer of the mucosa, the deeper layer being made up of gastric glands. In the fundus and body, the superficial layer occupies 25% (Fig. 5) of the total thickness of mucosa, whereas in the antrum it makes up 50% of that segment.

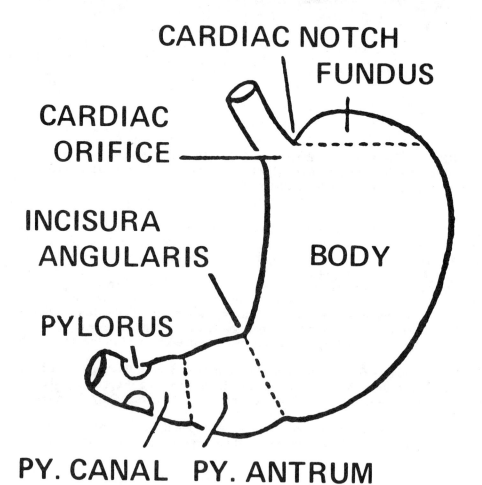

FIGURE 4   Diagram of the different regions of the stomach. (From Ref. 1. Reprinted with permission.)

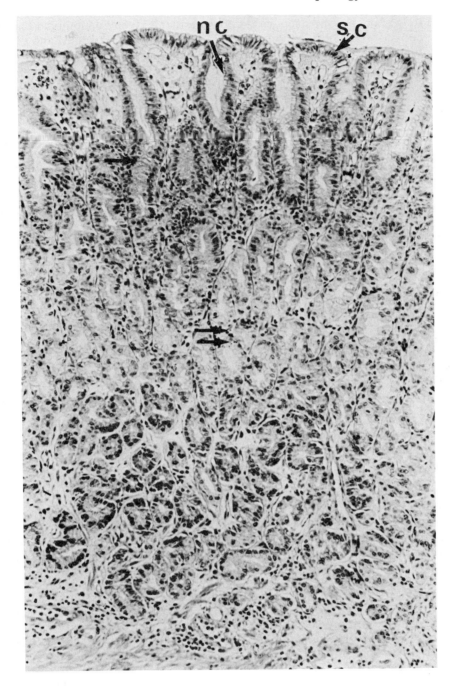

FIGURE 5   Stomach-fundic mucosa with narrow superficial zone (arrow) and deep wide layer (double arrow). Neck mucous cells (nc) are seen in the upper third; (sc) surface epithelial cells. Hematoxylin-eosin stain. Original magnification x 150.

The gastric glands of the deeper layer are branched tubular elements that are coiled in the fundus and body, and straight in the remaining areas. Each gland is made up of three segments: deep, middle, and upper, respectively called base, neck, and isthmus. The last is in continuity with the gastric pits. The neck region represents the active growth zone responsible for rapid cell proliferation (2).

The main epithelial cell types encountered in the gastric mucosa are: surface epithelium, parietal or oxyntic cells, neck mucous cells, and zymogen or chief cells (14).

The surface epithelial cells are uniform, tall, columnar, mucous-producing cells (neutral mucopolysaccharides) (15) with basal nuclei (see Fig. 5). As the name indicates these cells are encountered on the mucosal surface admixed with few parietal and chief cells; foveolae are also lined by these cells.

Parietal cells have a round or triangular shape, pink granular cytoplasm in the hematoxylin-eosin stain, and dark central nuclei (Fig. 6). These cells are responsible for secretion of hydrochloric acid and intrinsic factor, although other investigators consider the chief cells as the source of intrinsic factor (2).

The neck mucous cells are cells with pale, foamy cytoplasm, basal nuclei (see Fig. 5) containing PAS-positive, diastase-resistant mucus, and characterized by histochemical stains as an acid nonsulfated mucopolysaccharide. These cells are encountered in the neck portion of the gastric glands.

Chief cells have a pale cytoplasm with basal basophilic granules (see Fig. 6). These cells are responsible for secretion of pepsinogen, lipase, and renin.

The distribution of the different cells varies with the anatomical regions of the stomach and glandular site. Therefore, three different glands are considered: cardiac, fundic or body, and antral glands.

The cardiac glands, restricted to an area 1 cm distal to the cardioesophageal junction, are composed of cells similar to the surface epithelial cells. All types of cells are encountered in the fundic or body glands. The base of the gland contains chief and parietal cells. Neck mucous cells predominate in the neck, admixed with a few parietal cells, whereas the isthmus is made up of parietal and surface epithelial cells. The antral (pyloric) glands are not necessarily restricted to the pylorus. These are found immediately close to the pylorus at the greater curvature, but may extend to the incisura angularis along the lesser curvature (4). The appearance is similar to that of cardiac glands, being composed of neck mucous cells.

Less common but functionally very important cells deserve special mention: the immature and specialized cells. The former are found in the isthmus and neck region of the glands and give rise to the surface epithelial cells and probably to the neck mucous and parietal cells (1). The specialized type of cells are the neuroendocrine cells.

Gastrin-secreting cells (G cells) are encountered in the stomach predominantly in the antrum (7, 16), but also can be found in the cardia (17) and fundus. Considered argyrophilic by some (10), and an heterogenic group with silver-positive and silver-negative cells by others (8), they are identifiable by special staining procedures such as Herlant tetrachrome (8) or by immunoperoxidase techniques (18).

Most cells are of the ECL type and predominate in the body (7), and may be related to histamine production. Next in frequency are the D cells noted in the fundic and body mucosa. The EC cells are found in the antral mucosa only and S cells are present also in the antrum (11).

The remaining histological characteristics of the gastric wall include lymphoid follicles in the lamina propria of the antrum that increase in number with age; a muscularis mucosa made up of three layers of smooth muscle; a submucosa which might contain few glands close to the pylorus; a muscularis externa with three muscle layers—an internal oblique, a middle circular, and an outer longitudinal; and finally, an outer layer with the characteristics of the serosa.

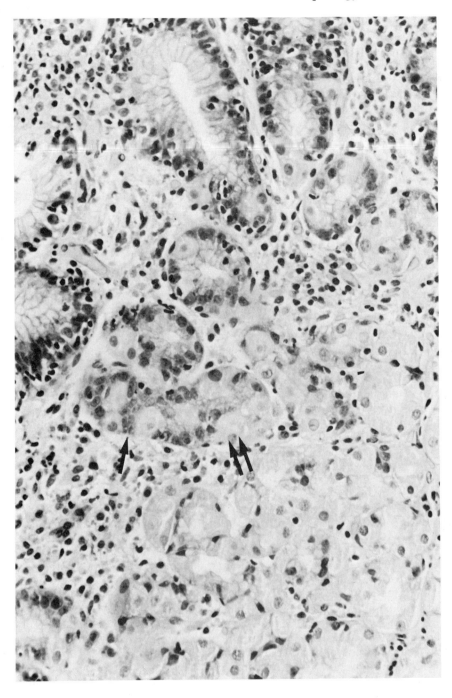

FIGURE 6   Stomach-fundic mucosa. Chiefs cells (arrow) stain dark and parietal cells, (double arrow) are lighter. Hematoxylin-eosin stain. Original magnification x 150.

SMALL INTESTINE

The mucous membrane of the small intestine is characterized by mucosal folds, plicae circularis or valves of Kerkring, and villi. Mucous folds, noted with the naked eye, are made up of mucosa and a portion of submucosa which forms the central core (Fig. 7). These folds persist with distention of the organ, are more developed in the jejunum, and decrease in size distally. They are absent in the lower ileum. Villi are mucosal folds visible only with a magnifying glass. They decrease in size distally and have different shapes, such as broad, short, and leaflike in the duodenum as a result of lateral fusion of two to three fingerlike villi; tonguelike in the jejunum; and more distally, fingerlike villi. The villous pattern may vary as well with different ethnic groups. Biopsies from Africans, Indians, South Vietnamese, and Haitians when compared with biopsies from North Americans and English (4), have shorter, thicker villi, an increased number of leaf-shaped villi, and more mononuclear cells in the lamina propria.

Various methods are suggested to determine the normal villous height. For practical purposes, the height of a normal villus should be more than half of the total thickness of the mucous membrane (20), or considering the villus/crypt ratio, the villi are three to five times as long as the crypts (Fig. 8). The villus has a fibrous connective tissue core with the general characteristic of a lamina propria and contains smooth muscle, one artery, a capillary meshwork, nerve fibers, and a central lymphatic or lacteal. The villi are covered by epithelial cells described next (see Figs. 8, 9).

Two types of glands are encountered in the small intestine: the Brunner glands and the Lieberkuhn crypts. The first are submucosal glands (Fig. 10) found specifically in the first portion of the duodenum and decrease in number in the distal duodenum. These glands also may be present in the pylorus and in the proximal jejunum, especially in children (21). The Brunner glands open into the Lieberkuhn crypts and morphologically resemble the pyloric glands. The Lieberkuhn are tubular glands that dip from the surface to the muscularis mucosa between the villi.

The main epithelial cell types are as follows: absorptive cells (also called columnar cells), goblet cells, Paneth cells, and enteroendocrine cells.

The absorptive cells are high columnar cells with oval, basal nuclei, eosinophilic cytoplasm with a PAS-positive free surface—the brush border (see Fig. 9). The goblet cells are oval or round, with a flattened basal nucleus and basophilic, metachromatic, PAS-positive cytoplasm (see Fig. 9), with sulfated and neutral mucoproteins. Paneth cells are flask-shaped, with a broad base against the basement membrane, and eosinophilic granular cytoplasm. The function of the Paneth cells is controversial. They contain zinc and secrete lysoenzymes, are considered as a nutritional unit for crypt epithelium and primitive goblet cells, and are said to have digestive functions (22).

The enteroendocrine cells found in the small intestine are S cells, Dl (K cells), EG, EC, H, and D cells, associated respectively with secretion of secretin, gastrin inhibitory polypeptide (GIP), enteroglucagon, motilin, 5-hydroxytryptamine, vasoactive intestinal polypeptide (VIP), and somatostatin (23-25). Intestinal I cells are linked to the production of cholecystokinin (CCK) (26), also known as pancreozymin, which is related to the control of pancreatic growth and gastric emptying. N cells are responsible for neurotensin secretion (27). Another peptide, bombesin, has been localized by immunofluorescence in the nonenterochromaffin P cells of the gastrointestinal tract, predominantly in the duodenal mucosa (27, 28). Bombesin controls gastric acid and pancreatic secretion.

The proportion of the above cells differs in the villi and crypt as well as in different segments of the intestine. Ninety percent of the epithelial cells of the villi are absorptive cells intermingled with some goblet and a few enteroendocrine cells. The proportion of the goblet to the absorptive cells increases towards the ileum.

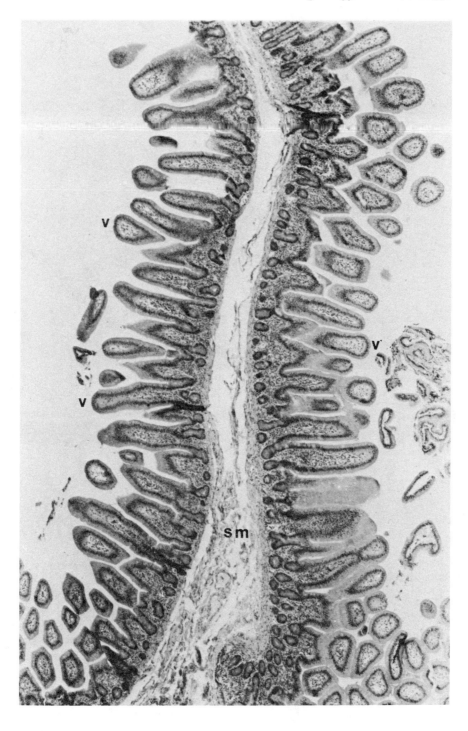

FIGURE 7   Ileum. Mucosal fold having as axis the submucosa (sm) and covered by villi (v). Hematoxylin-eosin stain. Original magnification x 39.

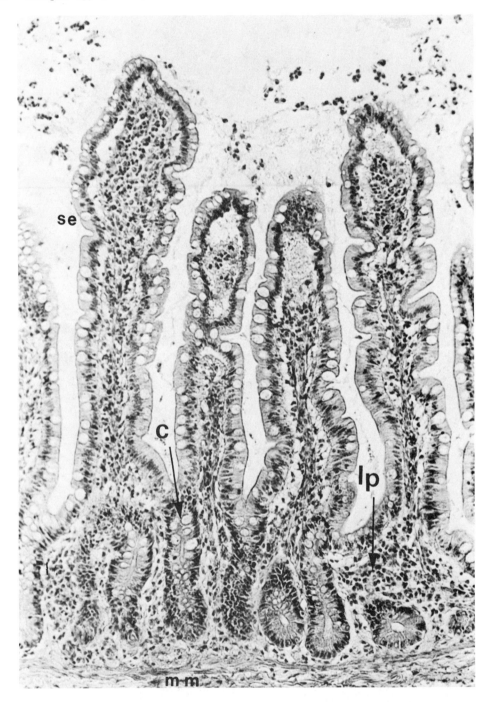

FIGURE 8   Jejunum. Fingerlike villi, three times as long as crypts: (Se) surface epithelium; (lp) lamina propria; (c) crypt; (mm) muscularis mucosa. Hematoxylin-eosin stain. Original magnification x 150.

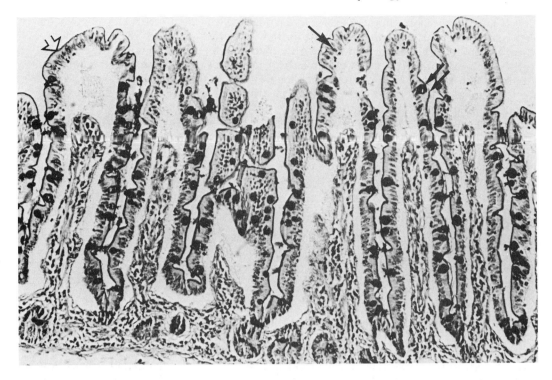

FIGURE 9 Ileum. Villi with absorptive cells (arrow) and goblet cells (double arrow). Brush border (open arrow). PAS stain. Original magnification x 150.

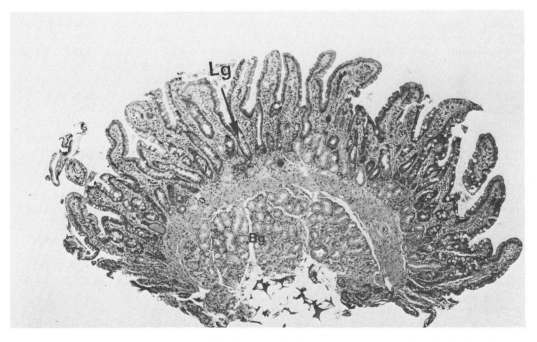

FIGURE 10 Duodenum. Brunner glands (Bg) and Lieberkuhn crypt (Lg). Hematoxylin-eosin stain. Original magnification x 39.

All four types of epithelial cells are encountered in the Lieberkuhn crypt. Paneth and cylindrical cells predominate in the base of the crypt. Above the base, absorptive cells are found with a few oligomucin cells giving origin to the goblet cells which predominate in the upper half of the crypt. Enteroendocrine cells are admixed with goblet cells. A few lymphocytes and other white blood cells, as well as globular leukocytes with basophilic granules similar to mast cells, are found between the epithelial cells.

Smooth muscle is encountered in the lamina propria of the small intestinal villus extending from the muscularis mucosa parallel to its axis. Plasma cells containing mainly IgA have been identified as well as a few associated with IgM and IgG production. Mast cells are present. Lymphoid tissue is prominent in the lamina propria as solitary nodules and as confluent masses, i.e., Peyer patches. They are seen in the submucosa as well. Peyer patches, distributed along the antimesenteric border, are more numerous in the terminal ileum and the number decreases with age (1).

No other special features are noted in the remaining layers of the small intestine.

LARGE INTESTINE

The mucous membrane of the large intestine is characterized by the presence of Lieberkuhn crypts, which are associated predominantly with goblet cells (Fig. 11) intermixed with a few cylindrical and enteroendocrine cells. These consist of H, EG, and EC cells secreting, respectively, VIP, enteroglucagon, and 5-hydroxytryptamine (12, 25). Paneth cells are scarce, noted only in the proximal colon especially in children. The lamina propria of the large intestine contains solitary lymphoid follicles extending into the submucosa. They are more developed in the rectum and decrease in number with age; confluent lymphoid tissue is present in the appendix. Macrophages predominate in the subepithelial portion of the lamina propria. These are weakly PAS-positive and are associated with stainable lipids (29). IgA-producing plasma cells are seen in the deeper portions.

The submucosal (Meissner) plexus in the rectum has been widely studied. Ganglion cells are distributed in two layers: a deep submucosal one adjacent to the inner muscular coat, and a superficial submucosal plexus close to the muscularis mucosa (30), which is accessible to rectal suction biopsy. Ganglion cells are scarce in a physiological hypoganglionic segment 1 cm above the anal margin. A suction biopsy for identification of these cells of the submucous plexus should therefore be taken proximal to this area. Ganglion cells usually are easily identified as large cells, isolated or grouped in small clusters, with an abundant basophilic cytoplasm, a large vesicular round nucleus, and a prominent nucleolus (see Fig. 11). In premature infants, ganglion cells may look like neuroblasts with scanty cytoplasm and a hyperchromatic nucleus. This can constitute a problem for their recognition. The normal submucosal plexus has a low acetylcholinesterase activity (6).

A well-developed myenteric plexus is seen between the circular and longitudinal layer of the muscularis externa.

The longitudinal layer of the muscularis condenses from cecum to rectum in longitudinal bands (the teniae coli) with sacculations (haustrae) between them. In the rectum the teniae fuse in anterior and posterior thick coats resulting in two transverse folds that protrude internally, the plicae transversalis.

The serosa separates focally in sacculations containing adipose tissue—the appendices epiploicae.

The anal canal has upper and lower demarcations (Fig. 12): proximally, the anorectal ring which is composed of the upper portion of the internal sphincter, the

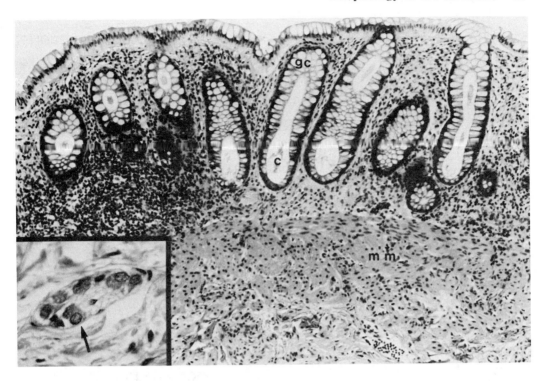

FIGURE 11   Colon. Mucosa with Lieberkuhn crypts (c). Note the predominance of goblet cells (gc) over absorptive cells: (Mm) muscularis mucosa. Hematoxylin-eosin stain. Original magnification x 150. Insert: ganglion cells of the superficial submucosal plexus (arrow). Hematoxylin eosin stain. Original magnification x 500.

longitudinal muscle of the large intestine, the deep portion of the external sphincter, and the puborectalis portion of the levator ani; and distally, the anal verge, consisting of the transition of anal skin to true skin. The internal landmarks can be divided into microscopic and gross anatomical. The first consists of three zones: proximal (P), intermediate or pecten (I), and distal (D) or anal skin. The proximal zone is lined by stratified cuboidal epithelium. The transition with the rectal mucosa, lined by high columnar mucous producing cells, is called the anorectal histological junction. The pecten is lined by stratified squamous epithelium not associated with adnexa. Its proximal margin, in contact with the proximal anal mucosa, is called the dentate line; its distal margin in contact with the anal skin constitutes the pectinate line, also referred to as the mucocutaneous junction. The anal skin is lined by squamous stratified epithelium associated with hair and sebaceous glands. The gross internal anatomical landmarks of the anal canal are the columns of Morgagni—six to 12 longitudinal mucosal folds in the microscopic proximal zone. Their distal fused ends are the anal valves. These are situated approximately at the level of the dentate line; branched tubular apocrine sweat glands open at this level—the anal glands.

The muscularis mucosa disappears in the anorectal canal, and the inner circular coat of the muscularis thickens, forming the internal anal sphincter. The sphincter ani externus muscle constitutes the external anal sphincter. It has a

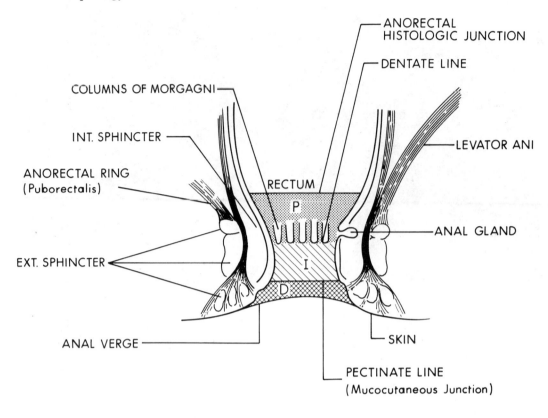

FIGURE 12   Schematic drawing of the anal canal: (P) proximal anal zone; (I) intermediate; (D) distal anal zone (see text).

superficial tendinous and a deeper muscular component, and surrounds the anal canal.

PANCREAS

The pancreas is both anatomically and physiologically related to the gastrointestinal tract. Its dual role as exocrine and endocrine gland, makes this organ a crucial center of the digestive system.

Two major components are found in the pancreas: stroma and parenchyma. The former is represented by the capsule and septae, the latter by the ducts and lobules.

Fibrous connective tissue covered by the peritoneum constitutes the capsule. Thin capsular extensions into the parenchyma form the interlobular septae, separating the parenchyma into lobules.

The ductal system is represented by the main pancreatic duct (the Wirsung duct) from which interlobular branches originate, the latter being located in the interlobular septae (Fig. 13). These branches are in continuity with the intralobular ducts that terminate in the ducts connecting the acini with the ductal system, the intercalated ducts. Those ducts that are of large diameter are surrounded by fibrous

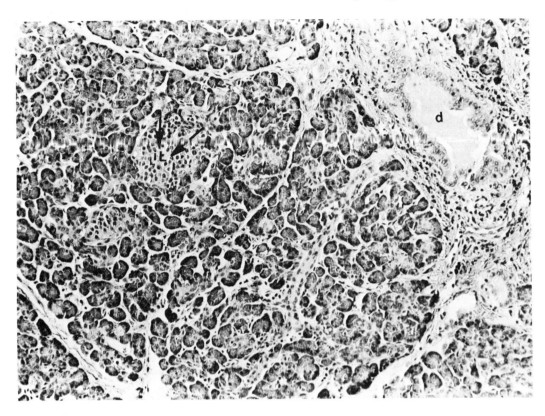

FIGURE 13   Pancreas.   Lobules at left with several islets of Langerhans (il) (arrows). Interlobular duct (d) at right. Hematoxylin-eosin stain. Original magnification x 150.

connective tissue and are associated with high columnar epithelium, a few goblet cells, and isolated glands near the duodenum. Interlobular ducts are lined by low epithelium with few goblet cells and enteroendocrine cells; cuboidal or flattened epithelium is encountered in the intralobular and intercalated ducts, respectively.

The lobules are composed of acini and islets of Langerhans, the exocrine and endocrine components of the pancreas (see Fig. 13). The acini are made up of a ring of pyramidal cells with bases adjacent to the basement membrane and an apex limiting a narrow lumen. Their basophilic cytoplasm contains eosinophil zymogenic granules and a basal nucleus. A few centrally located, flattened, pale cells, the centroacinar cells, represent the beginning of the ductal system in continuity with the intercalated ducts (31).

The islets of Langerhans constitute 1-2% of the parenchyma. More numerous in the tail (32), these appear in the hematoxylin-eosin stain as pale, round areas made up of cords of cells with pale cytoplasm and moderately chromatic, round nuclei, separated by capillaries (see Fig. 13).

Special stains, such as the aldehydefuchsin trichrome method of Gomori, allow the differentiation into four cell types: alpha or A, beta or B, C, and D cells. Sixty to seventy percent of the endocrine cells are B cells, with alcohol soluble granules, appearing blue by the Gomori stain (133). Alcohol insoluble, deep purple granules with the Gomori stain, characterize A cells (20-30% of the total). C cells are agranular cells, whereas D cells (2-8% of the total) are argentaffin. The A cells can be divided into two groups (34): A1 and A2. They are distinguished by localization, difference in cellular and nuclear size, cytoplasmic granules, and cytochemical characteristics. The A1 cells, for example, are argyrophilic, metachromatic, and have a high content of tryptophan (34).

D cells may represent degranulated to poorly granulated B cells (35). Others consider C and D cell variation in the secretory cycle (31) a degenerative stage of A and B cells, or equivalent to A1 cells (22). D, A, and B cells interrelate. The A cells predominate in the periphery of islets, associated with few D cells. The B cells are more numerous in the center, and as such are responsible for a stable release of insulin, whereas sudden release of insulin is related to the periphery (36).

Currently four or perhaps five types of islet cells are recognized by electron microscopy and are characterized by a certain shape and size of their neurosecretory granules and their hormone and polypeptide secretion (37). B and A (A2 cells), with 200-250 nm neurosecretory granules, secrete insulin and glucagon respectively. D (A1 cells), with neurosecretory granules of 300-350 nm, are linked to the secretion of somatostatin (38), and probably also to glucagon and gastrin. A fourth type of cell, PP cells, with neurosecretory granules in the range of 100-150 nm, produces human pancreatic polypeptide (HPP), and a not well-defined D1 cell is linked to the secretion of VIP. The hormone HPP seems to increase the bile duct tone and the secretion of bicarbonate, and to inhibit gallbladder tone and the output of pancreatic enzyme (39). Under pathological conditions, such as tumors, different polypeptides can be produced (40, 41).

REFERENCES

1. Ham, W.: Histology, 7th ed. J. B. Lippincott Co., Philadelphia, 1974.

2. Greep, R.O. and L. Weiss: Histology. McGraw Hill Book Co., New York, 1973.

3. Sobotta-Hammersten, F.: Histology—A Color Atlas of Cytology, Histology and Microscopic Anatomy. Lea & Febiger, Philadelphia, 1976.

4. Whitehead, R.: Mucosal Biopsy of the Gastrointestinal Tract, 2nd ed. W.B. Saunders Co., Philadelphia, 1979.

5. Morson, B.C. and J.H. Yardley: Inflammatory and Neoplastic Disease of the Gastrointestinal Tract. Williams & Wilkins, Baltimore, 1977.

6. Meier-Ruge, W.: Current topics in pathology. Ergeb Pathol 59:131, 1974.

7. Rubin, W.: Endocrine cells in the normal human stomach. A fine structural study. Gastroenterology 63:784, 1972.

8. Bencosme, S.A. and J. Lechago: Staining procedures for the endocrine cells of the upper gastrointestinal mucosa. Light-electron microscopic correlation for the gastrin-producing cells. J Clin Pathol 26:427, 1973.

9.   Polak, J. M., L. Grimelius, A. G. E. Pearse, S. R. Bloom and A. Arimura: Growth hormone release—inhibiting hormone in gastrointestinal and pancreatic D cells. Lancet 1:1220, 1975.

10. Pearse, A. G. E.: The APUD cell concept and its implication in pathology. Pathol Annu 9:27, 1974.

11. Chey, W. Y. and R. Escoffery: Secretin cells in the gastrointestinal tract. Endocrinology 98:1390, 1976.

12. Gould, R. P.: The APUD cell system. Rec Adv Histopathol 10:1, 1978.

13. Larsson, L. I.: Pathology of gastrointestinal cells. Scand J Gastroenterol 53 (suppl 14):1, 1979.

14. Padykula, H. A.: The Digestive Tract. in Histology. R. O. Greep and L. Weiss (eds.). McGraw-Hill Book Co., 1973, p. 643.

15. Gad, A.: A histochemical study of human alimentary tract mucosubstances in health and disease. Br J Cancer 23:52, 1969.

16. McGuigan, J. E., M. H. Greider and L. Grawe: Staining characteristics of the gastrin cell. Gastroenterology 62:959, 1972.

17. Jackson, B. M., D. D. Reeder, J. R. Searcy, L. C. Watson, F. M. Hirose, and J. C. Thompson: Correlation of the surface pH, histology and gastrin concentration of the gastric mucosa. Ann Surg 176:727, 1972.

18. Piris, J. and R. Whitehead: An immunoperoxidase technique for the identification of gastrin-producing cells. J Clin Pathol 27:798, 1974.

19. McGuigan, J. E. and M. H. Greider: Correlative immunochemical and light microscopic studies of the gastrin cells of the antral mucosa. Gastroenterology 60:223, 1970.

20. Fontaine, L. and J. Navarro: Small intestinal biopsy in cow's milk protein allergy in infancy. Arch Dis Child 50:357, 1975.

21. Landboe-Christenson, E.: The duodenal glands of Brunner in man, their distribution and quantity. Acta Pathol Microbiol Scand 52 (suppl):240, 1944.

22. Subbuswamy, S. G.: Paneth cells and goblet cells. J Pathol 111:181, 1973.

23. Polak, J. M., A. G. E. Pearse, J. C. Garaud, and S. R. Bloom: Cellular localization of vasoactive intestinal peptide in the mammalian and avian gastrointestinal tract. Gut 15:720, 1974.

24. Bolande, R.: The neurocrestopathies. A unifying concept of diseases arising in neural maldevelopment. Hum Pathol 5:409, 1974.

25. Welbourn, R. B., A. G. E. Pearse, J. M. Polak, S. R. Bloom, and S. N. Jaffee: The APUD cells in the alimentary tract in health and disease. Med Clin N Am 58:1359, 1974.

26.   Polak, J. M. , S. R. Bloom, P. L. Rayford, A. G. E. Pearse, A. M. J. Buchan, and J. C. Thomson: Identification of cholecystokinin-secreting cells. Lancet 2:1016, 1975.

27.   Holstein, J. : Gut endocrine tumor syndrome. Clin Endocrinol Metab 8:413, 1979.

28.   Polak, J. M. , S. Hobbs, S. R. Bloom, and E. Solcia: Distribution of a bombesin-like peptide in human gastrointestinal tract. Lancet 1:1109, 1976.

29.   Eidelman, S. and D. Lagunoff: The morphology of the normal human rectal biopsy. Hum Pathol 3:389, 1972.

30.   Aldridge, R. T. and P. E. Campbell: Ganglion cell distribution in the normal rectum and anal canal. A basis for the diagnosis of Hirschprung disease by anorectal biopsy. J Pediatr Surg 3:475, 1968.

31.   Ito, S. : The pancreas. in Histology. R. O. Greep and L. Weiss (eds.). McGraw-Hill Book Co. , New York, 1973, p. 747.

32.   Wittingen, J. and C. F. Frey: Islet concentration in the head, body and tail and uncinate process of the pancreas. Ann Surg 179:412, 1974.

33.   Thomson, O. F. : Staining of the beta-cells in pancreatic islets by an indirect immunofluorescence method on Bouin-fixed, paraffin-embedded tissue. Acta Pathol Microbiol Scand Sect A 79:497, 1971.

34.   Hellerstrom, C. and B. Hellman: Some aspects of silver impregnation of the islets of Langerhans in the rat. Acta Endocr (KBH)35:518, 1960.

35.   Warren, S. , P. Le Compte, and M. A. Logg: The Pathology of Diabetes Mellitus. Lea & Febiger, Philadelphia, 1966.

36.   Orci, L. and R. H. Unger: Functional subdivision of islets of Langerhans and possible role of D cells. Lancet 2:1243, 1975.

37.   Kostianovsky, M. : Endocrine pancreatic tumors, ultrastructures. Ann Clin Lab Sci 10:65, 1980.

38.   Orci, L. , D. Baetens, C. Rufener, M. Amherdt, M. Ravazolla, P. Studer, F. Malaisse-Lagae, and R. H. Unger: Hypertrophy and hyperplasia of somatostatin containing D cells in diabetes. Proc Natl Acad Sci 73:1338, 1976.

39.   Polak, J. M. , T. E. Adrian, M. G. Bryant, S. R. Bloom, P. Heitz, and A. G. E. Pearse: Pancreatic polypeptides in insulinomas, gastrinomas, vipomas and glucagonomas. Lancet 1:328, 1976.

40.   Bloom, S. R. , J. M. Polak and A. G. E. Pearse: Vasoactive intestinal peptides and watery diarrhea syndrome. Lancet 2:14, 1973.

41.   Larsson, L. I. : Human pancreatic polypeptides, vasoactive intestinal polypeptides and watery diarrhea syndrome. Lancet 2:149, 1976.

2

ULTRASTRUCTURE OF GASTROINTESTINAL CELLS

Saul Teichberg, Ph. D.

INTRODUCTION

Many of the relationships between the structure of cellular organelles and the organization of metabolic functions have been revealed by recent advances in cell biology (1). Some organelles undergo characteristic structural alterations that reflect altered function under pathophysiological conditions. Many of the typical cellular organelles and illustrations of the structure-function relationships seen in all cells of the gastrointestinal tract are found in intestinal absorptive epithelial cells. This discussion will begin with a detailed analysis of the ultrastructure of the intestinal epithelial cell, followed by a limited discussion of the key differentiating features of other prominent cell types of the intestinal tract.

BASIC ULTRASTRUCTURE OF INTESTINAL EPITHELIUM

Absorptive epithelial cells are filled with a variety of organelles including a nucleus, nucleolus, rough and smooth endoplasmic reticulum (ER), mitochondria, microbodies, Golgi apparatus, lysosomes, and fat droplets (Figs. 1, 2). The cell is surrounded by a plasma membrane that is specialized at different regions of the cell surface.

PLASMA MEMBRANE AND ITS SPECIALIZATIONS

Membrane Structure

The plasma membrane of the epithelial cell has a typical bimolecular lipoprotein "unit" structure (1-3). When studied by transmission electron microscopy, the membrane is 75-100 Å wide and appears as two electron dense lines separated by a clear space (Figs. 3, 4). It has now been shown that there are proteins, mucopolysaccharides, and glycolipids that extend out of either the extracellular or cytoplasmic surface of the plasma membrane or extend across the entire membrane (3, 4). Some of the proteins and other cell surface molecules serve significant receptor, enzymatic, transport, and antigenic roles (1,3,5). For example, cell

LUMEN

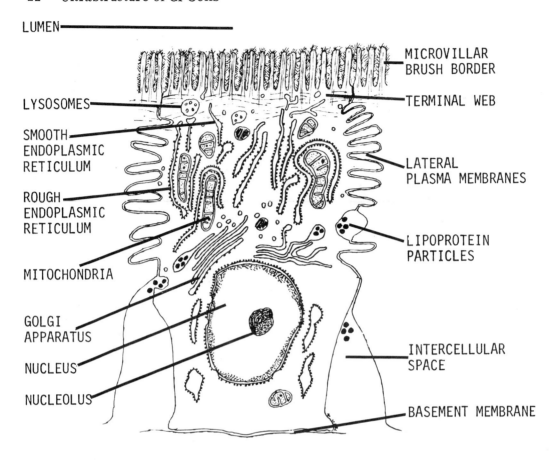

MICROVILLAR
BRUSH BORDER

TERMINAL WEB

LYSOSOMES

SMOOTH
ENDOPLASMIC
RETICULUM

LATERAL
PLASMA MEMBRANES

ROUGH
ENDOPLASMIC
RETICULUM

LIPOPROTEIN
PARTICLES

MITOCHONDRIA

GOLGI
APPARATUS

INTERCELLULAR
SPACE

NUCLEUS

NUCLEOLUS

BASEMENT MEMBRANE

FIGURE 1   Diagram illustrating the basic organization of the small intestinal absorptive epithelial cell.   The microvillar brush border with its fuzzy coat contains
digestive enzymes and is the principal site of absorption of dipeptides, amino
acids, monosaccharides, and fatty acids.   The lateral plasma membranes probably contain Na+-K+ ATPase activity and are also probably the site of cyclic nu-
cleotide (cAMP) metabolism.   Lipoprotein particles, synthesized on the endoplasmic reticulum are seen being packaged in the Golgi apparatus and released by exocytosis into the intercellular space.   Numerous cellular filaments form a meshwork in the terminal web region: these filaments interact with the fine actinlike
filaments of the microvilli and with junctional complex associated filaments.   The
absorptive cell nucleus is basally located.

surface receptors recognize and bind peptide hormones such as insulin, viral attachment to the surface of a particular cell is dependent upon appropriate surface
receptors, and transport enzymes such as the Na+-K+ATPase are thought to be
integrally incorporated into the plasma membrane.   Many of the proteins and lipids
within the plasma membrane may be laterally mobile within the basic bimolecular
lipid structure (3, 6, 7) a process beautifully illustrated in the case of lymphocyte
capping.

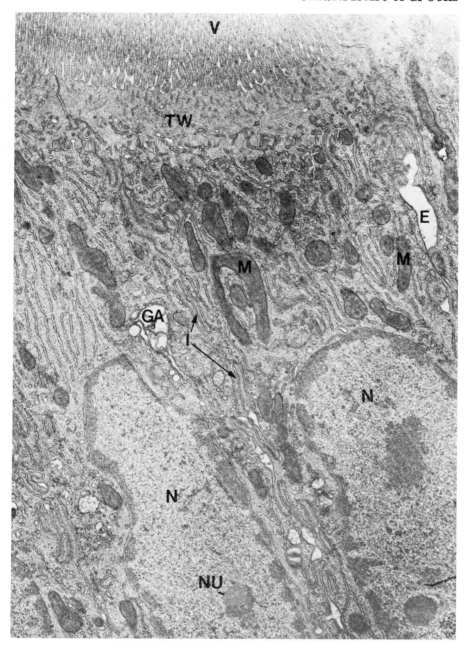

FIGURE 2   Low power electron micrograph of several jejunal absorptive epithelial cells: microvilli (V); terminal web (TW); smooth endoplasmic reticulum (SER);
rough endoplasmic reticulum (RER); mitochondria (M); Golgi apparatus (GA); nuclei (N); nucleolus (NU); interdigitating plasma membrane (I); extracellular space
(E). Original magnification x 10,500.

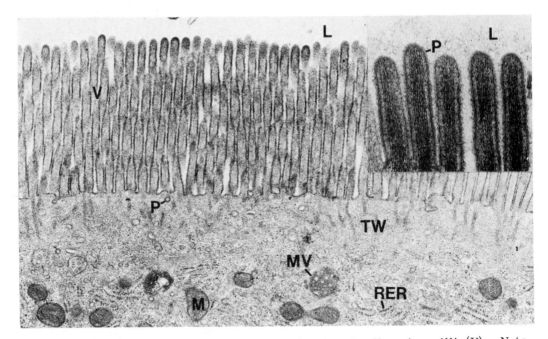

FIGURE 3   Apical portion of an absorptive epithelial cell: microvilli (V). Note the thin microvillar filaments that extend through the core of the microvilli and into the terminal web (TW) region: intestinal lumen (L); mitochondrion (M); rough endoplasmic reticulum (RER); pinocytotic vesicle (P); and a multivesicular body (MV). Original magnification x 17,500. Insert: tips of microvilli containing thin microvillar filaments. From the surface of the microvillar plasma membrane (P) there extend into the lumen (L) many fine branching filaments. These surface filaments contain intestinal disaccharidases and are composed of acid mucopolysaccharides. Original magnification x 30,000.

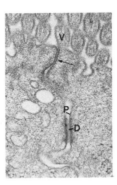

FIGURE 4   Two adjacent absorptive epithelial cells with a specialized junctional complex are seen. Immediately beneath the microvilli (V) the plasma membranes of the two cells appear to fuse at several points (arrow) to form a tight junction that is a barrier to the passage of macromolecules from the intestinal lumen. A desmosome is seen at D. Here the intercellular space widens but is filled with amorphous material that forms a single electron-dense line down the center. Cytoplasmic densities are seen immediately adjacent to the plasma membranes (P) and from these densities there extend numerous filaments. Original magnification x 40,000.

Microvilli

One surface of the absorptive epithelial cell faces the intestinal lumen. In this region the cell surface is thrown into an enormous number of microvillar folds (see
Figs. 1-5) which amplify the surface area (8).

Fine branching filaments, composed of acid mucopolysaccharides (8, 9) project
toward the intestinal lumen from the microvillar plasma membrane (see Fig. 3).
The microvillar surface is probably an important digestive site since it contains
most of the cells' disaccharidase activity as well as alkaline phosphatase (10, 11).
Inside the core of the microvilli there are fine filaments that run along the microvillar axis (see Figs. 3, 5). In addition to their obvious architectural function,
these filaments are composed of an actinlike protein and may be involved in microvillar motile processes (12).

Junctional Complexes

At the apical lateral margins of adjacent epithelial cells there is an elaborate
junctional complex (8, 13). Next to the intestinal lumen the plasma membranes of
adjacent cells come very close together to form a tight junction (see Figs. 4, 5)
that surrounds the cell like a belt (8). The tight junction is probably a morphological barrier to the passage of macromolecules from the intestinal lumen directly
into the circulation (8, 14). This barrier can break down under certain conditions
of experimental stress such as malnutrition (15), surgical trauma (16), luminal
hyperosmolality (17), or bile salt deconjugation in the upper small intestine (18)
(reviewed in Ref. 19). During early normal neonatal life and most of infancy, maternal milk antibodies and various antigens are able to selectively cross the intestinal epithelium (14); immunoglobulin G molecules particularly, are pinocytosed at
the luminal surface and exocytosed at the basolateral margins of the cell (14).
Immediately beneath the tight junction there is an intermediate zone where the intracellular space is filled with an amorphous material (8, 13) (see Fig. 5). This
is followed by a desmosomal region, which consists of distinct buttonlike attachment zones (see Figs. 4, 5) thought to function principally as cell-binding sites.
The intercellular space between plasma membranes in this region contains a characteristic thin electron-dense line.

Beneath the junctional complex, the lateral plasma membranes of adjacent cells
interdigitate over extensive distances (see Figs. 1, 2, 5). Occasionally, the intercellular space between adjacent cells widens and it may be filled with lipidlike particles (8, 20) (see Fig. 1). At the base of the epithelial cell there is a thin basement membrane.

In addition to tight junctions and desmosomes, cell-to-cell contact may occur
by means of "gap" junctions. In this region cells come into close contact (20-40 Å)
and appear to create a structural continuity sufficient for the passage of small
molecules. Cells which "communicate" by being able to exchange ions and small
molecules usually also have gap junctions (1, 4, 21). Communication through gap
junctions is a property of many epithelia (21).

NUCLEUS

Absorptive epithelial cells contain a basally located nucleus (see Figs. 1, 2). The
nuclei often contain a prominent nucleolus (see Figs. 1, 2). The nucleolus is the
site of ribosomal RNA synthesis, as well as the assembly with protein of ribosomal
subunits before their transport to the cytoplasm (22). Nuclear chromatin (DNA
plus protein) occurs in two morphological forms; electron-dense "heterochromatin"
represents DNA coiled and complexed with nuclear proteins and is inactive in RNA
synthesis (see Figs. 1, 2, 11, 12, 13). Euchromatin is much more electron lucent

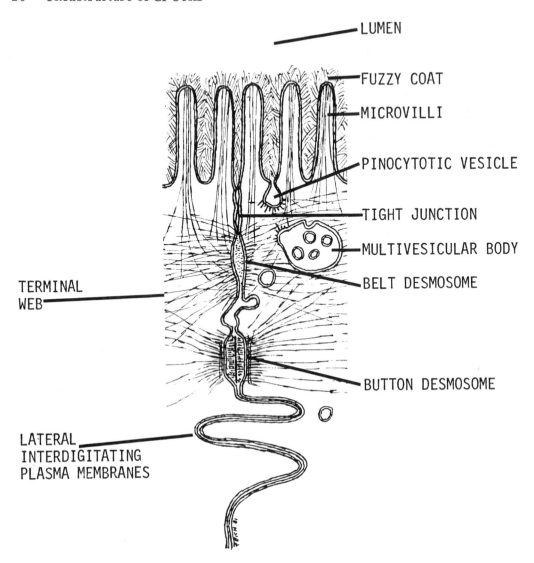

FIGURE 5   Schematic diagram of the structural features of the junctional complex found at the apex of adjoining intestinal epithelial cells. At the apical tight junction, plasma membranes appear as if fusing at a series of points. This is probably the result of a close apposition of intramembranous particles which form the tight junction. The belt desmosome which surrounds the cell and the button desmosomes probably play a role in holding the epithelium together. Numerous filaments from the terminal web insert into the desmosomal regions. Occasionally, macromolecules are absorbed into the intestinal epithelium via pinocytotic vesicles that bud into the terminal web zone. These vesicles either fuse with multivesicular bodies and eventually are digested, or they go around the tight junction and deposit their content into the intercellular space.

and probably represents uncoiled DNA, actively transcribing RNA (23). The nucleus is bounded by a double-membraned structure, the nuclear envelope (see Figs. 11, 13) that is perforated by "pores" thought to be the sites of molecular interchanges between the nucleus and cytoplasm. The nuclear envelope is also part of the cytoplasmic endoplasmic reticulum (ER); it contains ribosomes bound to its cytoplasmic face, and proteins synthesized on the ER also accumulate in the nuclear envelope.

ENDOPLASMIC RETICULUM

The endoplasmic reticulum (ER) is a membrane-delimited canalicular network that is very well developed in absorptive epithelia. The rough ER (see Figs. 1, 2) is primarily the site of synthesis of protein or lipoprotein destined for export out of the cell (1, 3, 24) (see Fig. 1). The first few amino acids on such a growing polypeptide appear to represent a "signal" binding the ribosome to the ER (3). Newly synthesized proteins are deposited into the lumen of the rough ER and transported by an energy-dependent process (24) to packaging sites, i. e. , Golgi apparatus, for eventual export. When the rate of protein synthesis exceeds the rate of intracellular transport, or a protein is not able to be transported because of some defect, it can accumulate in the lumen of the rough ER. Some proteins and enzymes are firmly bound to ER membranes; these enzymes include glucose-6-phosphatase, nucleoside diphosphatase, and cytochrome b_5. Such enzymes probably are inserted into preexisting ER membrane (5, 25) rather than entering the membrane while it is formed. Other cellular proteins, normally found "free" in the cell cytoplasm, e.g. , gluconeogenic enzymes, are synthesized on polyribosome complexes in the cytoplasm that are unattached to any membrane systems (1).

In addition to its role in protein synthesis, the enterocyte ER is the site of triglyceride synthesis from absorbed fatty acids and monoglycerides (26, 27). The ER of absorptive epithelia also contains enzymes for the metabolism of drugs such as phenobarbital; this function is similar to that which is classically seen in the liver (28, 29). As in the liver, drug metabolism in the epithelium of the small intestine is associated with a proliferation of smooth ER and an induction of "detoxification" enzymes such as NADPH diaphorase, cytochrome P_{450} and demethylation enzymes (30).

GOLGI APPARATUS AND SECRETION

The Golgi apparatus is a system of smooth, membrane-delimited sacs and small vesicles (see Figs. 1, 2, 7, 11). It functions in the processing and packaging of materials for secretion (1, 31). Secretion most often occurs by exocytosis (31, 32), the fusion of a membrane-delimited secretory granule with the plasma membrane of the cell permitting release of the contents of the granule into the extracellular space or blood. This is also the mechanism for the addition of new plasma membrane to the cell surface (1, 33). As in other cells, the Golgi apparatus plays a role in packaging materials for export in the absorptive epithelial cell. During fat absorption, electron-dense lipids first accumulate in the ER, then in Golgi saccules after which they are released into the extracellular space between the cells (34, 35). These fat droplets are able to enter the lymphatic circulation which contains an open endothelium that permits the passage of such a large complex (20, 26, 35).

MITOCHONDRIA

Absorptive epithelial cells contain numerous oval and filamentous mitochondria. These consist of both an outer and inner mitochondrial membrane (see Figs. 1-3) and a mitochondrial matrix. The inner membrane is thrown into numerous folds known as cristae (see Fig. 10). They are the site of the cytochrome electron transport chain and the enzymes for oxidative phosphorylation (36, 37). These molecules are geometrically arranged on the cristae in exact correspondence to their metabolic sequence, thus enhancing their efficiency (1, 36). The inner mitochondrial matrix surrounding the cristae contains the enzymes for the Krebs cycle. Mitochondria also contain their own DNA and RNA and genetically are considered semiautonomous organelles (38, 39). Recently, the complete sequence of human mitochondrial DNA has been determined (40). This mitochondrial DNA contains the genes for mitochondrial ribosomal RNA and several mitochondrial enzymes including cytochrome c oxidase. The inner mitochondrial matrix also contains several electron-dense granules that bind and sequester divalent cations such as calcium.

MICROBODIES (PEROXISOMES)

Microbodies (41) are round organelles with a single limiting membrane and a loose granular matrix (Fig. 6). Their function is poorly understood, although they are known to contain several enzymes including urate oxidase, catalase, and D-amino acid oxidase. Microbodies may be involved in lipid oxidations and in the breakdown of peroxides generated by some oxidative metabolism (42). A total absence of microbodies has been reported as a characteristic of the cerebrohepatorenal syndrome also known as Zellweger syndrome (43). In the absorptive intestinal epithelial cell, the peroxisomes are relatively small in size and the term microperoxisomes has been applied to them (44).

LYSOSOMES

Lysosomes are acid hydrolase-containing organelles of heterogeneous morphology. They are primarily concerned with intracellular digestion (1, 45, 46) and contain more than 30 enzymes such as acid phosphatase, ribonuclease, cathepsins, and deoxyribonuclease that split all classes of macromolecules. The morphology of lysosomes includes small "coated" vesicles or primary lysosomes that bud off the Golgi apparatus, multivesicular bodies in which foreign molecules are sequestered for eventual digestion, various residual bodies, and autophagic vacuoles concerned with the breakdown of intracellular organelles (45, 46).

The role of lysosomes in absorptive epithelial cells is poorly understood. Multivesicular bodies located in apical regions of the cell probably play a role in sequestering and degrading some of the macromolecules that may be endocytosed into the epithelial cells (see Figs. 1, 3, 6). In the neonatal, mammalian small intestine a paucity of multivesicular bodies and perhaps other lysosomes may in part account for the increased passage of macromolecules. Intestinal epithelia also contain variable numbers of dense bodies and autophagic vacuoles.

INCLUSIONS

Filaments—Terminal Web

The terminal web region (see Figs. 1-4, 6) lies beneath the microvilli and consists of a meshwork of fine filaments that mix with the microvillar filaments and attach to the junctional complex at the lateral margins of the cell (8). In the terminal

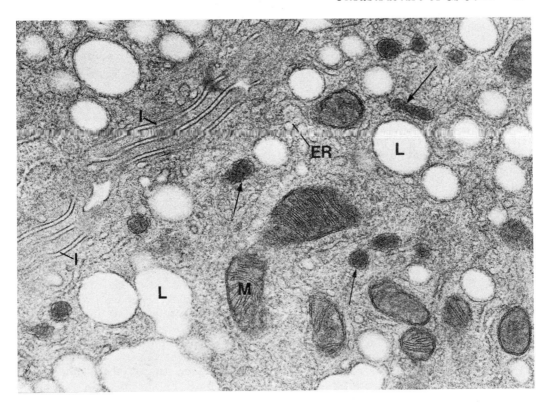

FIGURE 6   Electron micrograph of a portion of an absorptive epithelial cell from
an animal that had been fed a fatty meal. Note the numerous membrane-delimited
lipid droplets (L); endoplasmic reticulum (ER); and microperoxisomes (arrows);
intercellular space (I); and mitochondria (M). Original magnification x 25,000.

web there are also considerable amounts of smooth ER, pinocytotic vesicles, and
occasional multivesicular bodies (8, 26). As described previously the microvillar
filaments have actinlike properties (they bind myosin) and they probably play a
role in the motility or contraction of microvilli (12). Actinlike filaments (60 Å in
diameter), intermediate filaments (100 Å in diameter), and microtubules (240 Å
in diameter) are seen in a variety of cells including those of the small intestine.
In addition to their cytoskeletal role, these filamentous structures may have transport or other functions. Best understood are the microtubules which are the underlying structural basis of the mitotic spindle, centrioles, cilia, and flagella.
The organization of microtubules into more complex structures has been reviewed
in detail (47).

Fat Droplets

Droplets of fat are found in absorptive epithelial cells; particularly in the more apical cells of villi (20, 27, 35). These are formed, after absorption of fatty acids
and monoglycerides, in the endoplasmic reticulum. Under the electron microscope, fat generally appears in relatively homogeneous, smooth, round bodies that
may or may not be membrane-delimited; the electron density may vary with the

properties of the lipid (see Fig. 6). Occasionally two distinct densities of lipid are seen. Phospholipid also can form membranous structures that appear to form swirls. Such bodies accumulate in the lysosomes of patients with various hereditary lysosomal enzyme deficiency diseases that lead to a pileup of glycolipid materials (46).

Glycogen

Glycogen particles are present in absorptive epithelial cells although they are not nearly as prominent as in hepatocytes. Glycogen particles may associate to form larger clusters (B particles).

MUCOUS-PRODUCING CELLS

GOBLET CELLS

The goblet cells of the intestinal mucosa contain numerous secretory mucous droplets (8, 48) (Fig. 7), a basal nucleus, well-developed, stacked, rough ER and an elaborate Golgi apparatus that packages mucous droplets. Mucous protein is synthesized on the rough ER, sugars are added to the protein moiety in the rough ER and in the Golgi apparatus (48), and secretory granules accumulate in the apical portion of the cell. During secretion the membrane of the mucous droplet fuses with the plasma membrane, permitting release of the mucus. The functional role of intestinal mucus remains obscure. It has been suggested that this mucus may "wash" luminal antigen-antibody complexes off the surface of the epithelium (49).

STOMACH

The four major cell types on the mucosal epithelium of the stomach are (1) surface mucous cells, (2) neck mucous cells, (3) parietal or oxyntic cells, and (4) peptic or chief cells. In addition, there are also several chromaffin cell types (26).

MUCOUS CELLS

Surface mucous cells cover the entire surface of the stomach and line the gastric pits. These are columnar epithelial cells with apical secretory granules and a small amount of rough ER (50) (Fig. 8). Neck mucous cells contain clear, less dense secretory granules and a highly developed Golgi apparatus (26, 50, 51) (Fig. 9).

PARIETAL (OXYNTIC) CELLS

The parietal cells are acid-secreting cells principally located in the neck of gastric glands. The apical cell surface is extensively invaginated and contains numerous microvilli that form a secretory canaliculus (Fig. 10). There are also many large mitochondria. During acid secretion there is an increase in the apical surface area probably caused by the addition of intracellular membrane to the surface (26, 50, 51).

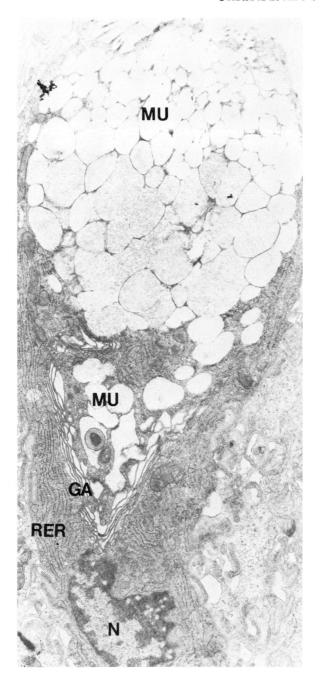

FIGURE 7   Goblet cell filled with mucous droplets. Note the polarized organization of the cell; basal nucleus (N); rough endoplasmic reticulum (RER); stacks of Golgi apparatus filling up with mucus (GA); newly formed and mature mucous droplets (MU). Original magnification x 8000.

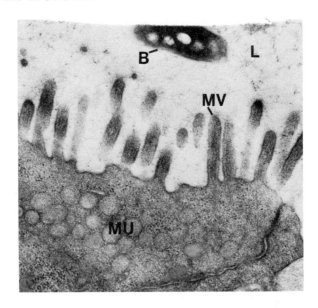

FIGURE 8   Apical region of surface mucous cell of the stomach of a rat. A bacterium (B) is seen in the lumen (L) which is also filled with fibrous material that is probably released from mucous droplets; intracellular mucous droplets (MU); microvilli (MV). Original magnification x 19,000.

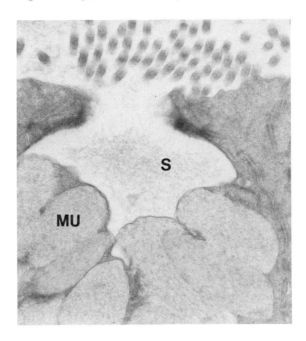

FIGURE 9   Apical region of a neck mucous cell in the stomach of a rat. The mucous granule (MU) in this type of cell is usually less dense than in the surface cells; secreted free mucous material (S); microvilli (MV); lumen (L). Original magnification x 14,000.

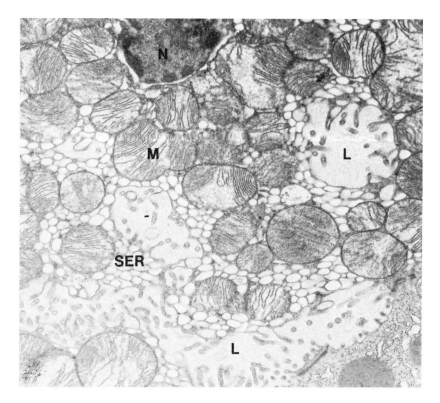

FIGURE 10   Portion of a parietal cell from the glandular stomach of the rat. Hydrochloric acid is thought to be released from the tubulovesicles of the extensive smooth endoplasmic reticulum (SER) into the elaborate surface lumen (L) of the gland that is lined with microvilli. Mitochondria (M) with numerous fine cristae are a characteristic of parietal cells.   Original magnification x 14,000.

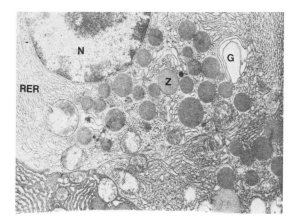

FIGURE 11   Chief cell from the rat stomach.   Chief cells produce zymogen granules (Z) with pepsinogen and other enzymes that are released by exocytosis into the gastric lumen.   These cells contain an elaborate rough endoplasmic reticulum (RER) and a well-developed Golgi apparatus (G).   Chief and parietal cells are seen in close association in the glandular stomach.   Original magnification x 8000.

CHIEF (PEPTIC) CELLS

Chief cells are zymogen-type cells with a well-developed rough ER and numerous secretory granules that form in the Golgi apparatus. Chief cells release pepsinogen and probably renin (26, 50, 51) (Fig. 11).

ENTEROCHROMAFFIN CELLS

The enterochromaffin cells of the stomach (Fig. 12) manufacture peptide hormones, amines (serotonin, histamine, catecholamines), gastrin, and enteroglucagon. There are four morphological types based on the secretory granule's appearance (52).

The enterochromaffinlike (ECL) cell contains small (0.1-0.15 μm), round moderately electron-dense granules that may contain histamine. G cells probably synthesize gastrin. They contain secretory granules that are approximately 0.25 μm in diameter and of varying electron density. D cells contain large (0.25-0.30 μm) granules with a homogeneous finely granular matrix. Enterochromaffin cells (EC) contain small, very dense pleomorphic granules, 0.05-0.1 μm in diameter. EC cells are thought to synthesize serotonin.

PANCREAS

ACINAR CELLS

The exocrine pancreas is principally composed of acinar cells. These cells contain numerous membrane-delimited, electron-dense, zymogen granules filled with digestive enzymes (Fig. 13) that are released by exocytosis into the pancreatic ducts (53). The digestive enzymes are synthesized on a very elaborate, stacked rough ER, and transported to the Golgi apparatus where they are packaged into secretory granules (24, 53).

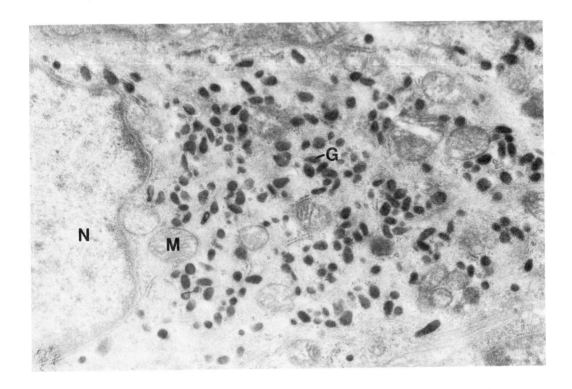

FIGURE 12   Enterochromaffin cell in the stomach of a rat. There are numerous pleomorphically shaped electron-dense secretory granules (SG). This type of enteric chromaffin cell is thought to produce serotonin: nucleus (N); mitochrondrion (M). Original magnification x 10,000.

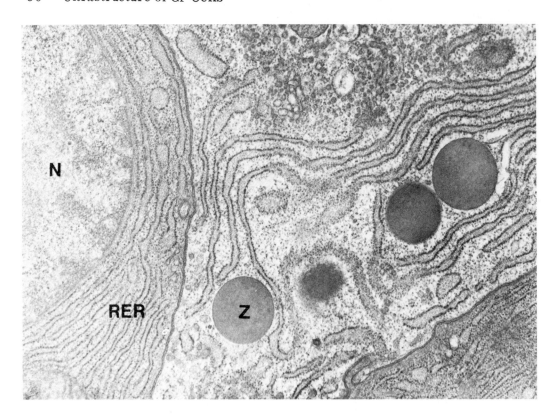

FIGURE 13   Portion of a zymogen-producing cell from the exocrine pancreas of the rat. Digestive enzymes (e.g., lipase, amylase) are synthesized on the rough endoplasmic reticulum (RER) and packaged in the Golgi apparatus (G) into membrane-delimited zymogen granules. Original magnification x 18,500.

REFERENCES

1.   Novikoff, A. B., and E. Holtzman: Cells and Organelles, 2nd ed. Holt, Rinehart and Winston, New York, 1976.

2.   Robertson, J. D.: Molecular structure of biological membranes. in Handbook of Molecular Cytology. A Lima de Faria (ed.). North Holland, Amsterdam, 1969, p. 1403.

3.   Rothman, J. E., and J. Lenard: Membrane asymetry. Science 195:743, 1977.

4.   Branton, D., and D. W. Deamer: Membrane Structure. Springer Verlag, Vienna, 1972.

5.   Bennet, H. S.: The cell surface: Components and configurations. in Handbook of Molecular Cytology. A Lima deFaria (ed.). North Holland, Amsterdam, 1969, p. 1261.

6. Schlesinger, J. , D. Axelrod, D. E. Koppel, W. W. Weff, and E. L. Elson:
    Lateral transport of a lipid probe and labeled proteins on a cell membrane.
    Science 195:307, 1977.

7. McIntyre, J. A. , M. J. Karnovsky, and N. B. Gilula: Intramembranous par-
    ticle aggregation in lymphoid cells. Nature 245:147, 1973.

8. Trier, J. S.: Morphology of the epithelium of the small intestine. in Hand-
    book of Physiology, Chapter 63, Soc. 6, Alimentary Canal Vol. III Intestinal
    Absorption. C. F. Code and W. Heidel (eds.). Am Physiol Soc, Washington,
    1968, p. 1125.

9. Ito, S.: The enteric surface coat on cat intestinal microvilli. J Cell Biol
    27:475, 1965.

10. Miller, D., and R. K. Crane: The digestive function of the epithelium of the
    small intestine. II. Localization of dissacharide hydrolysis. Biochim Bio-
    phys Acta 52:293, 1961.

11. Eichholz, A. , and R. K. Crane: Studies on the organization of the brush bor-
    der in intestinal epithelial cells. I. TRIS disruption of isolated hamster
    brush borders and density gradient separation from intestinal epithelium.
    J Cell Biol 71:417, 1976.

12. Mosseaker, M. S.: Brush border motility, microvillar contraction in Triton-
    treated brush borders isolated from intestinal epithelium. J Cell Biol
    71:417, 1976.

13. Staehlin, L. A.: Structure and function of intercellular junctions. Int Rev
    Cytol 39:191, 1974.

14. Walker, A. W. , and K. J. Isselbacher: Uptake and transport of macromole-
    cules by the intestine. Possible role in clinical disorders. Gastroenterology
    67:531, 1974.

15. Worthington, B. S. , E. S. Boatman, and G. E. Kenny: Intestinal absorption of
    intact proteins in normal and protein deficient rats. Am J Clin Nutr 27:276,
    1974.

16. Rhodes, R. S. , and M. H. Karnovsky: Loss of macromolecular barrier func-
    tion associated with surgical trauma to the intestine. Lab Invest 25:220,
    1971.

17. Cooper, M. , S. Teichberg, and F. Lifshitz: Alterations in rat jejunal per-
    meability to a macromolecular tracer during a hyperosmotic load. Lab In-
    vest 38:447, 1978.

18. Fagundes-Neto, U. , S. Teichberg, M. A. Bayne, B. Morton, and F. Lifshitz:
    Bile salt enhanced rat jejunal absorption of a macromolecular tracer. Lab
    Invest 44:18-26, 1981.

19. Teichberg, S.: Penetration of epithelial barriers by macromolecules: The
    intestinal mucosa. in Clinical Disorders in Pediatric Gastroenterology. F.
    Lifshitz (ed.). Marcel Dekker, New York, 1980, p. 185.

20.   Casely-Smith, J. R.: The identification of chylomicrons and lipoproteins in tissue sections and their passage into jejunal lacteals. J Cell Biol 15:259, 1962.

21.   Gilula, N. B.: Gap junctions and cell communication. in International Cell Biology, 1976-1977. R. Brinkely and K. R. Porter (eds.). Rockefeller University Press, New York, 1977, p. 61.

22.   Warner, J.: The assembly of ribosomes in Hela cells. J Mol Biol 19:383, 1966.

23.   Berendes, H., and W. Beerman: Biochemical activity of interphase chromosomes. in Handbook of Molecular Cytology. A. Lima de Faria (ed.). North Holland, Amsterdam, 1969, p. 500.

24.   Jamieson, J. D., and G. E. Palade: Intracellular transport of secretory proteins in the pancreatic exocrine cell IV. Metabolic requirements. J Cell Biol 39:589, 1968.

25.   Leskes, A., P. Siekevitz, and G. E. Palade: Differentiation of endoplasmic reticulum in hepatocytes. J Cell Biol 49:264, 1971.

26.   Padykula, H. A.: The digestive tract. in Histology, 3rd ed. R. O. Greep and L. Weiss (eds.). McGraw-Hill Book Co., New York, 1973, p. 573.

27.   Brindley, D. N., and G. Hubscher: The intracellular distribution of the enzymes catalyzing the biosynthesis of glycerides in the intestinal mucosa. Biochim Biophys Acta 106:495, 1965.

28.   Menard, D., A. Berteloot, and J. S. Hugon: Action of phenobarbital on the ultrastructure and enzymatic activity of the mouse intestine and the mouse liver. Histochemistry 38:241, 1974.

29.   Wattenberg, L.: Effects of dietary constituents on the metabolism of chemical carcinogens. Cancer Res 35:3326, 1975.

30.   Siekevitz, P.: Dynamics of intracellular membranes. Hosp Prac 8:91, 1973.

31.   Favard, P.: The Golgi apparatus. in Handbook of Molecular Cytology. A. Lima de Faria (ed.). North Holland, Amsterdam, 1969, p. 1130.

32.   Satir, B.: The final steps in secretion. Sci Am 233:28, 1975.

33.   Moore, D. J., H. H. Mollenhauer, and C. E. Bracker: Origin and continuity of Golgi apparatus. in Origin and Continuity of Cell Organelles. J. Reinert and H. Ursprung (eds.). Springer Verlag, New York, 1971, p. 82.

34.   Jones, A. L., N. B. Ruderman, and M. G. Herrera: An electron microscope study of lipoprotein production and release by the isolated perfused rat liver. Proc Soc Exp Biol Med 123:4, 1966.

35.   Palay, S. L., and L. J. Karlin: An electron microscopic study of the intestinal villus. II. The pathway of fat absorption. J Biophys Biochem Cytol 5:373, 1959.

36. Chance, B. , and D. F. Parsons: Cytochrome function in relation to inner membrane structure of mitochrondria. Science 142:1176, 1963.

37. Racker, E. , and L. L. Horstmann: Partial resolution of the enzymes catalyzing oxidative phosphorylation. XIII. Structure and function of submitochondrial particles completely resolved with respect to coupling factor. J Biol Chem 242:2547, 1967.

38. Kroon, A. M. , and C. Saccone: The Biogenesis of Mitochrondria. Academic Press, New York, 1974.

39. Roodyn, D. B. : Factors affecting the incorporation of amino acids into protein by isolated mitochrondria. in Regulation of Metabolic Processes in Mitochondria. J. M. Tagger, S. Paper, E. Quaglierillo, and E. C. Slater (eds.). Elsevier, Amsterdam, 1966, p. 383.

40. Anderson, S. , A. T. Bankier, and B. G. Barrell: Sequence and organization of the human mitochondrial genome. Nature 290:457, 1981.

41. De Duve, C. , and P. Baudhuin: Peroxisomes, microbodies and related particles. Physiol Rev 46:323, 1966.

42. Reddy, J. K. : Possible properties of microbodies (peroxisomes): Microbody proliferation and hypolipidemic drugs. J Histochem Cytochem 21:967, 1973.

43. Goldfischer, S. , C. Moore, A. B. Johnson, A. J. Spiro, M. P. Valsamis, H. H. Wisniewski, R. H. Ritch, W. T. Norton, I. Rapin, and L. M. Gartner: Peroxisomal and mitochrondrial defects in the cerebro-hepato-renal syndrome. Science 182:62, 1973.

44. Novikoff, P. M. , and A. B. Novikoff; Peroxisomes in absorptive cells in mammalian small intestine. J Cell Biol 53:532, 1972.

45. De Duve, C. , and R. Wattiaux: Functions of lysosomes. Ann Rev Physiol 28:435, 1966.

46. Holtzman, E. : Lysosomes: A Survey. Springer Verlag, New York, 1975.

47. Tilney, L. G. : Origin and continuity of microtubules. in Origin and Continuity of Cell Organelles. J. Reinert and H. Ursprung (eds.). Springer Verlag, New York, 1971, p. 222.

48. Neutra, M. , and C. P. LeBlond: Synthesis of the carbohydrate of mucus in the Golgi complex as shown by electron microscope autoradiography of goblet cells from rats injected with glucose H^3. J Cell Biol 30:119, 1966.

49. Walker, W. A. , M. Wu, and K. H. Bloch: Stimulation by immune complexes of mucus release from goblet cells of the rat small intestine. Science 197:370, 1977.

50. Ito, S. : Anatomic structure of the gastric mucosa. in Handbook of Physiology. C. F. Code and W. Heidel (eds.). Am Physiol Soc, Washington, 1967.

51.   Rubin, W. , L. L. Ross, M. H. Sleisenger, and G. H. Jeffries: The normal human gastric epithelia. A fine structural study.   Lab Invest 19:598, 1968.

52.   Rubin, W. : Endocrine cells in the normal human stomach.   Gastroenterology 62:784, 1972.

53.   Ito, S. : The Pancreas. in Histology. R. O. Greep and L. Weiss (eds.). McGraw-Hill Book Co. , New York , 1973, p. 645.

3

INTESTINAL SECRETION AND ABSORPTION

Raul A. Wapnir, Ph. D. , M. P. H.

INTRODUCTION

ONTOGENIC DEVELOPMENT OF THE SMALL INTESTINE

The gastrointestinal tract constitutes the one uninterrupted, open exchange surface between the environment and the inner milieu. It can also be visualized as the internal lining, or protective separation from the outside world for liquids and solids, in the way the respiratory apparatus is for the gaseous phase. In addition, the small intestine is the area of nutrient absorption. The surface available to achieve this role is exponentially increased by transverse ridges, fingerlike villi, and a thick carpet of microvilli which increase the surface another order of magnitude. The total absorptive surface of the small intestine can be estimated to be 200 times the body surface in the adult (1,2).

The small intestine has a vast absorptive potential. However, food reaching its lumen has to be physically and chemically pretreated to break down complex molecules into compounds available for absorption. This requirement is abridged only in very limited instances, particularly early in life, when large protein molecules may be absorbed.

Development of the gut begins during the third week of intrauterine life with a rudimentary tube formation. Further differentiation and tubal rotations occur during the second and earlier part of the third month of gestation. At that time, the fingerlike villi, about 1 mm long, appear initially in the proximal end of the small intestine and progressively extend through the distal ileum. A well-defined inner space, or lumen, is already observable by the thirteenth week. Between the villi, microscopic depressions, or crypts, contain specialized cells—goblet, argentaffin and Paneth cells, which are differentiable between the ninth and seventeenth week of intrauterine life (3).

Intestinal mucosal enzymes become detectable by the first trimester. Alkaline phosphatase and disaccharidases are measurable by the eighth week and peptide hydrolases during the following 2 weeks (4, 5). Enterokinase is detectable only after the 26th week of gestation (6). Active transport of glucose and amino acids have been demonstrated in tissues of fetuses 8-12 weeks old (7). All other enzymes tend to increase during the course of intrauterine development. Thus, the newborn infant starts extrauterine life with a full complement of intestinal mucosal enzymes and specialized transport mechanisms, as shown by in vitro assays. The potential for assimilation of nutrients at the intestinal level is comparable to that of an adult with appropriate allowances for the differences in absorptive surface capacity, which can be estimated to be one-twentieth that of the adult. The rate of development of absorptive functions early in life has been supported by animal studies that have contributed to clarifying the development of amino acid transport (8-10), and the kinetics of this phenomenon (11).

Wilson (2) has estimated that the active surface of the small intestine is 500 times larger than a simple tube of the same length. Such an increase results from the additive effect of the trebling due to the folds of Kerkring (valvulae conniventes), plus two orders of magnitude expansion of the absorptive surface due to the existence of villi and their submicroscopic hairlike projections, the microvilli (Fig. 1). Microvilli are approximately 1000 times smaller and constitute the ultimate interface between the lumen of the intestine and the intracellular space.

CELLULAR MORPHOLOGY

Two principal types of cells characterize the villi: the columnar, absorptive cells, and the goblet cells whose role is mucous secretion. In between villi, the Lieberkuhn crypts contain argentaffin and Paneth cells which play little part in absorption processes. The presence of a mucoid layer on the surface of the microvilli, the glycocalyx, introduces a passive factor in the free passage of substances between the external and the internal milieu and gives rise to an "unstirred layer" not directly affected by the flow of matter down the lumen.

The absorptive cells or enterocytes have all the organelles required for energy synthesis, catabolism, and transport (see Chap. 2). The blood capillaries in the lamina propria exhibit a simple layer of endothelial cells backed by a basement membrane. Lymphatic capillaries are thicker and possess no basement membranes or fenestrations.

FLUID AND ELECTROLYTE EXCHANGES IN THE INTESTINE

Intestinal absorption is a phenomenon that occurs with molecules in solution or in suspension in an aqueous medium. A continuous flow of water into the gastrointestinal tract is needed to ensure solubility of ingested food and its breakdown products entering the small intestine. Fluid also is required to fill the lumen of the intestine and allow contact of the microvilli with dissolved nutrients entering the absorptive region.

In the older child, daily water intake may exceed 1 Liter. However, this volume represents only 10-20% of the total fluid load imposed on the small intestine. The largest contributor is gastric juice, estimated as 35% of the total liquid volume circulating in the gastrointestinal tract. Pancreatic juice follows in importance, with about one-fourth of the amount, followed by the contribution of saliva, which is comparable to that of external sources. Bile participates with 5-10% of the volume. The effectiveness of the system to prevent water losses is such that only 50-150 ml of water are eliminated in the feces of the infant and the older child (1, 2) (Fig. 2).

In the infant who is breastfed or receives a milk formula, the external water load is proportionately much larger. A daily intake of 600-800 ml during the first few weeks of life is compensated by higher water losses in the excreta and through the skin, since the infant has a comparatively higher surface/weight ratio than the adult.

The intestinal cells constitute an essentially uninterrupted layer. So called tight junctions appear to form a closer seal then the interdigitating plasma membrane boundaries. However, there are good indications for the existence of

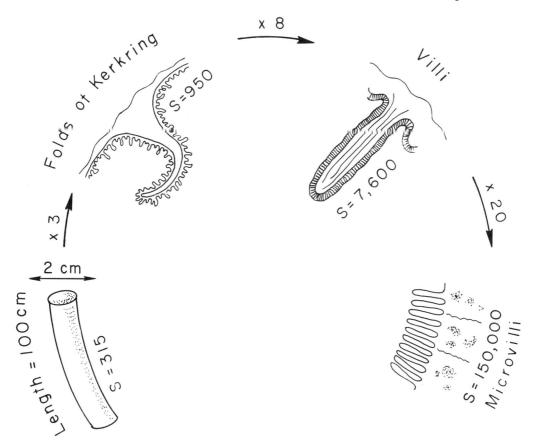

FIGURE 1   Schematic representation of the increase in available surface in the small intestine of an infant as a result of morphological differentiation. If the small intestine were a smooth tube, its effective surface would be only 315 cm². The presence of Kerkring folds increases the surface three times. Almost one order of magnitude is gained by the existence of villi. It is estimated that the microvilli upgrade the infant's absorptive surface another 20 times to a final surface about 500 times that of the simple tube.

ultramicroscopic pores, in the microvilli region, about 2-7 Å in diameter, permeable to water molecules and solutes with a molecular weight (mol. wt.) under 200, a size adequate to permit passage of electrolytes, monosaccharides, and most amino acids. Once inside the columnar cells, water may continue down the intracellular space and finally reach the capillary and lymphatic vessels (1, 2, 12, 13).

Each villus in the small intestine is heavily perfused and the blood flow in the adult is estimated at 1 L/min (1). This volume is sufficient to remove all substances traversing the intracellular space. The flow of lymph is much more limited—only about one-thousandth that of the blood. The absorptive capacity of the intestine exceeds the nutritional requirements of the human organism, as witnessed by the minimal nutritional deficiencies occurring even when a substantial segment of the small intestine is removed.

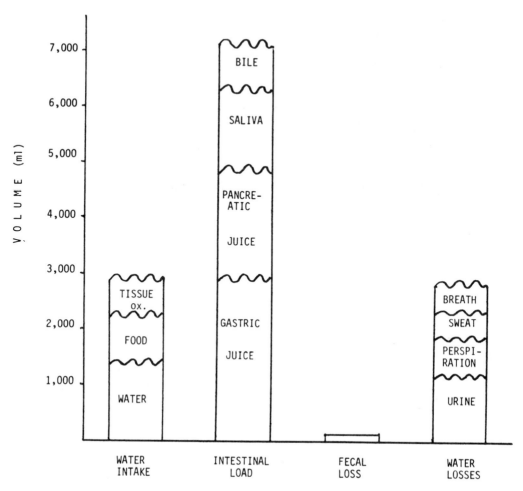

FIGURE 2   Overall water balances and intestinal water load in the older child and adolescent. The wavy line separation in the respective columns denote the expected normal variability. Water intake, urine volume, and sweat losses have the greatest range. Adapted from Refs. 1, 2.

Although water is absorbed together with solutes in the jejunum, a substantial reverse flow may occur when the alimentary mass in the stomach starts to be digested and solubilized. Under these conditions, elevated osmotic pressures can be generated in the lumen of the duodenum and the upper jejunum. In this case, water fluxes from the circulation to the intestinal lumen are accompanied by a proportional outflow of sodium. This phenomenon can be demonstrated easily by instilling into the gastrointestinal tract of a rat a hypertonic, nonabsorbable solution (Fig. 3). Within 2 hours, there is a 2.5-fold dilution of the original load and a near equalization of the nonabsorbable bolus with the intracellular tonicity (14).

As demonstrated in an experimental animal, the exchange of fluids across the small intestine is directed toward achieving isotonicity. When the stomach is presented a hypertonic load, a massive secretion of gastric juice contributes not only to digestion of food, but also to dilution of the hypertonic bolus. Solid food does not contribute to the osmotic pressure of gastric contents until its solubilization has taken place, either in the stomach or the jejunum. For teleological

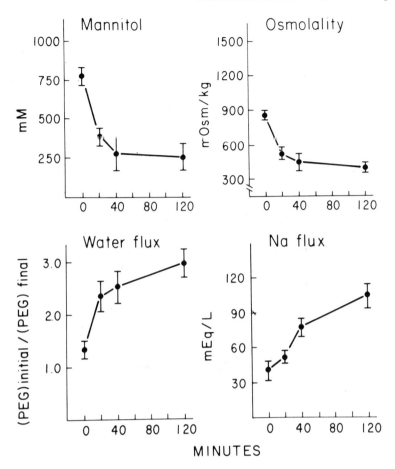

FIGURE 3   To follow water and electrolyte fluxes in the small intestine, at zero time rats were given 5 ml/100 g body weight of 20% (w/v) solution of mannitol, a poorly absorbed polyol, via gastric tube. The animals were sacrificed at the stated intervals and the contents of the jejunum were assayed. The water flux was estimated from the ratios of nonabsorbable marker concentrations (polyethylene glycol, PEG, mol wt 3000-3700). ^{3}H-mannitol was present as a tracer. Concentrations of this substance were determined by isotope dilution counting. (Data from Refs. 14 and 15, reproduced with permission.)

physicochemical reasons, the larger, initial breakdown products of complex carbohydrates and proteins contribute to the osmotic pressure of the chyme in inverse proportion to their molecular weight.

Fluxes of water in both directions occur in the stomach. However, no substantial net absorption takes place either in the stomach or the jejunum. As pointed out earlier, the regulated passage through the pylorus allows for progressive dilution to an osmolarity comparable to that of the plasma and the cytoplasm of the cells in the villi. Failure to achieve this equilibrium produces the dumping syndrome (16), commonly observed in individuals who undergo partial resection of the stomach or pyloroplasty. Tube feedings of hyperosmotic solutions directly into the small bowel can produce the identical effect, following massive transudation of extracellular fluid into the intestinal lumen, with consequent fall of arterial pressure and hypovolemia, nausea, abdominal pain, profuse sweating, and even loss of consciousness.

Diarrhea is essentially a breakdown in the balance of fluid exchange across the intestinal mucosa resulting in exaggerated losses of water. This condition, of special concern in infancy, is discussed in Chap. 14.

Small ions are surrounded by an "atmosphere" of water molecules. The four ions that constitute the largest share of small-intestine electrolytes are sodium, potassium, chloride, and bicarbonate. Sodium is generally present in the diet in substantial amounts. Since stools contain very little sodium, it is suggested that most of the intake is absorbed. The active mechanism that, in addition to simple diffusion, carries sodium into the cell and from there into the circulation, is counteracted by an energy-consuming process, the sodium pump (Fig. 4), that translocates sodium to the lumen and reduces intracellular concentration of this ion. Interactions of sodium with glucose and amino acid transport are discussed later.

On the other hand, electrochemical gradients appear to be the driving force for the membrane passage of potassium. The net effects that can be observed are the result of a bidirectional flux that varies as a consequence of local conditions. There are no substantial differences in the absorptive capacity of the jejunum and the ileum, but potassium is secreted by the colon. In general, absorption occurs when the luminal concentration is 1-2 mEq/L higher than in plasma.

Chloride is generally carried into the cells as a resultant of cation absorption and to maintain electroneutrality. However, the small-intestinal mucosa of man can absorb chloride against an electrochemical gradient.

If the jejunal concentration of bicarbonate is above 6mM, absorption occurs. However, secretion takes place in the ileum and the colon if the luminal concentration falls below 40-45 mM. This phenomenon is often coupled with chloride absorption and is one of the key mechanisms for the regulation of intraluminal pH (1, 16).

INTESTINAL SECRETION

The net absorptive function of the small intestine is the resultant of a bidirectional flux of water, salts, and other small molecules. In addition, there is a constant renovation of the intestinal epithelium. In the adolescent, over 100 billion cells are extruded every day into the lumen of the small intestine. Such a turnover implies the release of 50-80 g of protein. Only minimal amounts are normally lost through the feces, however (1).

The physiological properties of enterocytes vary during their migration from crypts to villi. Their enzymatic stores increase with their progression toward the tip of the villi and they acquire the mucous coat of the glycocalyx.

The duodenum is an area particularly rich in secretory glands. In man, these glands are generally grouped together in discrete sections and open into the bottom or sides of the crypts. The secretion produced is highly viscous, although isotonic with blood and of similar electrolyte composition. Enterokinase, alkaline phosphatase, and pepsin are present in the duodenal secretions. Hydrolytic enzymes (amylases, peptide hydrolases, and disaccharidases), also found in that fluid, are considered to be derived from desquamated duodenal cells. The limited buffer capacity of duodenal secretion is insufficient to neutralize digestion products from the stomach, but the high viscosity of the secretion is sufficient to prevent surface damage from contact with acid.

Secretion is regulated and stimulated by intramucosal hormones, namely gastrin, secretin, cholecystokinin, and glucagon, which in turn are activated by food reaching the gastrointestinal tract.

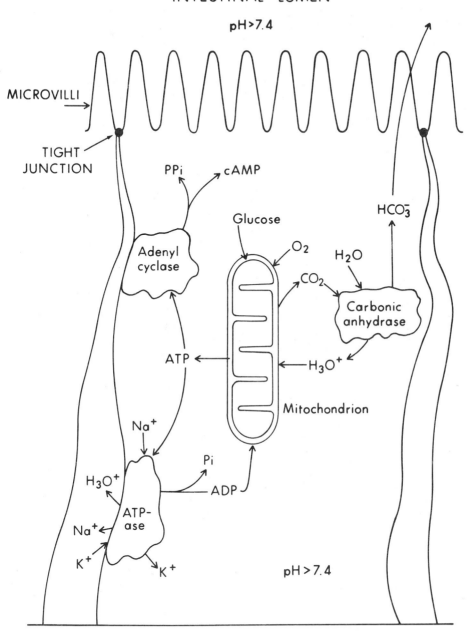

INTESTINAL LUMEN

pH>7.4

FIGURE 4   Schematic diagram of some of the principal energy-related mechanisms of the enterocyte. The sodium pump associated with membrane-bound
ATPase, adenyl cyclase, and carbonic anhydrase are linked to the metabolic activities occurring in the mitochondrion. Electrolyte exchange, water transport
and pH adjustment are thus intimately linked. (Adapted from Waddell, W.J.:
Role of membrane-bound enzymes in biological transport. in Intestinal Absorption
and Malabsorption, T.Z. Csaky (ed.), Raven Press, New York, 1975, p. 37.)

The colon also is an area where secretion occurs. No villi exist, and the crypts are rich in mucous-secreting goblet cells. The liquid portion of colonic secretion is alkaline due to an elevated concentration of bicarbonate (85-155 mEq/L). Sodium and potassium levels are reversed from the familiar figures of serum (K^+ 145-200 mEq/L; Na^+ 3-10 mEq/L) (1).

The normal fluxes of water and electrolytes along the alimentary canal can be severely disrupted by bacterial toxins. Vibrio cholerae produces an exotoxin which attaches to the enterocyte and activates adenyl cyclase, which converts adenosine triphosphate (ATP), the generally accepted "currency" for active transport across membranes, into cyclic adenosine monophosphate (cAMP). This substance specifically stimulates secretion, rather than simply inhibiting the normal absorptive process, thus resulting in a net loss of fluid. Theophylline, which prevents the enzymatic breakdown of cAMP, enhances these effects. The onset of the diarrhea may be fulminant and catastrophic (17). A similar series of events can follow infection by toxigenic strains of Escherichia coli, creating the familiar symptomatology experienced by tourists in areas of the world with inadequate sanitary facilities (18, 19).

There is no substantiation for the hypothesis that absorption and secretion are totally independent functions located in different cells, or cells with two kinds of receptors. A consensus is being reached on the reversibility of fluid passage across intestinal mucosal cells.

Several hormones affect intestinal secretion. Prostaglandins E_1 and F_{2a} have been shown experimentally to cause secretion of fluid. A substantial number of peptides normally present in the gastric antrum and the duodenal mucosa (gastrin, secretin) have definite action on the secretive process (Table 1). Certain pancreatic tumors, not affecting beta cells, synthesize inordinate amounts of active compounds, principally vasoactive intestinal peptide (VIP), secretin, and serotonin, which cause production of the alkaline secretion generally associated with severe diarrhea in those conditions (pancreatic cholera).

TABLE 1   Active Peptides of the Digestive Tract

Substances with Confirmed Hormonal Properties

Peptide	Number of amino acid residues	Action on gastrointestinal tract
The gastrin family Gastrin	"Big": 34 "Little": 17 "Mini": 14 Synthetic "penta": 5	Increases gastric acid secretion, plus other effects (see Table 2)
Cholecystokinin-pancreozymin (CCK-PZ)	33	Increases gallbaldder contraction and pancreatic enzyme secretion (see Table 3)
Caerulein	10	Like cholecystokinin, but 10-fold more potent

TABLE 1 (cont'd)

Peptide	Number of amino acid residues	Action on gastrointestinal tract
The secretin-glucagon family		
Secretin	27	Increases pancreatic water and electrolyte secretion
Vasoactive intestinal peptide (VIP)	28	Stimulates intestinal secretion; inhibits acid and pepsinogen secretion
Glucagon (enteroglucagon)	*	Identical to pancreatic glucagon or with similar immunoreactivity
Gastric inhibitory polypeptide (GIP)	43	Inhibits gastric secretion and motility; stimulates intestinal secretion and insulin release
Other "candidate" hormones		
Motilin	22	Increases motor activity of GI tract
Urogastrone	52	Inhibits gastric secretion (present in male human urine)
Chymodenin	40*	Stimulates secretion of chymotrypsinogen by the pancreas
Gastrone	80*	Inhibits gastric secretion (present in mucous fraction of gastric juice)
Entero-oxyntin	*	Stimulates acid production in the stomach
Bulbogastrone	*	Inhibits gastric secretion; released by acid
Duocrinin and enterocrinin	*	Stimulate intestinal secretion
Incretin	*	Releases insulin

TABLE 1 (cont'd)

Peptide	Number of amino acid residues	Action on gastrointestinal tract
Villikinin	*	Stimulates contraction of villi
Bombesin	*	Releases gastrin; regulates satiety (?)

*Exact number of amino acid residues and composition not entirely established.

The physiological activities of gastric, pancreatic, and intestinal secretions are finely regulated in the intact individual. In addition, recent knowledge accumulated on the structure of the active peptides present in the gastrointestinal tract, and their synthesis, has enabled the description of pharmacological activities of these substances. Classical experiments have discriminated between a cephalic and a specifically gastric phase of gastric digestion, associated with vagal and local stimuli, respectively.

The presence of a meal, or mechanical distention of the stomach, triggers the release of gastrin from the G cells in the glandular area of the pylorus and the duodenal mucosa (20). The most effective stimulants for gastrin release are peptides, neutral amino acids, and commercial meat extracts. Calcium salts and epinephrine also produce the same effect. Acidification of the luminal contents, as well as a variety of blood-circulating active peptides, namely, secretin, gastric inhibitory polypeptide (GIP), vasoactive intestinal peptide (VIP), glucagon, and calcitonin, inhibit further release of gastrin. In the case of gastrin, as well as other peptide hormones, a feedback mechanism closes the physiological circuit, i.e., products released by that hormone cause eventual inhibition of further gastrin production. There are several gastrins in man (see Table 1). Other species produce closely related compounds. A summary of the physiological and pharmacological effects of gastrin is presented in Table 2.

Another example of a positive-feedback mechanism is entero-oxyntin, a hormone secreted by the small intestinal mucosa which stimulates acid production by the stomach. A comparable effect is achieved as a consequence of another hormone from the intestinal mucosa, similar to bombesin, which stimulates gastrin release.

For the last 50 years it has been known that digestion products in the duodenum induce contraction of the gallbladder. The hormone responsible was designated cholecystokinin. The same stimulus was observed to provoke the secretion of pancreatic enzymes. The agent mediating this effect was initially called pancreozymin. Ultimately, both hormones have been proved to be the same substance. The first name has prevailed, and the initials CCK or CCK-PZ are frequent designations. A summary of its effects is listed in Table 3.

Another polypeptide, with a structure very close to glucagon, is secretin, which appears to act synergistically with cholecystokinin in pancreatic stimulation. Secretin is released as a result of acidification of the duodenum. Functionally related is caerulein, a substance first isolated from frog skin. Its high cholecystokininlike activity makes it a good pharmacological agent.

TABLE 2   Actions of Gastrins

Stimulatory	Inhibitory	Pharmacological
Acid secretion	Contraction of pyloric, ileocecal and Oddi sphincters	Water, bicarbonate, and electrolyte secretion by pancreas, liver, and small intestinal mucosa
Pepsinogen secretion		
Gastric blood flow	Gastric emptying	
Contraction of circular stomach muscle	Absorption of glucose, water, and electrolytes across the small intestinal mucosa	Enzyme secretion by pancreas and small intestinal mucosa
Growth of gastric and small intestinal mucosa and pancreas		Contraction of lower esophageal sphincter, gallbladder, small intestine, and colon
Release of insulin, glucagon, calcitonin		

TABLE 3   Actions of Cholecystokinin

Stimulatory	Inhibitory	Pharmacological
Contraction of the gallbladder and relaxation of the sphincter of Oddi	Gastric emptying	Poor stimulant of acid secretion in the absence of gastrin
Enzymatic secretion of the pancreas	Gastrin-stimulated acid secretion	Stimulates pepsinogen secretion
Synergistically with secretin for the alkaline secretion of pancreas and liver		Stimulates motility of the sigmoid colon
Growth of the pancreas		Stimulates secretion of duodenal glands
		Stimulates glucagon and insulin release
		Elicits satiety after a meal

A large group of peptides with hormonal properties have been isolated both from gut endocrine cells and from neuronal tissue. These substances may have a common embryological origin. Their physiological roles are still under investigation and present one of the most fascinating challenges in present day physiology and neurochemistry. A partial list of active peptides and "candidate" hormones is presented in Table 1 (21-24). For the microanatomical aspects of these peptide secreting cells, see Chapter 1.

TRANSPORT MECHANISMS

The passage of solutes across a biological membrane can be generally classified according to one of several mechanisms. One of them, diffusion, is a purely physicochemical phenomenon which can be described by mathematical expressions. The others, active transport, facilitated diffusion, and pinocytosis are biological processes comparable to other physiological events or to properties typical of the living cell.

DIFFUSION

Diffusion requires a concentration gradient between the two sides of the membrane. In simple terms, the rate of passage of solutes as a function of time is proportional to the difference of concentrations, to the area of the membrane, and inversely proportional to the thickness of the barrier. It does not assume expenditure of energy, and competition between solutes is negligible. Chemicals affecting active transport mechanisms have no influence on diffusion. Also, in theory at least, the transport capacity should not be saturable.

Negatively charged substances (anions) are poorly absorbed by the small intestine. Hence the cathartic properties of sulfates, tartrates, and citrates (2).

Molecular size and solubility are key factors in transport phenomena across membranes. The small intestine is fairly impervious to high-molecular-weight substances. The salient exception is the absorption of undigested proteins early in life. Also, the intestinal mucosa provides a good protective barrier against indigestible substances, either to the individual subjected to involuntary environmental hazards or to the child who mouths and swallows accessible objects and loose materials (pica).

ACTIVE TRANSPORT

Active transport is a property common to most living cells as a means to concentrate nutrients for protein synthesis, energy requirements, and replacement of other constituents lost by catabolism and breakage (Fig. 5). The "action" is triggered by energy-yielding reactions within the cell or in locations at or near the membrane. In consequence, substances interfering with those reactions can produce inhibition of transport.

An additional characteristic is the existence of saturation phenomena, comparable to those of enzymatic reactions. As generally expressed, K_t is the concentration at which the transport of a solute will reach one-half of the maximum attainable rate, or V_m. A substance with a low K_t will have greater affinity for the transport system than another with a higher K_t.

Active transport can be competitively inhibited by substances that share identical transport mechanisms. Changes in temperature also will affect strongly the velocity of active absorption, as in most biological processes. Active transport is an aerobic process. However, in experimental animals, energy derived from anaerobic glycolysis can drive active transport for amino acids, glucose,

time

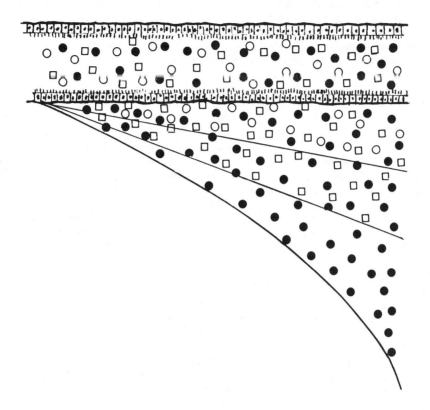

FIGURE 5   Idealized representation of the three most important types of transport mechanisms in the small intestine. A substance absorbed by diffusion only
(open circles) would traverse cells at a rate proportionate with time. Compounds carried across by facilitated transport (open squares) would enter cells at
a faster rate and be more abundant after a certain time than the first type of substances. Molecules absorbed by active transport mechanisms (closed circles)
would be appearing in the mucosal side at a rate generally faster than any of the
above, even against a concentration gradient, not indicated in the diagram, and be
relatively prevalent on the serosal side (below).

electrolytes, and other physiological substances in tissues obtained during the fetal period or early in life (9, 10). Young animals also show an accelerated rate of
transport, probably due to the presence of more active sites and hence have an apparent higher V_m (11). It stands to reason that if the active absorption capacity of
the small intestine would grow at the same rate as the mass of the individual there
would be exponential excess of sites available which would have no need to be functional.

FACILITATED TRANSPORT

Facilitated transport has been postulated by Danielli (25), as a working hypothesis stemming from his studies on membrane structures. It was noted that many substances crossed membranes very slowly, while others were allowed through them quite rapidly. Some substances such as urea, glycerol, and glucose, exceeded expectations by several orders of magnitude. It was shown that this movement will not take place against a concentration gradient. No energy expenditure is required for facilitated transport. However, enzyme poisons, such as cupric ions, can block this passage. This fact suggests that the transfer of those solutes takes place through pores that resemble seams of a mosaic in a schematic diagram of the membrane. The protein-lined channel is strong enough to prevent osmotic disruption, but with the capability of being hydrated and transversed. Some investigators have postulated a reorientation of those pores and a "flip-flop" mechanism to extrude solutes from one side to the other (26). The transport of glucose into the erythrocyte appears to be the most outstanding example of facilitated transport. Its role in absorption across the intestine may not be as important during the ingestion of nutritive substances. It should be realized that in the course of a substantial sugar load, all three mechanisms discussed so far may be in operation. The relative load carried by each is subjected to constant changes because of dynamic alterations and local concentration differences.

PINOCYTOSIS

The duodenum and the small intestine of mammals have been known to engulf colloidal and insoluble particles by a phagocyticlike process apparently similar to that operative in protozoans (27). However, more important is the absorption of native proteins (1) by the process of pinocytosis, particularly antibodies which are present in the globulin fraction of maternal colostrum. This phenomenon has been shown clearly in newborn rats (28), where a selective affinity favoring maternal proteins in preference to proteins from other species has been conclusively demonstrated.

In the infant, globulins are protected from digestion by an inhibition of trypsin and the relative lack of hydrochloric acid in the newborn stomach. The capacity to absorb native proteins drops sharply after the second day of life. The absorbed globulins are channeled into the lymph to the systemic plasma, bypassing portal circulation and the enzymatic assault of the liver. By this physiological device, the half-life of ingested antibodies is markedly extended (29).

Recently, attention has focused on pinocytosis phenomena occurring in older individuals when subjected to various forms of nutritional stress. In marasmic children, the intestinal mucosa presents large autophagosomes, characteristic organelles possessing proteolytic enzymes, among others (30). In experimental animals, protein deficiency may increase permeability to macromolecules (31). Ferritin (mol wt 650,000) and adenovirus type 5 (mol wt 1 million) are absorbed by pinocytosis in malnourished rats. Animals fasted for extended periods show electron-dense materials in the intercellular space of the intestinal epithelium and lamina propria, opening the possibility of large particles moving between cells, across the tight junction. This alternative has been confirmed recently in experiments where the intestine of rats was exposed to hyperosmotic, nonabsorbable solutions. Horseradish peroxidase, a medium-sized protein (mol wt 40,000) was shown to reach the intracellular space and the cytosol in the enterocytes of rats (14).

UNSTIRRED LAYERS

It has been shown that immediately next to every biological membrane there is a succession of unstirred layers of water through which solutes must move by simple diffusion.   Therefore, the apparent immobile liquid barrier can act as another membrane present between the lumen and the surface of the microvilli (32). The thickness of these layers has been estimated in vitro to reach 400 μ m.   However, it is considered that in vivo the presence of mucus can effectively increase the depth of the unstirred fluid to the millimeter range.   The realization of this physiological property of the intestinal mucosal membrane has forced investigators to reexamine values previously obtained for kinetic constants in active transport systems (33).   For instance, while a K_t as low as 1.4 mM was calculated from in vitro experiments for phenylalanine, concentrations as much as 70 times higher were still below the saturation point when the tests were performed in vivo.   Also, it appears that fatty acids and higher alcohols are slowed down so much by the immobile layer adjacent to the mucosa, that the permeation of the barriers constitutes the true limiting step for their absorption (34).

ABSORPTION OF PROTEINS (1, 35-38)

The role of the stomach in the absorption of protein is considered to be very limited.   A low pH denatures native proteins and activates various species of pepsinogens into proteolytically active pepsin, which is active as a proteolytic enzyme from pH 1-3.   When pH increases, pepsin is inactivated.

The organism requires the breakdown of proteins into polypeptides and amino acids to effect absorption.   Pancreatic enzymes are the key to this step.   Their lack can severely decrease net protein absorption and increase fecal protein losses.   Natural proteins consist of chains and cross-linked globular clusters containing hundreds or thousands of L-amino acids.   Proteolytic enzymes rapidly cleave those complex sequences into smaller pieces.   Another set of enzymes present on the mucosal surface and in the cytosol of enterocytes—peptide hydrolases—complete the task of reducing the fragments to smaller peptides and single amino acids.

ABSORPTION OF PEPTIDES

The digestion of proteins was believed to be essentially carried out to the final hydrolytic stage, i.e., amino acids, before absorption.   More recent studies showed that the mucosal surface is the main site of peptide hydrolase activity, to a greater extent than that of the intestinal lumen.   There appears to be a large variety of hydrolases.   Most of those in the cytosol of the columnar cells are active on dipeptides and to a minor extent on tripeptides.   Brush border enzymes hydrolyze peptides with both low and high numbers of residues.

Intact peptides are absorbed as such across the intestinal mucosa, independent of how the individual amino acids are absorbed.   This phenomenon can be due to either simple diffusion or to a carrier-mediated transport.   There are strong indications supporting the latter option, since saturation constants (K_t) for specific dipeptides have been determined in human intestinal mucosa.   They are, generally, one order of magnitude higher than for amino acids.   Thus dipeptides are less efficiently bound than neutral amino acids.   However, no competition between oligopeptides and single amino acids has been observed.

Since the rate of individual amino acid absorption is not parallel to that of protein breakdown, it is probable that the rate of transport of glycine, threonine,

serine, proline, hydroxyproline, aspartic and glutamic acids is dependent particularly on the absorption of small peptides (39). Additional evidence on the importance of the existence of transport mechanisms for di- and tripeptides is the
demonstration that individuals with specific, genetically determined abnormalities of neutral or dibasic amino acid transport, such as cystinuria, or Hartnup
disease, have no impairment in the absorption of either dibasic amino acids
(40, 41), or neutral amino acids, provided these amino acids are part of a
dipeptide. The ability to absorb peptides is a natural way to bypass genetically
determined limitations and possible nutritional disturbances due to competition
between individual amino acids. Since for the usual 20 L-amino acids there exists
the possibility of 380 dipeptides and 6840 tripeptides, there is a good likelihood of
overlapping transport mechanisms for a substantial number of them.

By judicious, simultaneous removal from the intestinal lumen of small peptides, as well as amino acids, the local accumulation of osmotically strong products is reduced. The therapeutic use of oral protein hydrolysates therefore
must be viewed with a certain caution. A product essentially consisting of free
amino acids is more likely to give rise to transport competition phenomena at the
intestinal mucosal level than another with a larger proportion of oligopeptides.
Animal studies have shown that a more rapid and normal growth is achieved with
native protein foods than with otherwise comparable semipurified diets, where the
protein had been substituted by an enzymatic hydrolysate.

ABSORPTION OF AMINO ACIDS

The intestinal mucosa is very effectively prepared to insure the entry of the ultimate breakdown products of protein—the amino acids. Studies in humans with
synthetic equimolar mixtures of amino acids have shown that the eight essential
amino acids are more rapidly absorbed than the nonessential amino acids. The
most poorly absorbed amino acids are aspartate and glutamate.

The unique nutritional position of protein makes its defective absorption a critical condition. Intake of essential amino acids is a cornerstone for growth and
for maintaining a positive nitrogen balance. A deficiency of brush border peptidases associated with villous atrophy and an absence of microvilli is characteristic of celiac sprue in children and nontropical (idiopathic) sprue in adults. A well
known relationship exists between these patients' intolerance to glutamine-rich
polypeptides present in gluten (one of the proteins of wheat, rye, oats, and bar-
ley), and the status of their disease. Since other sources of protein can successfully replace the noxious product, the condition of the patients can be easily controlled.

Neutral amino acids are transported into the cells by active, energy-requiring,
and saturable translocation mechanisms. They have been very extensively studied
in vitro and in vivo in human tissues and in experimental animals. The number of
carrier systems present in the intestinal mucosa has been generally considered to
be three—one for basic and diaminoamino acids (lysine, arginine, ornithine, and
cystine), one for neutral amino acids, and a third for imino acids (proline, hydroxyproline), glycine, and some of its substituted derivatives. Patients with inborn errors of metabolism have provided supporting evidence for the singularity
of the transport of lysine, arginine, ornithine, and cystine, since these amino
acids are poorly absorbed by cystinuric individuals (42). As indicated earlier,
the patient has recourse to alternate routes to offset these deficiencies. A majority of free, neutral amino acids are poorly absorbed in Hartnup disease (43), but
individual disturbances of amino acid transport have been reported in isolated cases, specifically for methionine (44), tryptophan (45), and proline (46). A genetically determined hyperaminoacidemia can be the cause of an abnormal rate of phenylalanine and tryptophan transport, as observed in phenylketonuria (47). A

reduction of blood phenylalanine levels by dietary means can control the defect and normalize rates of transport for both phenylalanine and tryptophan. These studies, together with comparable animal experiments, suggest that the intestinal absorption of free amino acids is not exclusively accomplished by a single neutral amino acid carrier system, but by a combination of specific and nonspecific transport mechanisms. This has been reinforced also by the demonstration of noncompetitive inhibitory effects caused by an excess ingestion of one neutral amino acid, phenylalanine, in in vivo experimental studies (48, 49) (Fig. 6).

In vitro studies have conclusively shown that the presence of sodium was mandatory for active transport of amino acids. The justification for this requirement has been postulated as due to the existence of the sodium pump (see p. 46), which maintains a critical electric potential gradient across the mucosa. Moreover, the absolute requirements of that ion for the activity of membrane adenosine triphosphatase—Na$^+$-K$^+$ ATPase, the key mechanism for energy-demanding intercellular transport, or the obligatory linkage of sodium to nonionized molecules—add to the pivotal role for sodium in the transfer of molecules across membranes (50, 51). However, under physiological conditions, sodium does not appear to be a limiting factor for the absorption of amino acids in the face of the free flow of electrolytes across mucosal pores as a response to osmotic changes and the almost constant fluxes of water.

There have been reports on the influence of monosaccharides on amino acid transport (52, 53). This could involve an interaction of both type of molecules at the level of membrane carriers. An excess of carbohydrate has been shown to reduce the absorption of glycine. Although these studies were performed in vivo in humans, it is questionable whether or not they could have physiological impact under normal conditions.

Environmental alterations can change amino acid absorption patterns. Experimental malnutrition has been shown to increase the absorption of tyrosine (54). It is not clear, however, if this effect is secondary to alterations in the intestinal mucosa that would reflect in an enhancement of membrane permeability, or in a decrease in the blood levels of that amino acid that would reduce the concentration, from lumen-to-blood gradient, and facilitate diffusion without additional contribution of the active transport mechanisms.

Another source of absorptive damage has been shown to be secondary to experimental lead poisoning (55). In this instance too, the oral intake of the heavy metal can cause a selective impairment of amino acid absorption in addition to a more generalized effect on glucose and sodium transport. The well-documented, frequent gastrointestinal complaints following pica and the ingestion of paint chips or dust containing lead, and sometimes associated with radiological evidence of duodenal damage, may coexist with a transport alteration in the small intestine. This physiological damage appears to be the counterpart of the aminoaciduria often existing in lead poisoning.

ABSORPTION OF CARBOHYDRATES (56-60)

While the small intestine has to cope with the uptake of 20 different amino acids and an astronomical number of peptides, one substance—glucose—has a key position in carbohydrate absorption parallel to the central role it plays in energy metabolism. Two other six-carbon oligosaccharides, galactose and fructose, follow in importance from a dietary and metabolic standpoint (Fig. 7).

There are remarkable similarities between amino acid and carbohydrate intestinal absorption as well as clear differences. One disaccharide—lactose—has preponderance in the diet early in life. The ingested carbohydrate will be split into equal amounts of glucose and galactose, most of which will be channeled into glucose.

COMMON CARRIER

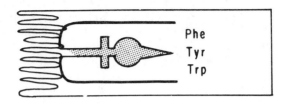

COMMON CARRIER WITH SPECIFIC SITES

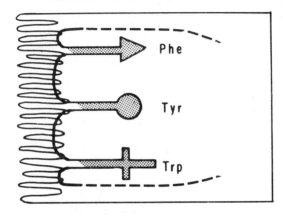

SPECIFIC CARRIER

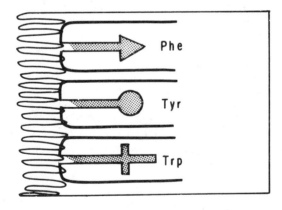

FIGURE 6   Schematic representation of possible configurations of the "neutral amino acid carrier system. " The case of phenylalanine (Phe), tyrosine (Tyr), and tryptophan (Trp) intestinal transport provides an appropriate example of the possibilities open.   Either a "common carrier" has a single site for the three amino acids (upper panel), or the same carrier has different sites for Phe, Tyr, and Trp (center panel).   The third option is the existence of entirely separate and specific carriers for each of these amino acids (lower panel).   The experimental evidence suggests that more than one of those forms may coexist in vivo.

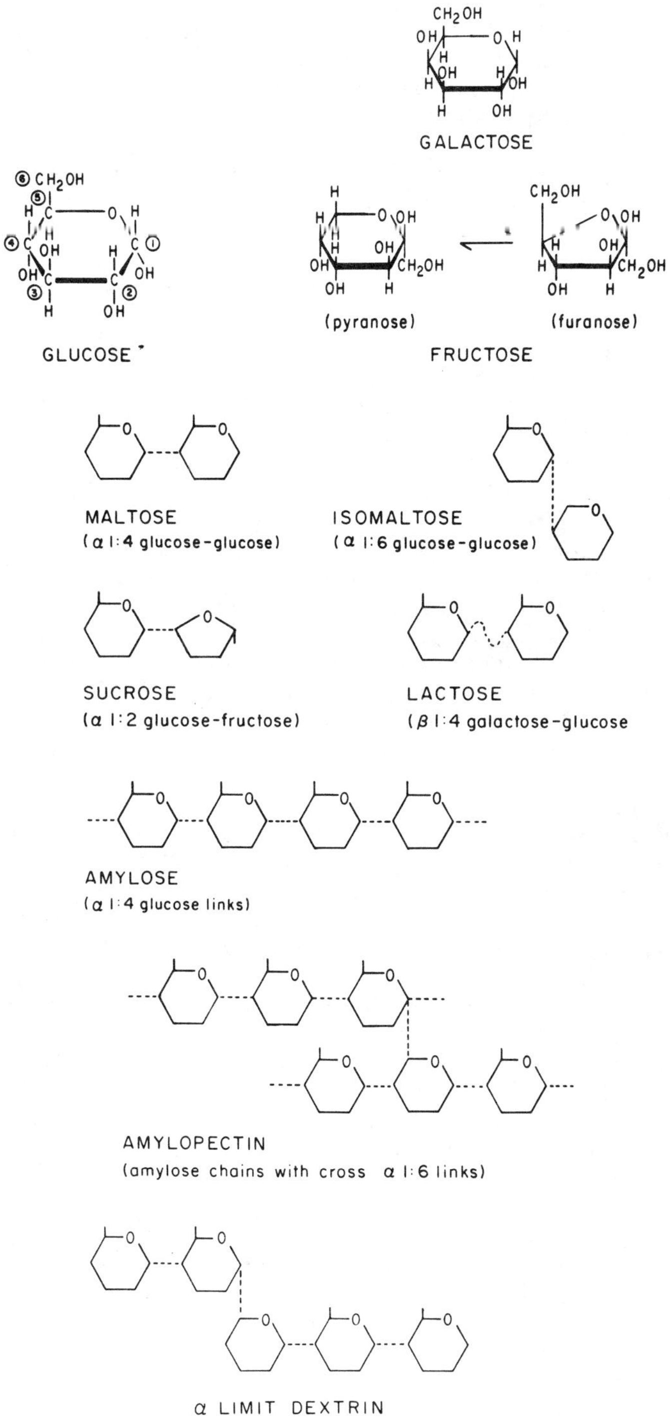

FIGURE 7   Chemical structure of the mono-, di-, and polysaccharides of major significance in human nutrition.

In contrast, it has been estimated that in the older child ingesting a typical North American or Western European diet, the contribution of glucose and its precursor starch is about 70% of the carbohydrate intake, while only one-tenth of that amount is derived from milk sugar—lactose—with the remainder coming from sucrose, one of the very few products that man has added to his diet in an essentially pure chemical form.

Although the very young infant is spared the challenge of breaking down complex disaccharides, e. g. , starch, it is equipped with the enzymes needed to perform the scaling-down transformation. Salivary amylase initiates the splitting of starch, but the bulk of the hydrolysis is carried out by pancreatic amylase. This is a very efficient enzyme (low K_m) and is active even at very low concentrations of substrate irrespective of the size of the starch molecule. Cooking helps starch hydrolysis since it unfolds the native starch molecules and exposes more linkages for amylase action. The results of this enzymatic cleavage are a mixture of oligosaccharides—maltose, maltotriose, and α-limit dextrins. Disaccharides, namely sucrose or lactose, are not digested by enzymes present in the lumen of the duodenum or upper jejunum. This is the role of a complex group of enzymes, the disaccharidases, which are located at the absorptive surface of the microvilli and are intimately linked to the process of absorption.

In this broad category of enzymes, maltases (glucosidases) split the α-1:4 glucose-glucose bond of maltose at the end of chains of short or extended length. They are activated by sodium ions, but are independent of other electrolytes. One of these glucosidases has hydrolytic activity vis-à-vis sucrose and isomaltose and is generally referred to as sucrase-isomaltase. Its individuality has been confirmed since a genetic deficiency has been associated with its absence.

Of more clinical relevance is the existence or absence of lactase activity. An enzyme with well-defined biochemical characteristics is present in the brush border and is responsible for the bulk of lactose hydrolysis. Its absence is linked to primary lactase deficiency occurring in a wide spectrum of ethnic groups as a genetically determined enzymatic defect. Other intracellular lactases (lysosomal) are less specific and have only marginal importance. The widespread lactose intolerance in ethnic groups of non-Caucasians has brought a new awareness of the social and nutritional limitations linked to a whole family of dietary products (61).

Since the absorption of glucose is the key to the assimilation of carbohydrates, it has been questioned whether or not disaccharide hydrolysis is the limiting factor in this phenomenon. A second point in dispute is whether or not the bulk of this chemical simplification occurs inside or outside the absorptive cells. Investigations in the last decade have indicated that disaccharides reach an area in the surface of the microvilli where the probability of being hydrolyzed and almost immediately absorbed is maximum, with only a small proportion having the chance to escape out to the lumen (Fig. 8). Other experiments have demonstrated that absorption is closely related to disaccharidase levels and that when the intestinal mucosa is damaged by disease not only the disaccharidases, but the "glucose pumps" are affected (62, 63).

Glucose also may cross the intestinal mucosa membrane by simple diffusion since the mucosal pores are large enough to allow free passage of that solute, and a large concentration gradient is possible during digestion. However, active transport is a far more efficient mechanism which is independent of concentration once the active sites are saturated (64).

Crane and co-workers (56, 58, 59, 65), as well as other investigators (66-68), have shown that when sufficient sodium is present, glucose is tightly bound to a carrier (low K_m), but when sodium concentration falls the affinity for glucose decreases. This is what happens on the luminal side and in the immediate proximity of the microvilli, where a "microecological" environment rich in sodium exists, provided by an active translocation of this ion from the absorptive cell outwards.

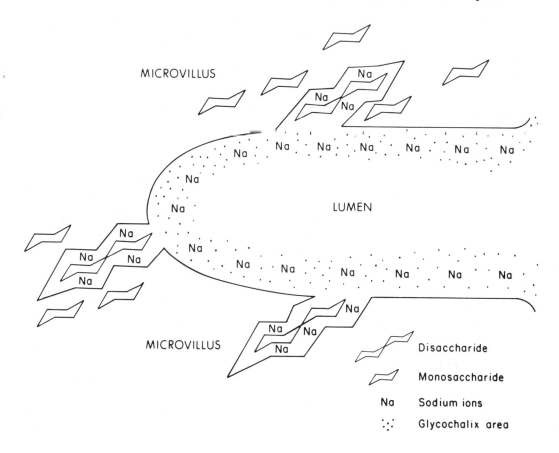

MICROVILLUS

LUMEN

MICROVILLUS

Na   Sodium ions

Disaccharide

Monosaccharide

Na   Sodium ions

:·:   Glycochalix area

FIGURE 8   Visualization of the interaction between disaccharidases and transport mechanisms on the surface of the microvilli. Disaccharides traverse the glycocalyx area where a slower diffusion mechanism prevails and where they acquire an "atmosphere" of sodium ions. The disaccharides are attached to the active sites of disaccharidases and the absorption of the resulting monosaccharides occurs immediately afterward under conditions very favorable for active transport.

Conversely, the cellular cytoplasm has a lower level of sodium and the glucose can become unbound from the carrier and be removed from the cell to the circulation. A small part of the glucose may be metabolized in situ and thus provide energy for ATP synthesis and other energy-rich compounds. Although the abolition of sodium pump activity does not terminate glucose absorption (69), it is now well-established that the translocation of both substances under physiological conditions is intimately linked (58, 70). Other physical parameters, such as the presence of salts (71) or diuretics (72) all can affect glucose absorption. There also may be a diurnal rhythm modulating the rate of transport of the key carbohydrate (73).

   Galactose appears to be transported by the same mechanisms as glucose (74, 75). Fructose, for a long time considered to cross the mucosa only by diffusion, has been shown to possess an independent carrier, which requires sodium (76). Xylose follows the glucose path, although it is difficult to demonstrate saturation mechanisms for it. Xylose was earlier considered to be absorbed only by diffusion. However, there is now experimental evidence of active transport (77). The administration of oral xylose and follow-up of excretion as an index of mucosal damage is nevertheless still valid. Contrariwise, a polyol traditionally assumed to be nonabsorbable, mannitol, has been demonstrated more recently to cross the intestinal mucosa (78).

ABSORPTION OF LIPIDS (79-82)

The large majority of dietary lipids are triglycerides, that is, esters of glycerol with three identical or dissimilar long-chain fatty acids. The physicochemical properties of these substances is dependent on the identity of the fatty acids. Saturated, long-chain fatty acids, i. e. , palmitic and stearic acids, will originate fats that are solid at room or body temperature, and are primarily from animal sources. Nonsaturated (oleic, linoleic, linolenic acids), hydroxylated (ricinoleic acid), or shorter chain (lauric, miristic acids) are generally liquid under these conditions and usually are derived from vegetable sources. Medium-chain triglycerides (MCT) have fatty acids with eight to twelve carbons and have found a specific role in therapeutic formulas (83). Minor components of the diet are cholesterol, the fat-soluble vitamins A, D, E, and K (84), and phospholipids. The latter are structurally similar to triglycerides, with a nonpolar carbon chain, but with a terminal carbon of glycerol attached to a phosphate linked to a nitrogenous base (choline, ethanolamine). Therefore, these substances have both hydrophylic and hydrophobic properties.

A key to the solubilization and absorption of lipids are bile acids. They are biosynthetically derived from cholesterol and may contain two (deoxycholic, chenodeoxycholic), or three (cholic) hydroxyl groups (Fig. 9). In human bile they exist as peptide conjugates with taurine or glycine. In the infant, taurine conjugates predominate (85, 86); in older children, the glycine/taurine ratio becomes 3:1. Conjugation increases the degree of ionization of bile acids at physiological pH, as well as their water solubility, thus becoming effective detergents for the stabilization of oil-water interfaces. Part of the molecule in all bile salts is nonpolar or hydrophobic, while the part containing the conjugated amino acid is polar or hydrophylic. At high dilutions, bile salts (the ionized form of bile acid conjugates) exist as monomers, but above a specific concentration, they form molecular aggregates or micelles (87), i. e. , the critical micellar concentration, or CMC (Fig. 10). Micelles are spherical conglomerates with a diameter between 30-100 Å. It also has been postulated that the lipolytic products of triglyceride hydrolysis and phospholipids such as lecithin can incorporate water molecules (88) and enter in the formation of "mixed" micelles together with bile salts.

Human liver synthesizes cholic and chenodeoxycholic acids. These substances are considered the primary bile acids. Bacteria in the gut dehydroxylate those compounds and produce, respectively, deoxycholic acid and lithocholic acid, the latter a monohydroxy bile acid. These two derivatives are secondary bile acids (see Fig. 9). The turnover of bile salts in the organism is delicately balanced. Only 3-5% of the conjugated bile salts secreted by the liver is lost in the stools and has to be replaced by synthesis de novo. After accomplishing their role as physiological solubilizers, bile acids are reabsorbed in the distal portion of the ileum, in part after undergoing deconjugation by the intestinal flora. The portal vein system returns the free bile acids to the liver for recycling. This essentially closed circuit is known as the enterohepatic circulation of bile salts (Fig. 11).

Fat ingestion in childhood varies from 30-80 g/day, according to diet and age. The adult diet may contain double these amounts. Dietary cholesterol probably accounts for less than 1 g, although the gastrointestinal tract also deals with endogenous cholesterol from bile, gastric juice, desquamated cells, and saliva.

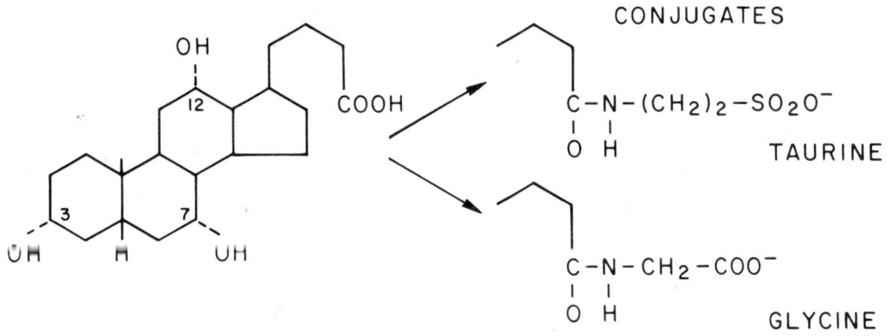

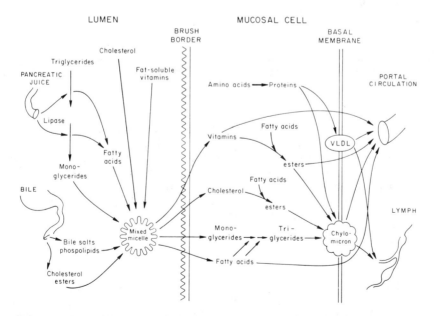

CONJUGATES

$$C-N-(CH_2)_2-SO_2O^-$$
O   H   TAURINE

$$C-N-CH_2-COO^-$$
O   H   GLYCINE

BILE ACIDS

	HYDROXYL GROUPS	PRIMARY	SECONDARY
TRIHYDROXY	→ 3α 7α 12α	Cholic	—
DIHYDROXY	→ 3α 7α	Chenodeoxycholic	Deoxycholic
	→ 3α 12α	—	
MONOHYDROXY	→ 3α	—	Lithocholic

FIGURE 9   Chemical structure of physiologically significant primary and secondary bile acids and their conjugated derivatives with taurine and glycine. The dashed arrows indicate the biological linkage between primary bile acids and their derived secondary homologues produced in the gut by bacterial action.

FIGURE 10   Summarized view of the intestinal transport of lipids and fat-soluble compounds. VLDL = very low-density lipoprotein.

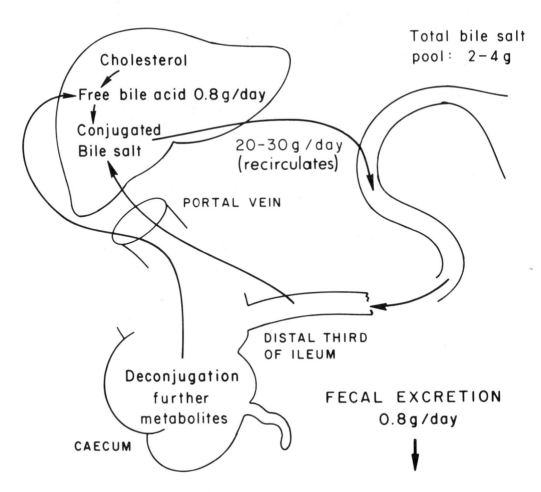

FIGURE 11   Diagrammatic summary of the enterohepatic circulation of bile salts. The amounts indicated correspond to adolescents. Estimates for children are closer to the lower range of the figures.

A normal individual over the age of 1 year absorbs more than 95% of the triglycerides ingested. In the younger infant, the amount absorbed is 80-95% varying with age and gestational maturity. Even under unusual overload circumstances, cholesterol absorption does not exceed 50%. The absorption of fat-soluble vitamins is generally fairly efficient. The interrelationship between vitamin D and calcium absorption and metabolism deserves special consideration elsewhere (see p. 66).

Digestion in the stomach and the presence of a gastric lipase has a limited effect on dietary fats and amounts to the formation of a crude emulsion, or chyme. After entering the duodenum, the increase in pH plus the addition of bile salts and lecithin to the products of triglyceride hydrolysis produces a well-dispersed emulsion, with particles ranging in size from 0.2-5 μm. The key enzyme in lipolysis is pancreatic lipase. Its secretion is triggered by a hormonal mechanism located in the duodenal mucosal cells, cholecystokinin-pancreozymin, released following contact of fat and other foodstuffs with active sites in the mucosa. Lipase splits successively the two outside fatty acids of triglycerides and the resulting 2-monoglyceride is either absorbed or slowly isomerized to the physiologically more stable 1-monogly-

ceride. Cholesterol often exists as an ester with long-chain fatty acids, and
a specific enzyme (esterase) is present in pancreatic juice and in mucosal cells
that can liberate free cholesterol or reesterify that compound.

The upper intestine thus contains mostly mixed micelles, free and esterified
cholesterol, mono- and diglycerides, free fatty acids, and unhydrolyzed triglycerides. After a rich meal, the contents of the upper jejunum can be separated
physically into an oily fraction, a micellar phase, and a heavier, less soluble
layer, rich in cholesterol and strongly adhesive to the mucosal membrane (87, 89).

There are various possibilities that can be envisioned for the passage of lipids
from micelles onto the absorptive cells. One of them is the extrusion of the lipid
from the inside of the micelle into the cell surface. A second possibility is that
the whole micelle would make contact with the brush border, at which point the
micelle would break into its molecular constituents and penetrate the brush border
membrane. According to recent experimental work (33, 34), the unstirred water
layer and the glycocalyx may regulate the rate of absorption, since they would
act also as an electrostatic barrier affecting the integrity of the micelles.

Fatty acids can be absorbed at a slower rate in the absence of bile, but cholesterol or lipid-soluble vitamins are essentially unabsorbed under these conditions
and this is important in the bile-salt deficiency syndromes.

Although early studies had advanced the notion that pinocytosis was the process
through which lipids were absorbed, more exhaustive work in the late 1960s (90)
has negated this view.   Since it has been shown that lipid uptake can occur at low
temperatures, the initial uptake of polar fats may be dependent upon binding to the
membrane of the microvilli or to the glycoproteins in the matrix immediately adjacent to it.   Nonpolar substances may pass by a diffusion process. Since during
digestion the local concentration at the membrane interface may be far higher than
that prevailing in the lumen, simple diffusion is a likely mechanism.

It is estimated that 75% of dietary lipid is absorbed as the 2-monoglyceride
rather than as di- or triglycerides. Once inside the cell, the partially hydrolyzed
glyceride can be either totally hydrolyzed to free fatty acids and glycerol or reesterified to triglycerides.   This is dependent on the relative concentrations of
each type of component. Most of the cholesterol is esterified also and absorbed
through lymph.

Biosynthesis of glycerides is achieved through two pathways: (1) activation of
of free fatty acids through enzymatic mechanisms which consume energy (ATP and
coenzyme A) and act on long-chain fatty acids, resulting in fatty acyl CoA, a highly reactive compound. (2) Glycerophosphate is mostly derived from glycolysis and
the phosphate attached to the glycerol skeleton can be readily exchanged for activated fatty acids. Quantitatively, however, 2-monoglycerides are the backbone
for the synthesis of triglycerides, carried out step by step through "activated"
(fatty acyl CoA) fatty acids. These newly synthesized triglycerides now combine
with specific proteins, also synthesized in the enterocyte, to form lipoproteins
that leave the cell through the lateral plasma membranes of the absorptive cells,
probably by a process of exocytosis. Cholesterol is also part of this complex that
leaves the cell as chylomicrons or as very low-density lipoproteins (91). Chylomicrons contain 81-97% triglycerides, 2-9% phospholipids and a small amount of
β -lipoprotein in a covering layer of the chylomicron. The small intestine is the
apparent origin of the lipoproteins circulating in the lymph. The intracellular origin of these proteins has been demonstrated with protein synthesis inhibitors and
by the accumulation of fat in genetically determined hypobetalipoproteinemia. In
this condition, lack of mature, low-density β -lipoprotein impairs transport of lipid into lymph (92).

Short- and medium-chain fatty acids (12 carbons or less) are not reesterified in
the mucosal cells and enter the circulation through the portal vein tributaries.
Longer fatty acids, when transported by this route are generally adsorbed to albumin molecules.

Fat-soluble vitamins may enter mixed micelles after hydrolysis of their esters which are often present in dietary products (Fig. 12). This step is indispensable in the case of vitamin A and is carried out by pancreatic hydrolases. In contrast to most nutrients, it appears as if intestinal absorption of vitamins D, K, and E is only partial, and that 10-50% of the intake is lost to bacterial degradation. The proximal and middle regions of the small intestine are most important for the absorption of liposoluble vitamins. There may be an active mechanism for two of the substances with vitamin K activity (84), although for other related compounds, simple diffusion through the lipid microvillar membrane prevails (93). Once inside the enterocyte only vitamins K and E remain unesterified and may enter lymph ducts as part of chylomicrons. Synthetic vitamin K_3 (menadione) can enter the portal circulation directly. In contrast, most vitamin A is reesterified with long-chain fatty acids. A fraction of the total vitamin D undergoes the same fate before its entrance into chylomicrons and eventual absorption via lymphatics. Only minor amounts of vitamins A and E are absorbed through the venous network.

ABSORPTION OF MINERALS

CALCIUM (94, 95) (See also Chap. 6)

The absorption of calcium is indispensable for life. It takes place in the proximal regions of the intestine, and is intimately related to an adequate availability of vitamin D. However, a primary, exclusive, calcium malabsorption syndrome is not known in man, although osteoporosis can be experimentally produced by a diet low in calcium.

Body homeostatis for this ion is maintained through the equilibrium between bone formation and resorption, as well as by the regulation of urinary excretion (Fig. 13). In addition, hormonal mediation has a direct influence on the active transport mechanism involved in the translocation of calcium across the intestinal mucosa.

In addition to vitamin D, parathormone and possibly calcitonin are operative in the translocation of calcium. Experimental work has indicated that the absorption of calcium is impaired by an alkaline pH and the presence of organic and fatty acids that can produce insoluble salts or soaps, as in steatorrhea. Conversely, a lowering of pH below 7 and the presence of bile salts enhance calcium uptake.

The study of calcium absorption in vivo is complicated by the contribution of this ion derived from the endogenous pool. The only effective way to discriminate the input from diverse sources is by the use of the radioisotopes ^{45}Ca or ^{47}Ca and requires a computerized analysis to solve the multiple variables of a credible model of absorption (96).

The role of vitamin D appears to take place at the serosal side of the cell, stimulating calcium absorption by repressing the flux of this ion from the circulation to the cell. It also influences the synthesis of a specific protein that binds calcium to the surface of the microvilli, in preference to nonspecific cellular debris (97).

The direct effects of vitamin D in the treatment of rickets are very clear. Untreated children with this condition have a negative calcium balance, which is reversed with minimal doses of vitamin D (98), although therapeutic levels may be as high as 100,000 units/day. Excess vitamin D can produce hypercalcemia because of increased intestinal absorption rather than as a consequence of bone resorption.

Parathormone action on calcium absorption has been demonstrated in experimental animals and in man suffering from parathyroid adenomas or other forms of hyperparathyroidism (99). The cellular basis for this effect may be related to an

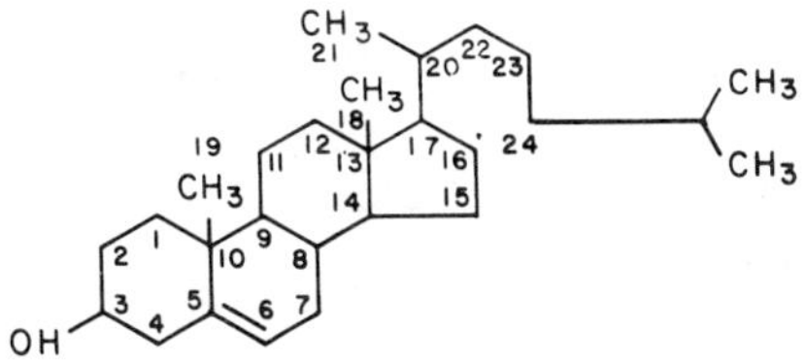

CHOLESTEROL

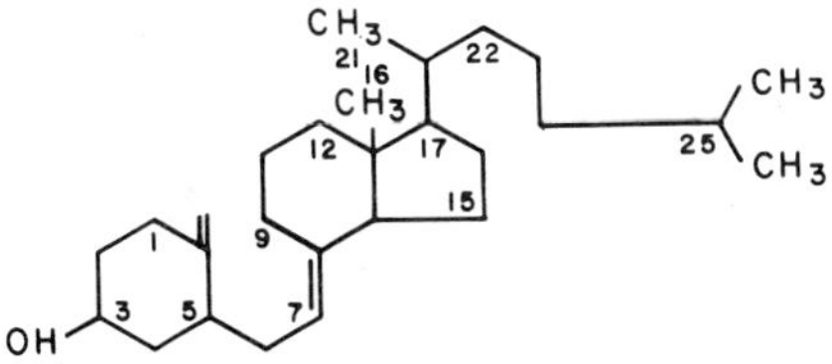

VITAMIN D_3 (Cholecalciferol)

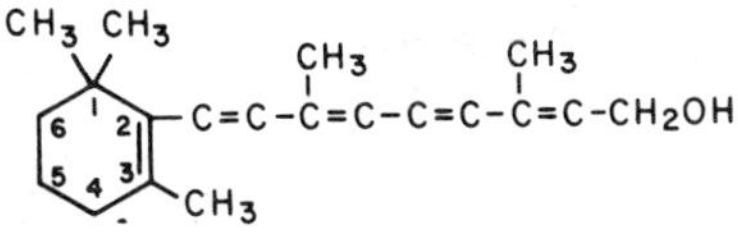

VITAMIN A_1 (Retinol)

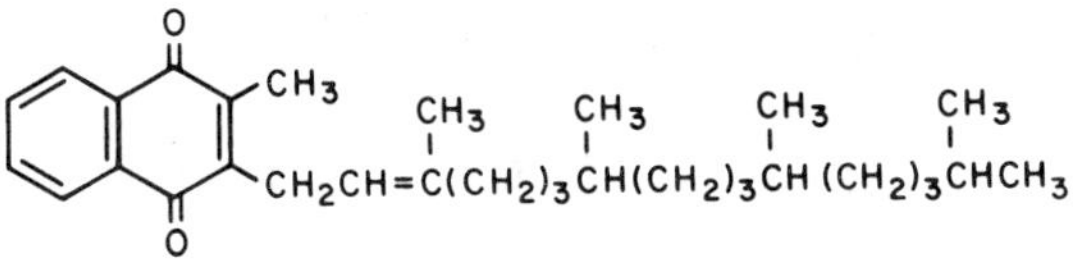

VITAMIN K_1 (Phylloquinone)

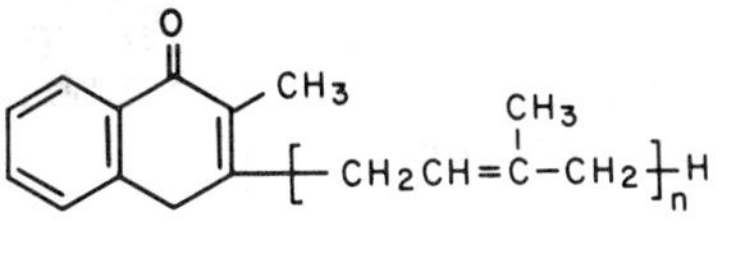

VITAMIN K_2

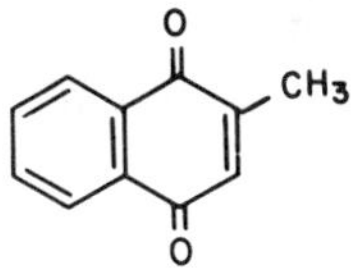

VITAMIN K_3 (Menadione)

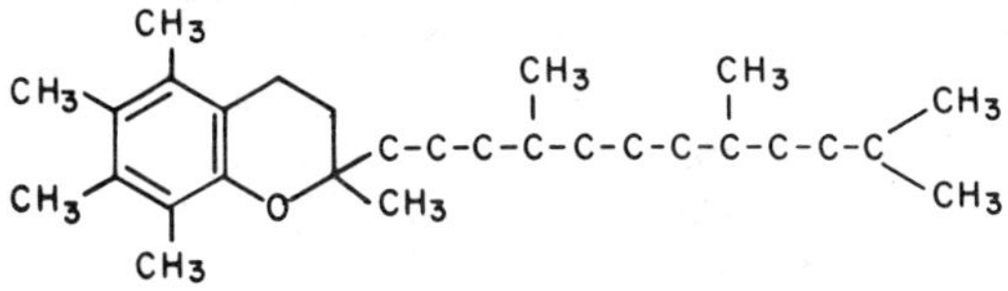

VITAMIN E (Alpha-Tocopherol)

FIGURE 12 Chemical structure of cholesterol and fat-soluble vitamins.

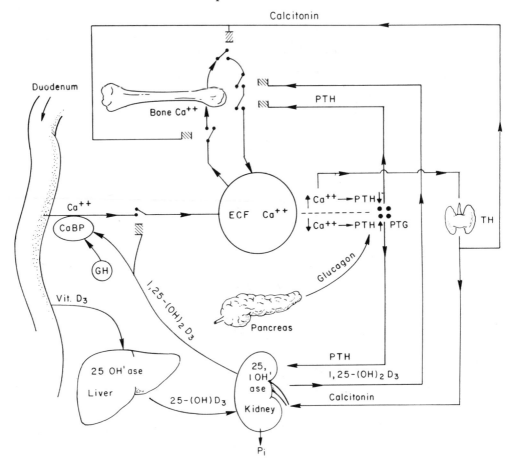

FIGURE 13   Homeostatic mechanisms for calcium:(CaBP) calcium-binding protein; (ECF) extracellular fluid; (GH) growth hormone; (PTH) parathormone; (PTG) parathyroid; (TH) thyroid.   Hormonal action on calcium absorption by the small intestine, as well as calcium deposition and secretion from bone are represented as relays, opening or closing the corresponding circuits.

increased synthesis of carrier protein.   The active form of vitamin D, 1, 25-di-hydroxycholecalciferol $(1,25-(OH)_2D_3)$ is the chemical vehicle that regulates the absorption of calcium and, together with parathyroid hormone, determines mobilization of calcium stores from bone (100).   Parathyroid hormone secretion, in turn, is regulated by calcium; a lowering in circulating concentrations of calcium brings about a stimulation of kidney $25-OH-D_3$ 1-hydroxylase.   Hence, parathormone and the active vitamin D derivative act on bone stores to release additional free calcium.   At the same time, $1,25-(OH)_2D_3$ increases the absorption of calcium at the level of the intestinal mucosa (101).   These complex interactions are summarized in Fig. 13.

Other hormones also have been shown to act on intestinal calcium absorption. Corticosteroids exert an inhibitory action on this function, as demonstrated in man and experimental animals (94).   Growth hormone has, on the contrary, a stimulating effect on calcium uptake by the intestine that can be demonstrated in hypophysectomized animals and in clinical studies carried out with patients suffering acromegaly (94). Calcitonin, which is capable of inducing hypocalcemia by stimulating bone uptake, acts on absorption of calcium indirectly as a result of the stimulation of parathyroid hormone caused by the reduction of circulating calcium concentration.

At a different level of events, calcium absorption can be disrupted by magnesium, as well as of other ions of no nutritional importance, probably through competition for sites on a common transport mechanism. Another divalent ion, lead, can interact with calcium. An apparent dietary calcium deficiency may stimulate craving for nonfood substances (pica) and increase susceptibility to lead intoxication (102-106).

A dietary history of low calcium intake can induce a higher proportion of absorption for this ion. That was the concept embodied in the "endogenous factor" proposed in the 1940s. Since recent advances in the biochemistry of vitamin D have indicated that kidney-synthesized $1,25-(OH)_2D_3$ stimulates the absorption of this ion, the identity of the classical "endogenous factor" now may have been settled (105). Moreover, there has been a good demonstration that the efficiency of calcium absorption varies inversely with intake. Recent studies have shown that at least part of the effective absorption of calcium is independent of control mechanisms (106).

Bile salts also have a favorable effect on the absorption of calcium, linked to their ability to form soluble calcium complexes from bound calcium products (107). Sugars, particularly lactose, have been found to enhance uptake of calcium by the small intestine. Recent studies suggest that its mode of action is not a direct interaction with calcium in solution, but with the absorptive cells of the intestine which may become more permeable to the ion (108). Contrariwise, the presence of fat has been long known to depress absorption of calcium possibly through formation of insoluble calcium soaps (94).

IRON (109, 110)

The intestinal absorption of this element is a complex phenomenon. Iron may be presented to the proximal portions of the small intestine at two stages of oxidation and either as inorganic salts, or as organic compounds bound to proteins. According to the redox potential and the pH, the equilibrium between ferrous and ferric ions can shift. At the low pH of the stomach, inorganic iron salts are well dissociated and its covalent bonds attached to water. Following passage to the duodenum and an increase in the pH, iron tends to be oxidated to trivalent ferric ion and to become insoluble. Many organic substances, including proteins, can form strong covalent compounds with iron. The heme molecule, for instance, has the iron atom extremely tightly bound, to the point of insensitivity to sharp pH alterations.

Iron absorption occurs mostly in the duodenum and the proximal parts of the jejunum which are the most active sites for the function. There is also absorption, but to a lesser extent, along distal portions of the small intestine. Apparently, once the iron enters the absorptive cell, it goes to a rapid turnover compartment where it probably is combined with the receptor protein to form ferritin. Gastric and intestinal juices partially solubilize and denature proteins to which iron may be attached, increasing its absorption by the mucosal cells. The efficiency of this process is variable. Once inside the absorptive cells, iron combines with a specific protein, apoferritin, with which it forms an organometallic compound, ferritin. The synthesis of apoferritin is stimulated apparently by the entry of iron into the enterocyte (111, 112). The iron in the circulation is bound to another protein, transferrin, with which it is distributed throughout the body. At this step, a feedback mechanism, sensitive to iron body stores and the rate of erythropoiesis, controls the effective absorption rate.

The most accurate way to determine iron absorption is by the use of either ^{59}Fe or ^{55}Fe, which are relatively low-penetration radioisotopes. The use of radioisotopes not only improves the reliability of measurements, but also allows the detection of tagged iron in the circulation, the red blood cells, or the feces. When using radioactive iron, total body counts taken shortly after the administration of the dose, minus the amount remaining 10-14 days later will give the true retention of this element. This technique, in spite of its elegance, has not been applied to pediatric studies.

Because of iron's chemical properties, foods rich in substances that may precipitate it, namely organic phosphates or phytates, will have a negative effect on iron absorption. Certain small organic molecules, such as ascorbate, cysteine, sorbitol, or mannitol have a favorable influence, since they can form stable, soluble complexes with iron. Alcohol may stimulate iron absorption by the enhancement of hydrochloric acid secretion in the stomach and consequent fall of the pH. Conversely, stimulation of exocrine pancreatic function by CCK-PZ and secretin appears to have an inhibitory effect on iron absorption. It has been noted that children with cystic fibrosis who receive long-term treatment with pancreatin may develop iron-deficiency anemia (113). However, it has not been elucidated whether the enzymes themselves, or the mere increase in pH due to bicarbonate secretion, are responsible for the reduction in iron uptake.

Absorption of pharmacological dosages of inorganic iron is different from iron present in foodstuffs. As noted above, ferrous sulfate or gluconate are absorbed best in the absence of solid food and in conjunction with organic acids that favor the solubility of the ferrous ion, e. g. , fruit juices (114, 115). Food intake can reduce this proportion by half. The presence of ethylenediamine tetraacetate (EDTA), frequently added to foods as a stabilizer for iron-enriched products and as a general preservative, can reduce substantially the absorption of this element and diminish the true availability of iron (116). It has been established that only 5-10% of dietary iron normally is absorbed (117). The best nutritional results according to these estimates derive from natural iron present in veal muscle or liver, from which 15-20% of the total element is available. In contrast, the proportion of absorbable iron in eggs or cereals is less than 5% and barely exceeds 1% in vegetables and rice (118, 119). Studies with ^{59}Fe ferrous ion in adult men have demonstrated conclusively that the relationship between the dosage of iron ingested and the amount absorbed is directly proportional. The mean rates of iron absorption in infants have been estimated to be approximately 23% (120) with doses under 1 mg, but only 7% when the dose was higher (113). Premature babies have more efficient iron absorption rates (29-32% with low dosages) and 11-22% with higher levels of administration. These figures are comparable to those observed in adults (120, 121).

COPPER (122)

The absorption of copper occurs in the upper segment of the small intestine, with only a small proportion of the estimated intake being absorbed. Neither mechanisms for the translocation of copper nor the chemical forms from which it is most effectively absorbed are known. Ceruloplasmin and amino acids bind 95% of all the body copper in circulation and act as its vehicle through the organism. A genetically determined deficiency of ceruloplasmin, as in Wilson disease, may produce the accumulation of this element in various tissues. Conversely, the congenital inability to absorb copper from the intestinal tract is considered to be the primary disorder associated with the Menkes "kinky hair" syndrome.

MAGNESIUM

It has been estimated that 40-50% of the normal magnesium intake is absorbed. This may represent as much as 100 mg/day in adults. Absorption takes place along the whole length of the intestine and continues for hours after the ingestion of a tagged tracer (1). Magnesium crosses the intestinal mucosa by simple diffusion and follows water displacement. Much of the magnesium ingested is derived from the chlorophyll of green vegetables. However, the endogenous turnover into the intestinal lumen is considerable and represents about 1% of the total body pool in physiological conditions and even more during surgical trauma and gastrointestinal disease. In addition, the proportion of magnesium ion absorbed can vary as a function of mucosal integrity in chronic diseases of the bowel (123).

PHOSPHATE

Inorganic and organic phosphates are absorbed all along the small intestinal tract both by passive and active translocation mechanisms (1). An excess of cations capable of forming insoluble phosphates can reduce the absorption rates for this ion. An identical deficiency can occur after therapeutic use of aluminum hydroxide gels or diets exceptionally rich in calcium, magnesium, or iron. Vitamin D stimulates duodenal transport of phosphate in the presence of calcium. In the jejunum, calcium has no effect, but the more active vitamin D derivatives, 25-OH-D_3 and 1,25-$(OH)_2$,D_3 stimulate passage of phosphate across the intestinal mucosa in vitro (124).

WATER-SOLUBLE VITAMINS (125)

VITAMIN B_{12}

While other water-soluble B vitamins are absorbed by simple diffusion across the intestinal mucosa, vitamin B_{12} is a very large molecule (mol wt 1357) and requires a special pathway. The key element involved in its intestinal absorption is the intrinsic factor (IF) needed for its uptake by the ileum. The IF is a glycoprotein (mol wt 55,000) which is released from the gastric parietal cells under stimulation by gastrin. In addition, stomach acidity contributes to solubilize vitamin B_{12} (deoxyadenosylcobalamine), or its analogues present in the diet. The complex with IF is taken up by specific receptor sites in the ileum. Calcium and magnesium are also required for this process. Gastric atrophy will lead to absence of IF and cause typical vitamin B_{12} deficiency—pernicious macrocytic anemia. Only parenteral doses of the cobalamins can substitute for the natural absorption across the ileum. The complex with IF is dissociated at the mucosal surface, since no IF appears in the circulation. The vitamin is transferred to portal circulation attached to a carrier protein, transcobalamin (1). Vitamin B_{12} contains about 4% cobalt; this vitamin is the main vehicle for this element. In addition, cobaltous ions, in free form, may have a direct role in erythropoiesis (126).

FOLACIN

Under this nomenclature are now included various derivatives of monopteroylglutamic acid (folic acid). Naturally occurring pteroylglutamates are generally absorbed in the jejunum. Excess glutamic acid fragments are hydrolyzed by a specific enzyme in the enterocyte.   Only the monoglutamate enters the circulation and is further reduced and methylated in the liver.   The deficiency in folacin observed in patients with enteric diseases has been re lated to the existing destruction of the mucosa rather than to a specific defect of transport (127, 128).

ACKNOWLEDGEMENT

Supported in part by USPHS Grant # SO8 RR 09128-03.

REFERENCES

1.   Davenport, H. W.: Physiology of the Digestive Tract, 4th ed.   Year Book Medical Publishers, Chicago, 1977, Part II, III, p. 129 ff.

2.   Wilson, T. H.: Intestinal Absorption. W. B. Saunders Co., Philadelphia, 1962, p. 1 ff.

3.   Hamilton, W. J., and H. W. Mossman (eds.): Human Embryology. Williams & Wilkins, Baltimore, 1972, p. 291.

4.   Dahlqvist, A., and T. Lindberg: Development of the intestinal disaccharidase and alkaline phosphatase activities in the human foetus.   Clin Sci 30:517, 1966.'

5.   Lindberg, T.: Intestinal dipeptidases. Characterization, development and distribution of intestinal dipeptidases of the human foetus.   Clin Sci 30:505, 1966.

6.   Antonowicz, I. and E. Lebenthal: Developmental pattern of small intestinal enterokinase and disaccharidase activities in the human fetus.   Gastroenterology 72:1299, 1977.

7.   Levin, R. J., O. Koldovsky, J. Hoskova, V. Jirsova, and J. Uher: Electrical activity across human foetal small intestine associated with absorption processes.   Gut 9:206, 1968.

8.   Wilson, T. H., and E. C. C. Lin: Active transport by intestines of fetal and newborn rabbits. Am J Physiol 199:1030, 1960.

9.   Pratt, R. M., and C. Tenner: Development of amino acid transport by the small intestine of the chick embryo.   Biochim Biophys Acta 225:113, 1971.

10.   Ferdinandus, L. D., J. F. Fitzgerald, and S. Reiser: Metabolic properties of neonatal transport.   Pediatr Res 8:884, 1974.

11.   Reiser, S., J. F. Fitzgerald, and P. A. Christiansen: Kinetics of the accelerated intestinal valine transport in 2-day-old rats. Biochim Biophys Acta 203:351, 1970.

12.   Sidorov, J. J.: Intestinal absorption of water and electrolytes. Clin Biochem 9:117, 1976.

13. Edmonds, C.J.: Salts and water. in Biomembranes, Vol. 4B, D.H. Smyth (ed.). Plenum Press, New York, 1974, p. 711.

14. Teichberg, S., F. Lifshitz, R. Pergolizzi, and R.A. Wapnir: Response of rat intestine to a hyperosmotic feeding. Pediatr Res 12:720, 1978.

15. Wapnir, R.A.: Intestinal osmotic and kinetic effects of carbohydrate malabsorption. in Carbohydrate Intolerance in Infancy. F. Lifshitz (ed.). Marcel Dekker, New York, 1982, p. 121.

16. Sessions, R.T., V.H. Reynolds, J.L. Ferguson, and H.W. Scott: Correlation between intraduodenal osmotic pressure changes and ^{51}Cr blood volumes during induced dumping in lumen with normal stomachs. Surgery 52:226, 1962.

17. Field, M.: Intestinal secretion. Gastroenterology 66:1063, 1974.

18. Gorbach, S.L., B.H. Kean, D.G. Evans, D.J. Evans, Jr., and D. Bessudo: Traveler's diarrhea and toxigenic Escherichia Coli. N Engl J Med 292:933. 1975.

19. Sachs, D.A., M.H. Merson, J.G. Wells, R.B. Sack, and G.K. Morris: Diarrhoea associated with heat-stable enterotoxin-producing strains of Escherichia Coli. Lancet 2:239, 1975.

20. Walsh, J.H., and M.I. Grossman: Gastrin. N Engl J Med 292:1324, 1377, 1975.

21. Grossman, M.I., et al.: Candidate hormones of the gut. Gastroenterology 67:730, 1974.

22. Barrington, E.J.W., and G.J. Dockray: Gastrointestinal hormones. J Endocrinol 69:299, 1976.

23. Dockray, G.J.: Comparative biochemistry and physiology of gut hormones. Ann Rev Physiol 41:83, 1979.

24. Snyder, S.H.: Brain peptides as neurotransmitters. Science 209:976, 1980.

25. Danielli, J.F.: The bilayer hypothesis of membrane structure. Hosp Prac 8:63, 1973.

26. Stein, W.D.: The transport of sugars. Br Med Bull 24:146, 1968.

27. Clark, S.L., Jr.: The ingestion of proteins and colloidal materials by columnar absorptive cells of the small intestine in suckling rats and mice. J Biophys Biochem Cytol 5:41, 1959.

28. Halliday, R.: The absorption of antibodies from immune sera by the gut of the young rat. Proc R Soc (London) Ser. B 143:408, 1955.

29. Morris, I.G.: Gamma globulin absorption in the newborn. in Handbook of Physiology, Sec. 6, Alimentary Canal. Vol. III. Intestinal Absorption. C.F. Code and W. Heidel (eds.). Am Physiol Soc, Washington, 1968, p. 1491.

30.   Brunser, O. , C. Castillo, and M. Araya: Fine structure of the small in-testinal mucosa in infantile marasmic malnutrition. Gastroenterology 70: 495, 1976.

31.   Worthington, B. S. , E. S. Boatman, and G. E. Kenny: Intestinal absorption of intact proteins in normal and protein-deficient rats. Am J Clin Nutr 27:276, 1974.

32.   Dietschy, J. M. , and H. Westergaard: The effect of unstirred water layers on various transport processes in the intestine. in Intestinal Absorption and Malabsorption. P. Z. Csaky (ed.). Raven Press, New York, 1975, p. 197.

33.   Winne, D. : Unstirred layer, source of biased Michaelis constant in mem-brane transport. Biochim Biophys Acta 298:27, 1973.

34.   Westergaard, H. , and J. M. Dietschy: Delineation of the dimensions and per-meability characteristics of the two major diffusion barriers to passive mu-cosal uptake in the rabbit intestine. J Clin Invest 54:718, 1974.

35.   Wiseman, G. : Absorption of amino acids. in Handbook of Physiology, Sec. 6, Alimentary Canal. Vol. III. Intestinal Absorption. C. F. Code and W. Heidel (eds.). Am Physiol Soc Washington, 1968, p. 1277.

36.   Holdsworth, C. D. : Amino acids and proteins. in Transport Across the In-testine. A Glaxo Symposium. W. L. Burland and P. D. Samuel (eds.). Williams & Wilkins, Baltimore, 1972, p. 136.

37.   Wiseman, G. : Absorption of protein digestion products. in Biomembranes, Vol. 4A. Intestinal Absorption. D. H. Smyth (ed.). Plenum Press, London, 1974, p. 363.

38.   Adibi, S. A. : Intestinal phase of protein assimilation in man. Am J Clin Nutr 29:205, 1976.

39.   Nixon, S. E. , and G. E. Mawer: The digestion and absorption of protein in man. 2. The form in which digested protein is absorbed. Br J Nutr 24:241, 1970.

40.   Asatoor, A. M. , M. R. Crouchman, A. R. Harrison, F. W. Light, L. W. Loughridge, M. D. Milne, and A. J. Richards: Intestinal absorption of oligo-peptides in cystinuria. Clin Sci 41:23, 1971.

41.   Asatoor, A. M. , B. Cheng, K. D. Edwards, A. F. Lant, D. M. Matthews, M. D. Milne, F. Navab, and A. J. Richards: Intestinal absorption of two peptides in Hartnup disease. Gut 11:380, 1970.

42.   McCarthy, C. F. , J. L. Borland, H. J. Lynch, E. E. Owen, and M. P. Tyer: Defective uptake of basic amino acids and L-cystine by intestinal mucosa of patients with cystinuria. J Clin Invest 43:1518, 1964.

43.   Shih, V. E. , E. M. Bixby, D. H. Alpers, C. S. Bartsocas, and S. O. Thier. Studies of intestinal transport defect in Hartnup disease. Gastroenterology 61:445, 1971.

44. Hooft, C. , J. Timmermans, J. Snoeck, I. Antener, W. Oyaert, and C. van den Hendre: Methionine malabsorption syndrome. Ann Paediatr (Basel) 205:73, 1965.

45. Drummond, K. , A. Michael, A. Ulstrom, and R. Good: Blue diaper syndrome: Familial hypercalcemia with nephrocalcinosis and indicanuria. Am J Med 37:928, 1964.

46. Goodman, S. I. , C. A. McIntyre, and D. O'Brien: Impaired intestinal transport of proline in a patient with familial aminoaciduria. J Pediatr 71:246, 1967.

47. Wapnir, R. A. , and F. Lifshitz: Intestinal transport of aromatic amino acids, glucose and electrolytes in a patient with phenylketonuria. Clin Chim Acta 54:349, 1974.

48. Wapnir, R. A. , and F. Lifshitz: L-phenylalanine interactions with structurally related substances at the intestinal mucosa. Biochem Med 11:370, 1974.

49. Wapnir, R. A. , and F. Lifshitz: Inhibition of intestinal absorption of L-phenylalanine in vivo by L-alanine. Proc Soc Exp Biol Med 152:307, 1976.

50. Skou, J. C. : Enzymatic basis for active transport of sodium and potassium across cell membranes. Physiol Rev 45:596, 1965.

51. Spencer, R. P. : Intestinal absorption of amino acids. Am J Clin Nutr 22:292, 1969.

52. Reiser, S. , and P. A. Christiansen: Intestinal transport of amino acids as affected by sugars. Am J Physiol 216:915, 1969.

53. Cook, G. C. : Comparison of intestinal absorption rates of glycine and glycylglycine in man and the effect of glucose in the perfusing fluid. Clin Sci 43:443, 1972.

54. Wapnir, R. A. , and F. Lifshitz: Absorption of amino acids in malnourished rats. J Nutr 104:843, 1974.

55. Wapnir, R. A. , R. A. Exeni, M. McVicar, and F. Lifshitz: Experimental lead poisoning and intestinal transport of glucose, amino acids and sodium. Pediatr Res 11:153, 1977.

56. Crane, R. K. : Absorption of sugars. in Handbook of Physiology, Sec. 6, Alimentary Canal, Vol. III, Intestinal Absorption. C. F. Code and W. Heidel (eds.). Am Physiol Soc, Washington, 1968, p. 1323.

57. Fordtran, J. S. , and F. J. Ingelfinger: Absorption of water, electrolytes and sugars from the human gut. in Handbook of Physiology, Sec. 6, Alimentary Canal. Vol. III, Intestinal Absorption. C. F. Code and W. Heidel, (eds.). Am Physiol Soc, Washington, 1968, Ch. 74, p. 1457.

58.   Crane, R. K.: Intestinal absorption of glucose. in Biomembranes, Vol. 4A. D. H. Smyth (ed.). Plenum Press, London, 1974, p. 541.

59.   Gray, G. M.: Carbohydrate digestion and absorption. New Engl J Med 292: 1225, 1975.

60.   McMichael, H. B.: Absorption of carbohydrates. in Intestinal Absorption in Man. I. McColl and G. E. Sladen (eds.). Academic Press, New York, 1975, p. 99.

61.   Bayless, T. M.: Recognition of lactose intolerance. Hosp Prac 11:97, 1976.

62.   Hamilton, J. D., and H. B. McMichael: Role of the microvillus in the absorption of disaccharides. Lancet 2:154, 1968.

63.   Caspary, W. F.: Ionic dependence of glucose transport from disaccharides. in Intestinal Ion Transport. J. W. L. Robinson (ed.). University Park Press, Baltimore, 1976, p. 153.

64.   Capraro, V., G. Esposito, and A. Faelli: Intestinal transport of monosaccharides. in Intestinal Absorption and Malabsorption. T. Z. Csaky (ed.). Raven Press, New York, 1975, p. 67.

65.   Crane, R. K., G. Forstner, and A. Eichholz: Studies on the mechanism of the intestinal absorption of sugars. X. An effect of Na^+ concentration on the apparent Michaelis constants for intestinal sugar transport in vitro. Biochim Biophys Acta 109:467, 1965.

66.   Swaminathan, N., and A. Eichholz: Studies on the mechanism of active intestinal transport of glucose. Biochim Biophys Acta 298:724, 1973.

67.   Alvarado, F.: Sodium-driven transport. A re-evaluation of the sodium-gradient hypothesis. in Intestinal Ion Transport. J. W. L. Robinson (ed.). University Park Press, Baltimore, 1976, p. 117.

68.   Kimmich, G. A.: Active sugar accumulation by isolated intestinal epithelial cells. A new model for sodium-dependent metabolite transport. Biochemistry 9:3669, 1970.

69.   Gracey, M., V. Burke, M. Storrie, and A. Oshin: Dissociation of intestinal active sugar transport from (Na^+-K^+)-ATPase activity. Clin Chim Acta 36:555, 1972.

70.   Goldner, A. M.: Sodium-dependent sugar transport in the intestine. Metabolism 22:649, 1973.

71.   Bieberdorf, F. A., S. Morawski, and J. S. Fordtran: Effect of sodium, mannitol, and magnesium on glucose, galactose, 3-0-methylglucose, and fructose absorption in the human ileum. Gastroenterology 68:58, 1975.

72.   Huang, K. C., M. A. Dinno, and D. R. Gelbart: Effect of diuretics on intestinal transport of electrolytes, glucose and amino acid. Proc Soc Exp Biol Med 151:779, 1976.

73.   Fisher, R. B. , and M. L. G. Gardner: A diurnal rhythm in the absorption of glucose and water by isolated rat small intestine. J Physiol 254:821, 1976.

74.   Naftalin, R. , and P. F. Curran: Galactose transport in rabbit ileum. J Membr Biol 16:257, 1974.

75.   Debnam, E. S. , and R. J. Levin: Influence of specific dietary sugars on the jejunal mechanisms for glucose, galactose and α -methyl glucoside absorption: Evidence for multiple sugar carriers Gut 17:92, 1976

76.   Gracey, M. , V. Burke, and A. Oshin: Active intestinal transport of D-fructose. Biochim Biophys Acta 266:397, 1972.

77.   Alvarado, F.: D-xylose active transport in the hamster small intestine. Biochim Biophys Acta 112:292, 1966.

78.   Nasrallash, S. M. , and F. L. Iber: Mannitol absorption in man. Am J Med Sci 258:80, 1969.

79.   Johnston, J. M.: Mechanism of fat absorption. in Handbook of Physiology, Sec. 6: Alimentary Canal. Vol. III. Intestinal Absorption. C. F. Code and W. Heidel (eds.). Am Physiol Soc, Washington, 1968, p. 1353.

80.   Borgstrom, B.: Fat digestion and absorption. in Biomembranes, Vol. 4B. D. H. Smyth (ed.). Plenum Press, London, 1974, p. 555.

81.   Brindley, D. N.: The intracellular phase of fat absorption. in Biomembranes, Vol. 4B. D. H. Smyth (ed.). Plenum Press, London, 1974, p. 621.

82.   Clark, M. L. , and J. T. Harries: Absorption of lipids. in Intestinal Absorption in Man. I. McColl and G. E. Sladen (eds.). Academic Press, New York, 1975, p. 187.

83.   Jackson, M. J.: Transport of short chain fatty acids. in Biomembranes, Vol. 4B. D. H. Smyth (ed.). Plenum Press, London, 1974, p. 673.

84.   Berdanier, C. D. , and P. Griminger: In vitro and in vivo absorption of three vitamin K analogs by chick intestine. Intern Z Vit Forschung 38:376, 1968.

85.   Poley, J. R. , J. C. Dower, J. Owen, and G. B. Stickler: Bile acids in infants and children. J Lab Clin Med 63:838, 1964.

86.   Watkins, J. B. , D. Ingall, P. Sczepanik, P. Klein, and R. Lester: Bile salt metabolism in the newborn. New Engl J Med 288:431, 1973.

87.   Knoebel, L. K.: Intestinal absorption in vivo of micellar and non-micellar lipid. Am J Physiol 223:255, 1972.

88.   Carey, M. C. , and D. M. Small: Micelle formation by bile salts. Arch Int Med 130:506, 1972.

89.   Simmonds, W. J. , A. F. Hofmann, and D. Theodor: Absorption of cholesterol from a micellar solution. Intestinal perfusion studies in man. J Clin Invest 44:426, 1966.

90. Cardell, R. R. , S. Baden Hauser, and K. R. Porter: Intestinal triglyceride absorption in the rat. An electron microscopical study. J Cell Biol 34:123, 1967.

91. Levy, R. I. , R. S. Lees, and D. S. Fredrickson: The nature of pre-beta (very low density) lipoproteins. J Clin Invest 44:426, 1966.

92. Sabesin, S. M. , and K. J. Isselbacher: Protein synthesis inhibition mechanism for the production of impaired fat absorption. Science 147:1149, 1965.

93. Hollander, D. , E. Rim, and K. S. Muralidhara: Mechanism and site of small intestinal absorption of α tocopherol in the rat. Gastroenterology 68:1492, 1975.

94. Holdsworth, C. D. : Calcium absorption in man. in Intestinal Absorption in Man. I. McColl and G. E. Sladen (eds.). Academic Press, New York, 1975, p. 223.

95. Harrison, H. E. , and H. C. Harrison: Calcium. in Biomembranes, Vol. 4B. D. H. Smyth (ed.). Plenum Press, London, 1974, p. 793.

96. Birge, S. J. , W. A. Peck, M. Berman, and G. D. Whedon: Study of calcium absorption in man: A kinetic analysis and physiologic model. J Clin Invest 48:1705, 1969.

97. Emtage, J. S. , E. M. Lawson, and E. Kodicek: The response of the small intestine to vitamin D. Biochem J 140:239, 1974.

98. Harris, F. , R. Hoffenberg, and E. Black: Calcium kinetics in vitamin D deficiency rickets. II. Intestinal handling of calcium. Metabolism 14:1112, 1976.

99. Root, A. W. , and H. E. Harrison: Recent advances in calcium metabolism. I. Mechanism of calcium homeostasis. J Pediat 88:1, 1976.

100. DeLuca, H. F. : Recent advances in our understanding of the vitamin D endocrine system. J Lab Clin Med 87:7, 1976.

101. Garabedian, M. , Y. Tanaka, M. F. Holick, and H. F. DeLuca: Response of intestinal calcium transport and bone calcium mobilization to 1. 25-dihydroxyvitamin D_3 in thyroparathyroidectomized rats. Endocrinology 94:1022, 1974.

102. Six, K. M. , and R. A. Goyer: Experimental enhancement of lead toxicity by low dietary calcium. J Lab Clin Med 76:933, 1970.

103. Mahaffey, K. R. : Nutritional factors and susceptibility to lead toxicity. Env Health Persp 7:107, 1974.

104. Snowdon, C. T. , and B. A. Sanderson: Lead pica produced in rats. Science 183:92, 1974.

105. DeLuca, H. F. : The kidney as an endocrine organ for the production of 1,25-dihydroxyvitamin D_3, a calcium mobilizing hormone. N Engl J Med 289:359, 1973.

106. Heaney, R. P. , P. D. Saville, and R. R. Recker: Calcium absorption as a function of calcium intake. J Lab Clin Med 85:881, 1975.

107. Webling, D. and E. S. Holdsworth: Bile salts and calcium absorption. Biochem J 100:652, 1966.

108. Armbrecht, H. J. , and R. H. Wasserman: Enhancement of Ca^{++} uptake by lactose in the rat small intestine. J Nutr 106:1265, 1976.

109. Crosby, W. H. : Iron absorption. in Handbook of Physiology, Sec. 6, Alimentary Canal, Vol. III, Intestinal Absorption. C. F. Code and W. Heidel (eds.). Am Physiol Soc, Washington, 1968, p. 153.

110. Brozovic, B. : Absorption of iron. in Intestinal Absorption in Man. I. McColl and E. G. Sladen (eds.). Academic Press, New York, 1975, p. 263.

111. Cumming, R. L. C. , J. A. Smith, J. A. Millar, and A. Goldberg: The relationship between body iron stores and ferritin turnover in rat liver and intestinal mucosa. Br J Haematol 18:653, 1970.

112. Brittin, G. M. , and D. Raval: Duodenal ferritin synthesis in iron-replete and iron-deficient rats: Response to small doses of iron. J Lab Clin Med 77:54, 1971.

113. Tonz, O. , S. Weiss, H. W. Strahm, and E. Rossi: Iron absorption in cystic fibrosis. Lancet 2:1096, 1965.

114. Brise, H. , and L. Hallberg: Effect of ascorbic acid on iron absorption. Acta Med Scand 171 (suppl 376):51, 1962.

115. Callender, S. T. , S. R. Marney, Jr. , and G. T. Warner: Eggs and iron absorption. Br J Haematol 19:657, 1970.

116. Cook, J. D. , and E. R. Monsen: Food iron absorption in man. II. The effect of EDTA on absorption of dietary non-heme iron. Am J Clin Nutr 29:614, 1976.

117. Moore, C. V. : Iron nutrition and requirements. Ser Heamatol 6:1, 1965.

118. Martinez-Torres, C. , and M. Layrisse: Effect of amino acids on iron absorption from a staple vegetable food. Blood 35:669, 1970.

119. Martinez-Torres, C. , and M. Layrisse: Iron absorption from veal muscle. Am J Clin Nutr 24:531, 1971.

120. Heinrich, H. C., H. Bartels, C. Goetze, and K. H. Shafer: Normal bereich der intestinaler eisenresorption bei Neugeborenen und Sauflingen. Klin Wochenschr 47:984, 1969.

121. Gorten, M. K. , R. Hepner, and J. B. Workman: Iron metabolism in premature infants. J Pediatr 63:1063, 1963.

122. O'Dell, B. : Copper. in Present Knowledge in Nutrition, 4th ed. D. M. Hegsted, et al. (eds.). The Nutrition Foundation, Washington, 1976, p. 302.

123. Shils, M. E. : Magnesium. in Present Knowledge in Nutrition, 4th ed. D.M. Hegsted, et al. (eds.). The Nutrition Foundation, Washington, 1976, p. 247.

124. Chen, T. C. , L. Castillo, M. Korycka-Dahl, and H. F. DeLuca. Role of vitamin D metabolites in phosphate transport of rat intestine. J Nutr 104: 1056, 1974.

125. Rose, R. C. : Water-soluble vitamin absorption in intestine. Ann Rev Physiol 42:157, 1980.

126. Underwood, E. J. : Cobalt. in Present Knowledge in Nutrition, 4th ed. D.M. Hegsted, et al. (eds.). The Nutrition Foundation, Washington, 1976, p. 317.

127. Rosenberg, I. H. , and H. A. Goodwin: The digestion and absorption of dietary folate. Gastroenterology 60:445, 1971.

128. Gerson, G. D. , and N. Cohen: Folic acid absorption in regional enteritis. Am J Clin Nutr 29:182, 1976.

DIAGNOSTIC APPROACH

Arnold Schussheim, M. D.

HISTORY

No outline can substitute for a knowledgeable and organized approach to a pediatric patient with a gastrointestinal problem. Nevertheless, Table 1 has been a useful intake outline for hospital and ambulatory practice. As in most other medical specialties, a thorough history contributes greatly to accurate and rapid diagnosis. In a large percentage of cases an accurate history alone leads to an initial reasonable diagnosis. The growing child is a very dynamic and changing organism and provides the history-taker with the opportunity to view the full spectrum of events in many illnesses. It is remarkable how frequently and accurately even young children can fully describe their complaints in their own words. The gastrointestinal history starts with antenatal and neonatal events such as infections (TORCH), drugs, smoking, prematurity and maternal bleeding. Neonatal anoxia and a history of umbilical vessel manipulation should be elicited. Maternal hydramnios should suggest high intestinal obstruction in the neonate. The fact that a neonate had to be rectally stimulated to produce the first bowel movement may not be volunteered by the parents except on specific questioning, but may be of great importance in evaluating even an older child with chronic constipation. Later, the temporal relationships of symptoms to the introduction of new foods into the diet may clarify a number of cases of diarrhea or vomiting without further elaborate investigations.

Interference with growth and development is of vital interest to the physician taking care of children, and the gastrointestinal system should always be considered when presented with a child with growth failure. All previous heights and weights should be plotted on a growth grid. A recent falling off the growth curve, as well as absolute percentiles must be considered. Food faddism, severely restricted diets and psychosocial deprivation deserve attention as environmental factors in gastrointestinal disorders. In a world grown smaller by rapid transportation, it is wise to inquire about recent family travels. Epidemiological factors such as illness in family, friends, or the community is vital, as illustrated in newspaper headlines telling of "epidemic appendicitis" that was shown to be gastroenteritis caused by Yersinia enterocolitica. The most common cause of pancreatitis in children is trauma; thus, the history of a recent bicycle handlebar blunt trauma may often be crucial to diagnosis.

TABLE 1   Pediatric Gastroenterology Intake Sheet

Name: Date:

Address: Requested by:

Phone #:   Religion: Chart #:

Date of birth: Race: Sex:

Problems - 1.
        2.
        3.
        4.

Present illness (onset, course, missed school days, etc.)

GI ROS - weight loss: Appetite: Borborygmi-gas:
  Fever: Distention:
  Pruritus: Jaundice: Mouth sores:
  Vomiting-dysphagia:
  Skin or joint problems: Trauma:
  Travel: Allergies (pets):
  Pain:

Stool pattern (blood, mucus, nocturnal, soiling):

Diet (results of dietary manipulations):

ROS - Milestones: CNS:
  Growth (grid):   EENT:
  Toilet training: Other:
  Menses:
  Psychiatric:
  School:
  Cardio-resp:
  Urinary:

Past medical history (previous hospitalizations, neonatal and first year) - surgery:

Family history:

Physical exam - Ht: Wt: BP: Temp:
  General condition:
  Pubertal changes: (Tanner staging)   Edema: Skin:
  Clubbing:
  Abdomen:

  Perianal: Rectal:

Other (emotional evaluation):

Laboratory (past and present summary)
  Hematological (anemia, bleeding, iron, CBC):
  ESR: Urine:
  Blood (total protein, liver function, immunoglobulins):

TABLE 1 (cont'd)

Stool: (culture, blood, O & P, pH, and reducing substances)

Absorption: (e.g., 72-hr stool fat analysis)

Other:

Radiographic:
    Upper GI and small bowel:
    Barium enema:
    Other (bone age, IVP, chest, radionuclide scans):

Endoscopy:

Biopsy- motility-intubation-sonography-breath tests:

Hospital course (results pending):

Differential diagnosis:

Summary (subj., obj., and assessment):

Plan (tests):

Treatment: Next visit:

The family history is of great importance. Hereditary disorders of the liver, pancreas, and gastrointestinal tract are numerous (1). Functional disorders have a high family incidence and this specific historical fact may be of help in supporting the diagnosis as well as making it acceptable to the parents.

PHYSICAL EXAMINATION

The general physical as well as the abdominal examination should be complete. One should not underestimate the therapeutic value of a careful physical examination. A normal physical examination does not eliminate major gastrointestinal pathology. Subtle extra abdominal signs such as facies, nutritional status, digital clubbing, edema, pigmentations, eye abnormalities or neurological abnormalities may in some cases point the way to a gastrointestinal tract disease. The emotional evaluation of both the child and the family may be done concurrently with the physical examination. When feeding technique is thought to be responsible for the problem, a demonstration feeding is often most enlightening.
    Abdominal examination (Fig. 1) should be gentle and thorough, not omitting the perianal and digital rectal examination. Bimanual (rectal, vaginal) examination is helpful in some cases. The examiner should be comfortable and may sit next to the child. The entire abdomen should be exposed so that any fullness or even a lump down at the inguinal ring may be seen. Visual inspection should always precede "laying on of the hands." The infant's abdomen shows the characteristic abdominal respiratory pattern. Abnormal peristaltic waves or scars of previous surgery may be seen. In the newborn, the umbilical stump should be examined for infection and to make certain that three major vessels are present, i.e., two arteries and a

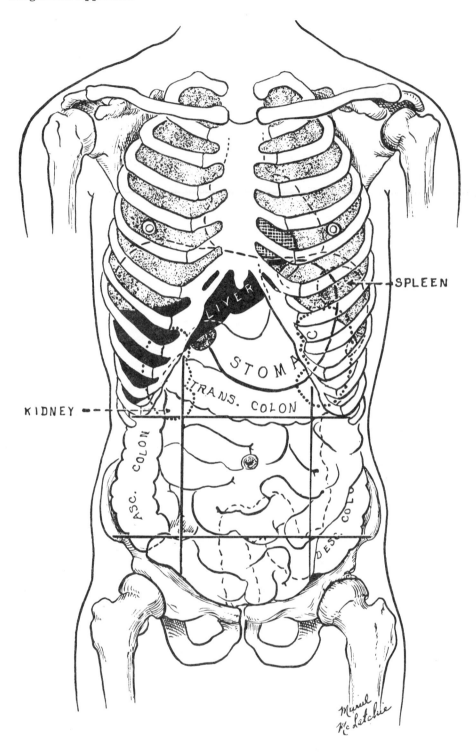

FIGURE 1   Topography of the abdomen showing arbitrary divisions including skeletal landmarks and surface orientation of related structures lying at a deeper level.

vein. Up to 5 years of age the abdomen normally appears full and may, after meals or air swallowing, even seem to be distended. Indeed a scaphoid abdomen in early infancy may indicate pathology, such as a diaphragmatic hernia or eventration. Absent abdominal musculature ("prune belly"), jaundice, rashes, and prominent abdominal venous patterns, e.g., caput medusae, as well as epigastric and umbilical hernias, should be noted. It is useful to have the child voluntarily pull in or protrude the abdomen maximally.

Auscultation of a silent belly or the high-pitched sounds of obstruction are helpful. Occasionally, an abdominal bruit may be heard over an aneurysm or vascular malformation. Percussion is used to determine liver size, presence of liver dullness, outline a mass, or confirm free (shifting) peritoneal fluid.

Palpation of the abdomen must be thorough and adjusted to the age of the child. At times, it may be necessary to place this at the beginning of the general physical examination to achieve adequate cooperation. An infant may be more cooperative while being held by its mother or by the judicious use of a pacifier. Older children usually appreciate a full explanation of what is going to happen. The examiner's hands should be warm, the child comfortable, supine, and with flexed knees. A rigid abdominal wall often may be found to be quite soft between episodes of crying. In cases of local abdominal pain it is wise to commence the palpation remote from that area.

The clinical act of examining the abdomen must be carefully practiced. It is no less important than many more elaborate diagnostic studies. Indeed a classical diagnosis of infantile pyloric stenosis may be confidently made solely by the appropriate history together with the physical findings of visible and reverse peristalsis, and the palpation of a typical "olive" pyloric tumor.

In assessing organomegaly, one should remember that the liver is normally palpable up to 3 cm below the right costal margin in the midclavicular line during the first 2 years of life (2). Hepatomegaly should be verified by percussion of the upper liver border, which should be at the level of the sixth intercostal space, to make certain the liver is not being displaced downward, e. g. , by overinflated lungs. Measurement of liver span and size on liver radionuclide scan are also useful in irregularly enlarged or difficult to palpate livers. The spleen tip may be felt in asthenic children. Palpable loops of bowel in the right or left lower quadrants have questionable significance when mobile and not tender. Prominent lumbar vertebral and aortic pulsations may be felt normally.

When examining a child with abdominal pain one should be very gentle to maintain the cooperation of the patient. The history helps a great deal in directing the examination and it may be amplified simultaneously while noting tenderness, rigidity, and rebound. An older child will point quite accurately if asked to "place one finger on the spot where it hurts most." Data, when investigating a child with abdominal pain, should include: onset, progression, time of occurrence (day or night), intervals between pain, character (cramplike), location, radiation, factors making it worse or better, as well as response to palpation. This last point may be judged well from facial expression and from verbal response. The examiner should estimate the child's general pain threshhold and be aware that state of consciousness, analgesics, and corticosteroids may blunt some responses.

When confronted by a child with abdominal enlargement, the components that might contribute should all be brought to mind. The normal protuberance of the preschool child's abdomen has already been mentioned. Lumbar lordosis and relatively weak abdominal musculature contribute to this. Fluid, feces, flatus, fat, fetus, tumor, organomegaly, or combinations of these are causative. Ascitic fluid may be due to chyle, bile, exudate, or transudate. Shifting dullness is diagnostic of free peritoneal fluid. Fecal masses within intestinal loops are often identified by their ability to be indented and may assume very large proportions. In young children, the sigmoid colon may enlarge as far as the right lower quadrant with a fecal mass. Air is characteristically tympanitic. Tumors may be cystic or solid and their usual characteristics of mobility, crossing the midline, point of origin, movement with respiration, or attachment to contiguous structures should be noted. Ovaries are not pelvic organs in young females and their enlargement may be discerned abdominally. All organs may be involved in mass formation, i. e. , hydronephrosis, distended bladder, hematocolpos, duplications of the bowel, omental cysts, etc. Although intestinal obstruction ranks high as a cause of abdominal enlargement, high obstruction may be seen in a child with a scaphoid abdomen. Malabsorptive states and aganglionic bowel are a frequent cause of nonobstructive abdominal distension. Transillumination of the abdomen can be used to distinguish solid from cystic masses (3). Abdominal enlargement due to an unsuspected pregnancy should be considered in adolescent females. Many abdominal masses may be felt only intermittently or may disappear quickly. An example of the former is an inguinal hernia, of the latter, a full bladder.

RECTAL EXAMINATIONS

Rectal examinations should never be omitted because of misplaced modesty on the part of the examiner or the patient or because of concern over possible induced psychic trauma. The procedure should always be preceded by adequate explanation. It should commence with a careful perianal examination. The well-lubricated index finger (or the fifth finger, below 6 months of age) is then gently introduced with a rotary motion. It is well to note that the average adult index finger can reach to the rectosigmoid junction in an infant (4). Supine, left lateral, or knee-chest position may be selected according to the age of the patient. Tenderness, stenosis, intra- and extraluminal masses, as well as the character of the stool and sphincters, are the main information to be gleaned. The stool on the glove should be tested for occult blood and stained for leukocytes when diarrhea or mucus is present.

DIAGNOSTIC PLAN

It is at this point that an assessment should be made of the case and a differential diagnosis composed, keeping in mind the frequency of occurrence of the various diagnostic considerations relative to the patient's age, sex, race, and geographical origin, as well as the above historical data and physical findings. The number of laboratory tests and procedures that may be employed subsequently are increasing rapidly, and at times the problem of which test to select is replaced by the question of when to call a halt to a reasonably complete diagnostic workup. In selecting a diagnostic plan, one has to make an early appraisal as to whether or not the problem is a primary gastrointestinal disease or a systemic condition with secondary gastrointestinal manifestations. Conversely, silent gastrointestinal disorders may present exclusively with extraintestinal symptomatology, e. g. , arthritis with inflammatory bowel disease. Table 2 lists some of the tests and procedures available. In the absence of severe illness or other compelling reasons for immediate hospitalization, it is remarkable how far one can proceed in diagnosis before hospitalization and by how much the hospital stay can be shortened by proper use of reliable ambulatory facilities. Tests should follow a phasic pattern, both in ambulatory and hospital settings. The sequence of testing is important to shorten the hospital stay and obtain accurate results. When indicated, sigmoidoscopy and mucosal biopsy followed by barium enema, then upper gastrointestinal series, is the customary order. An upper gastrointestinal series done as the

TABLE 2   Laboratory Aids

Phase IA: Ambulatory facility
   Medical tests as indicated
   CBC
   Urine
   Sedimentation rate
   Stool occult blood
   Stool microscopy
   Stool pH & reducing substances
   Pinworm Scotch Tape test
   Infectious mononucleosis screen
   Dietary trials
   Sigmoidoscopy
   Transillumination

Phase IB: Referred samples from patient
   72-hour stool collection for total fat
   Stool culture, and ova and parasites
   Blood screening tests, i. e. , cholesterol, anemia investigation, etc.

Phase IC: Ambulatory patient referral
   Sweat test
   Radiographic studies, i. e. , flat plate, bone age
   Rectal suction biopsy
   Some motility studies

Phase II: Hospital
   Blood studies: protein electrophoresis, clotting, etc.
   Stool studies, i. e. , trypsin, electrolytes, etc.
   Tolerance tests
   Histological: bowel; liver (light and electron microscopy)
   Motility studies
   Intestinal intubation for enzymes, culture, parasites, bile salts
   Radiographic studies: angiographic and radionuclide studies, IVP, GI contrast
     studies
   Sonography
   Endoscopy: fiberoptic and rigid
   Therapeutic trials: diet and drugs
   Miscellaneous medical and surgical tests: breath-analysis, peritoneoscopy,
     etc.

---

initial test can scatter a subsequent sonogram, quelch a radioisotopic study, delay an IVP or angiogram and make routine stool cultures and parasite examinations unreliable. Tests should be carefully selected on the basis of usefulness, safety, patient discomfort, and test availability. The age of the child may impose certain technical difficulties and safety restrictions. To be properly interpreted, tests must be done under standard controlled conditions. For example, testing the stool for reducing substances when the suspected offending sugar already has been removed from the diet will falsely give normal results.

Many physicians have found that proctosigmoidoscopy can be readily performed without difficulties under ambulatory circumstances (5, 6). Prehospitalization studies can be augmented by referring either the patient or samples from the patient to more sophisticated facilities. In the hospital during a 72- to 96-hour stool collection for fat, very few other tests can be done at that same time. Frequently, this type of collection as well as dietary trials may be equally well performed at home. In-hospital tests include an almost limitless number of sophisticated and complex procedures. Miniaturization of equipment and use of microchemical methods have greatly broadened the number of available tests in children (7, 8).

REFERENCES:

1.   McConnell, R. B. (ed.): Clinics in Gastroenterology—Genetics of Gastrointestinal Disorders. Vol. 2, No. 3. W. B. Saunders Co., Philadelphia, 1973.

2.   Younoszai, M. K. , and S. Mueller: Clinical assessment of liver size in normal children. Clin Pediatr 14:378, 1975.

3.   Mofenson, H. , and J. Greensher: Transillumination of the abdomen in infants. Am J Dis Child 115:428, 1968.

4.   Schapiro, S. : Proctologic problems in children. Lancet 1:134, 1964.

5.   Vanderhof, J. A. , and M. E. Ament: Proctosigmoidoscopy and rectal biopsy in infants and children. J Pediatr 89:911, 1976.

6.   Fenton, T. R. , J. A. Walker-Smith, and D. R. Harvey: Proctoscopy in infants with reference to its use in necrotizing enterocolitis. Arch Dis Child 56:121, 1981.

7.   Cadranel, S. , P. Rodesch, J. P. Peeters, and M. Cremer: Fiberendoscopy of the gastrointestinal tract in children. Am J Dis Child 131:41, 1977.

8.   Walker, W. A. , W. Krivit, and H. L. Sharp: Needle biopsy of the liver in infancy and childhood. Pediatrics 40:946, 1967.

5

CONGENITAL MALFORMATIONS OF THE
GASTROINTESTINAL TRACT

David L. Schwartz, M.D.

INTRODUCTION

The majority of the newborn gastrointestinal anomalies are the result of a development defect or an intrauterine accident. Several of these anomalies have had their etiology proved by a laboratory model, while others are only conjectural. Intestinal obstruction is the most frequent and the earliest component of the clinical presentation. The neonate with an intestinal anomaly will manifest signs and symptoms within hours or days from the time of birth. The alimentary tract may be obstructed not only by an intrinsic problem, but also by an extraintestinal or intraluminal condition which secondarily affects the gut. These entities include defects in abdominal wall formation, diaphragmatic hernias, and meconium ileus.

As is so often the case, many of these infants are critically ill, and the earlier the need for surgery is recognized the better the immediate prognosis. As a result of recent advances in postoperative support, anesthesia, antibiotics, nutrition, and surgical techniques, many neonates can be successfully nursed through a variety of postoperative crises which would have caused their death in the past. This markedly improved early survival rate has made even more imperative the need to make an accurate and rapid diagnosis of intestinal obstruction to avoid the long-term complications associated with massive bowel resection and the resultant "short-gut syndrome."

With the advent of intrauterine radiocontrast and grey scale sonography studies in high-risk mothers, some surgically correctable gut anomalies may be diagnosed during fetal life. It should be stressed that polyhydramnios, a single umbilical artery, and meconium staining are early indications of possible intestinal obstruction. This data is readily available in the delivery room. As more delivery room personnel become aware of acute surgical problems of the neonate, these babies are being referred earlier for surgery. For example, in a newborn a low Apgar score, cyanosis, and a scaphoid abdomen should suggest a diaphragmatic hernia. A chest x-ray film soon after birth can confirm the diagnosis, with certainty. A frequent practice is to pass a nasogastric tube into the stomach of all newborns, not only in those with excessive oral secretions. The inability to pass a relatively rigid tube into the stomach should alert the physician or nurse to consider an esophageal atresia. A simple x-ray of these patients with the tube in place and without the injection of any contrast material may confirm the diagnosis.

There are a number of congenital lesions which are readily apparent on simple inspection, including omphalocele, gastroschisis, and imperforate anus. The long-term care of these patients is often difficult, but the initial diagnosis is straightforward.

In the investigation of a suspected case of intestinal obstruction, there are several other aspects which require emphasis. A good family history is essential. For example, pyloric atresia, pyloric stenosis, and meconium ileus with cystic fibrosis often are inherited traits. Many other obstructing lesions, although not thought to be predictably inherited, have familial tendencies. It is important to recognize that there are clinical associations such as trisomy 21 or Down syndrome, and duodenal obstruction. Intestinal obstruction can be only one of a constellation of developmental anomalies associated with a complex list of autosomal derangements, e. g. , cleft palate, skeletal deformities, and craniofacial dysplasias.

OMPHALOCELE AND GASTROSCHISIS

The confluence of four ectodermal and mesodermal folds, cephalic, caudal, and two lateral, form the anterior abdominal wall. Failure of the lateral folds to fuse in the midline, between 2-4 weeks of embryonic development results in an anterior abdominal wall hernia, or omphalocele. The incidence of these abdominal wall defects is about 1:5000 births.

CLINICAL FEATURES

The omphalocele (Fig. 1), or exomphalos, is a congenital hernia involving the umbilicus, and is usually covered by an avascular sac composed of the fused layers of amnion and peritoneum. A small occult omphalocele may be missed, and therefore it usually is recommended that clamping of the umbilical cord in the delivery suite be at least 5 cm from the abdominal wall (1). Close inspection of the umbilical cord before clamping will avoid this serious complication. Gastroschisis (Fig. 2), is a full thickness complete abdominal wall defect, usually to the right of the normal umbilicus; the extruded intestine is never covered by a membrane. An omphalocele may rupture in utero and then may be indistinguishable from gastroschisis. Although the treatment is the same for a ruptured omphalocele and gastroschisis, there are several important clinical differences. The newborn with gastroschisis is premature in 40% of the cases and the nonrotated midgut appears to be abnormally short. In the large omphalocele, the liver and spleen are frequently outside of the abdominal cavity, whereas, this is never observed in a gastroschisis. Other anomalies rarely accompany gastroschisis, but the omphalocele patient frequently has other problems (60%) including incomplete intestinal rotation, intestinal obstruction, exstrophy of the bladder, vesicoenteric fistulas, renal anomalies, and cardiovascular defects. Infants with Beckwith-Wiedemann syndrome have an omphalocele associated with macroglossia, microcephaly, renal hyperplasia, macrosomia, and episodic, severe hypoglycemia.

The mode of treatment and the prognosis in these patients depends upon the size of the hernia, the presence or absence of a covering sac, and the severity of any associated anomalies. In the case of a small omphalocele in the base of the umbilical cord with an intact membrane, closure is easily achieved in a single-stage, primary reduction and abdominal wall repair. It is common practice to open the sac of the small omphalocele, and inspect any bowel that may be entrapped. This

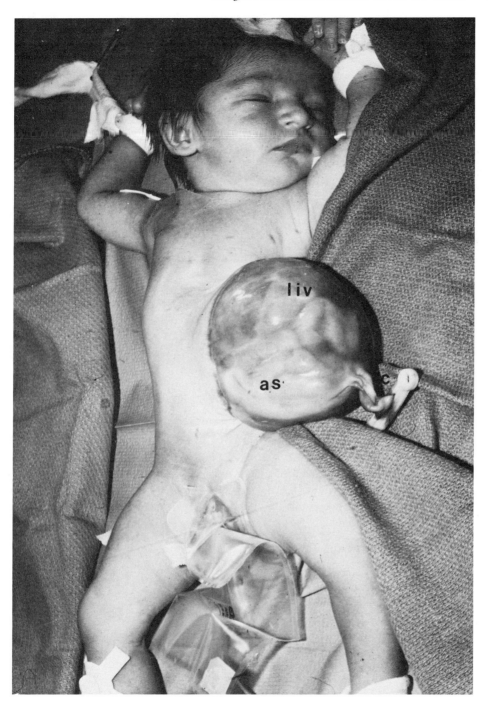

FIGURE 1   Omphalocele.   Amniotic sac (as) containing liver (liv) and umbilical
cord (c) at distal end.

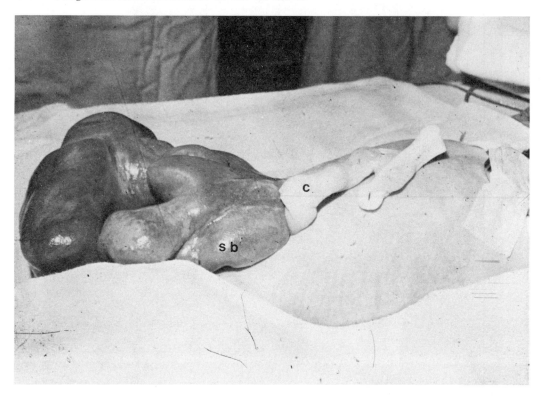

FIGURE 2   Gastroschisis. Abdominal defect lateral to base of cord (c) lying over lower abdomen. (sb = fused loops of small bowel). Head of the infant is to the right.

is imperative, particularly in the cases that demonstrate dilated intestine, either clinically or by x-ray examination. Intestinal atresia can be present within the small sac, and this obstructed gut must be identified and repaired at the time of omphalocele closure.

The goal of the surgeon is to achieve reduction of the extruded abdominal content into the peritoneal cavity. The basic problem hinges on the fact that the abdominal cavity is underdeveloped, and any forceful attempt at reduction produces very high intraabdominal pressure and resultant respiratory and circulatory compromise. It should be mentioned only in condemnation, that in the past, intestinal resections, splenectomy, and even partial hepatectomy were performed in an attempt to achieve closure of the abdominal wall.

In the neonate too ill to undergo surgery, 2% aqueous Mercurochrome can be applied on the intact sac producing an eschar (2). The eschar is then elevated by the ingrowth of epithelium from the edges of the hernial defect. However, this technique has several drawbacks: (1) 8-16 weeks of treatment, (2) mercurism has been reported, and (3) significant intestinal anomalies may persist undiagnosed. The problem of mercurism can be avoided by using silver nitrate as the eschar-producing agent. In 1948 Gross described a technique of abdominal wall closure using massive skin flaps (3). This operation left the surgeon with a very difficult secondary closure and for this reason is generally no longer used.

The surgeon may construct an extracoelomic silo (siliconized nylon) which houses the contents of the omphalocele (4) (Fig. 3a). This artificial housing is gradually closed, allowing the abdominal contents to return to the peritoneal cavity

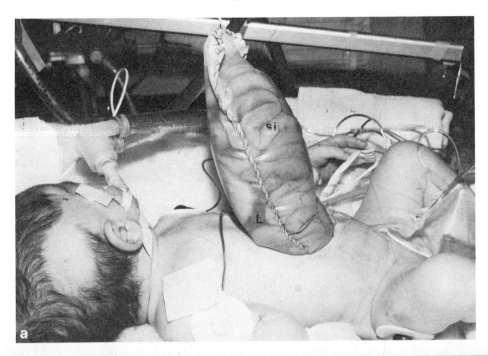

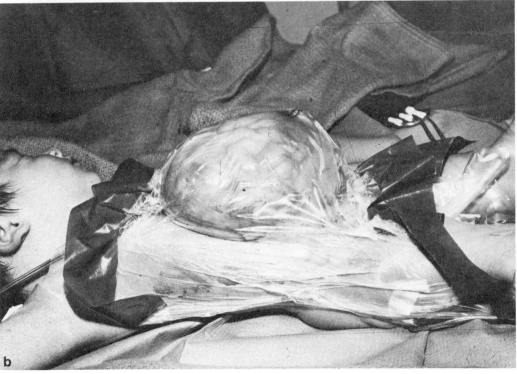

FIGURE 3   (a) Omphalocele in newborn, postoperatively, showing Silon housing, small intestine (si), liver (L).   (b) Op-site, a semipermeable synthetic membrane covering omphalocele.   (T. J. Smith & Newphew Ltd. , Welwyn Garden City and Hull, England)

without increasing intraabdominal pressure. This reduction is a bedside procedure which usually is completed within 10 days, following which the abdominal
wall is closed. This technique is particularly useful in treating gastroschisis
where there is no membrane and a surface cover is mandatory. The operation
can be simplified by using a transparent silicone bag which can be pulled over the
exposed bowel (5). Synthetic semipermeable membranes and xenographs of skin
are now being used in therapy of large omphaloceles (6) (Fig. 3b).

The exposed intestine, particularly in a gastroschisis, is edematous, brawny,
matted together, thick-walled, and foreshortened. It should be emphasized that
even though techniques are now available to achieve abdominal wall closure, the
return to normal function of this damaged bowel may take several weeks. Adhesive intestinal obstruction is a frequent complication. With the advent of total parenteral alimentation these infants survive. The changes affecting the eviscerated
intestine are completely reversible.

VITELLOINTESTINAL DUCT REMNANTS

The persistence of the duct communication between the intestine and the yolk sac
beyond the embryonic stage results in the most common malformation of the gastrointestinal tract—a blind omphalomesenteric duct or Meckel diverticulum.
Classically, a Meckel diverticulum is described as an antimesenteric outpouching
of the ileum, approximately 2 ft from the ileocecal junction (Fig. 4). It is found
in 2% of the population, with males predominating (75%). Ectopic gastrointestinal
mucosa or aberrant pancreatic tissue is present in nearly 50% of the cases, and
80-85% of the ectopic tissue found in the diverticulum is gastric. The length of the
diverticulum varies from 1-10 cm. A long omphalomesenteric duct that remains
patent throughout its length results in an umbilical-intestinal fistula. This is a
rare complication, and these patients present with fecal drainage from the umbilicus. The anatomical variations of the duct include its complete obliteration, and
in this circumstance there is a fibrous cord extending from the ileum to the umbilicus. Occasionally, the duct is closed at both ends, but patent in the center, producing a central cystic dilatation. This "cyst," lined by a secreting mucosa, has
the potential of reaching sizes large enough to present as abdominal masses.

CLINICAL FEATURES

The majority of Meckel diverticula cause no symptoms. They are usually incidental findings at laparotomy; however, 2% are associated with complications, two-
thirds of which occur under 2 years of age. The major complications include
hemorrhage, obstruction, diverticulitis, perforation, and pain. Umbilical dis-
charge, an abdominal mass, and incarceration in an indirect hernia sac (Littre
hernia) are less common features.

Ulceration of the ileal mucosa adjacent to the ectopic gastric mucosa of the diverticulum is the usual mechanism responsible for hemorrhage. Bleeding occurs
in 50% of symptomatic cases; it is usually painless, and varies in degree from
minimal recurrent occult bleeding, to sudden massive bright red or wine-colored
rectal bleeding and shock (7, 8). Tarry stools are uncommon. Hypotensive patients require immediate preparation for surgery without the undue delay associated with diagnostic workup. Patients with chronic blood loss should have a coagulation profile, upper gastrointestinal series, proctosigmoidoscopy, and radionuclide
scan. 99m Tc-pertechnetate is taken up and excreted and imaged by gastric
mucosa (Fig. 5). False-positive and false-negative scans have been reported,
but the reliability of the scanning is considered 60-80% accurate. Gastric tissue too small to be detected by this test may account for some of the false-neg-

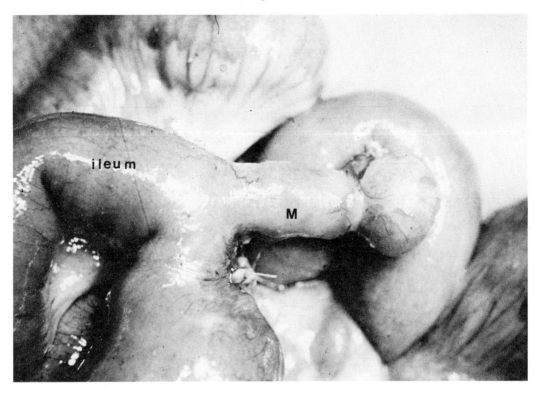

FIGURE 4   Meckel diverticulum (M) in 2-year-old male with rectal bleeding. Tip
is constricted by ulceration, which has perforated along upper margin.

ative results.   Ulceration with perforation of the Meckel diverticulum does occur
in infancy, and mortalities up to 50% are recorded.   Intestinal obstruction is caused by two principal mechanisms: (1) intussusception with the diverticulum as a
lead point; (2) herniation through, or volvulus around, a persistent fibrous cord
remnant of the vestigial vitelline duct.   Diverticulum-related intestinal obstruction
can occur at any age.   Volvulus around a vitelline duct cord does occur in the neonate.

DIAPHRAGMATIC HERNIA

At 8 weeks of embryonic life, the septum transversum forms beneath the heart and
extends posteriorly to join the dorsal mesentary of the foregut thus forming the
central tendon of the diaphragm.   Membranous pleuroperitoneal folds, one on each
side of the septum transversum, expand laterally and posteriorly to form the rest
of the diaphragm.   The last portions of the diaphragm to close are the posterolat-
eral triangular pleuroperitoneal canals (foramen of Bochdalek hernia).   The left
hemidiaphragm closes later than the right side and this explains the preponderance
of left-sided cases (80-90%).   At the same time the diaphragm is forming, the
midgut is undergoing rapid elongation and is returning into the abdominal cavity
from its extracoelomic position in the yolk sac.   While the intestine is rotating

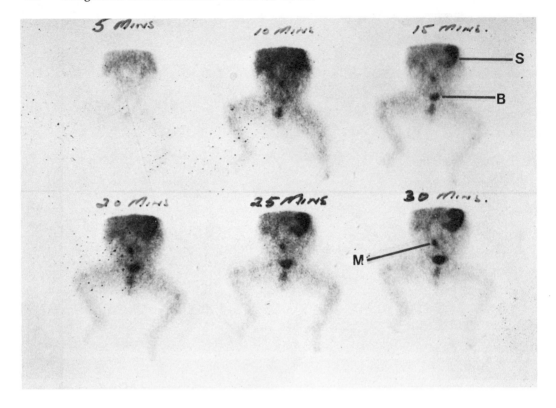

FIGURE 5   99m Tc-pertechnetate scan showing stomach (S), bladder (B) and
Meckel diverticulum (M), containing ectopic gastric mucosa.

counterclockwise, if there is a defect in the diaphragm, the gut will take the path
of least resistance and the intestine will enter the chest.

CLINICAL FEATURES

The amount of intestine in the thorax is variable. It is not unusual to find the entire small bowel in the chest; the liver, spleen, stomach, and transverse colon
may also be components of the hernia (Fig. 6).

The neonate with a diaphragmatic hernia, who is cyanotic, tachypneic, hypox-
emic, acidotic, and in shock, is an absolute surgical emergency. In the delivery
room the infant often will have an empty scaphoid abdomen and a barrel chest. The
affected hemithorax is dull to percussion and breath sounds are absent. Bowel
sounds are occasionally auscultated in the chest.

It is of interest to note that not all diaphragmatic hernias present in the newborn
period. Cases have been described at all ages. Patients that survive beyond the
neonatal period often present with a history of "chronic lung congestion" and frequent "colds." A routine screening chest x-ray reveals the unsuspected diaphragmatic hernia.

Clinical examination, chest x-ray studies, pulmonary function tests, and lung
scans of patients followed up to 21 years, demonstrated that lungs that were hypo-
plastic at birth remained underdeveloped, but the patient was usually able to live a
normal life.

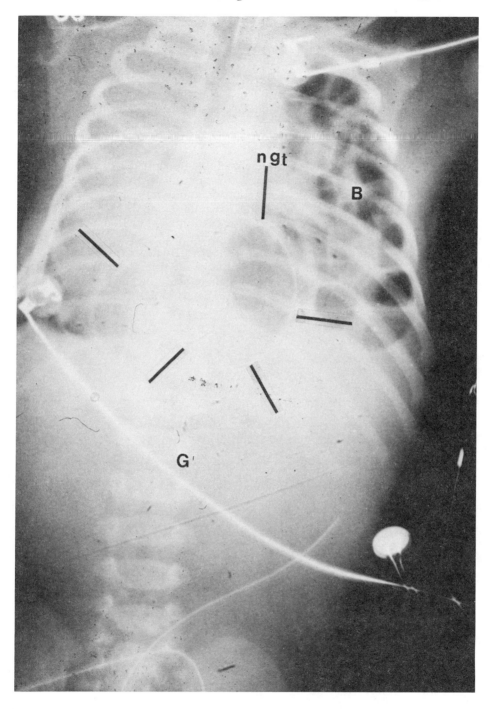

FIGURE 6   Left diaphragmatic hernia.   Bowel loops within left hemithorax (B), gasless abdomen (G), outline of coiled nasogastric tube in stomach which is also in the chest (ngt).

Survival statistics correlate with the time when respiratory distress first appears. If respiratory distress occurs within the first 12 hours of life, the mortality is 60%, whereas with symptoms occurring after 24 hours of life there is 38% mortality.   The most prevalent autopsy findings in those patients succumbing to diaphragmatic hernia include: (1) nonexpansion of the ipsilateral lung, (2) severe developmental hypoplasia of the contralateral lung; and (3) marked reduction of bronchial branching and consequently decreased numbers of functioning alveoli.

TREATMENT

The immediate steps before surgery should include endotracheal intubation and oxygenation, insertion of a nasogastric tube to prevent further distension of the loops of bowel in the chest, arterial cannulation and monitoring of blood gases, and the initiation of attempts to correct or abate the acidosis.

A large variety of additional intestinal anomalies have been described, and they should be identified and repaired at the time of herniorrhaphy.   The defect in the diaphragm (Fig. 7) can usually be closed without difficulty.   In cases where a large amount of the abdominal content is found in the chest, the abdominal cavity may not accommodate the reduced intestine without dangerously increasing intraabdominal pressure.   In this circumstance, the abdominal wall can, in most instances, be

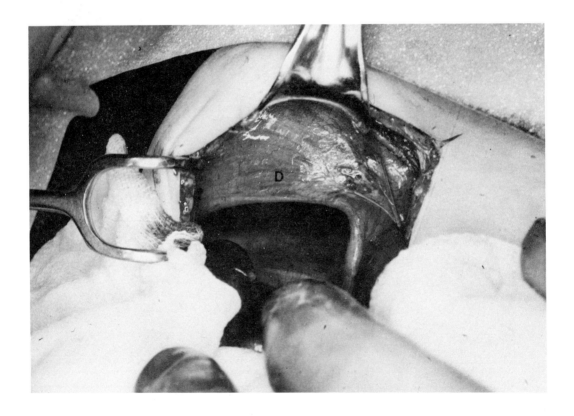

FIGURE 7   Diaphragmatic defect encompassing entire posterior half of the left hemidiaphragm revealing posterior rib cage; anterior half of left diaphragm (D).

sufficiently stretched to allow a comfortable abdominal closure. A Silon pouch
may be used which contains the gut extraperitoneally, as a temporary measure to
prevent high intraabdominal pressure (9). Skin flaps also have been used to a-
chieve the same results. Both of these techniques require a second procedure to
close the ventral abdominal wall hernia.

When repairing a diaphragmatic hernia there are several important considerations: (1) There is 2% incidence of bilaterality. (2) Complete agenesis of the hemidiaphragm does occur and successful repairs with synthetic mesh have been reported (10)   (3) Postoperatively, air may have to be removed or added into the
thorax to keep the mediastinum in the midline.

There is often an unexpected mortality in newborns that appeared to be doing
well in the immediate postoperative period (11-13). It is suggested that these patients develop pulmonary hypertension, resulting in a persistent fetal circulation
and right-to-left shunting through the ductus arteriosus. By measuring PaO_2
above and below the ductus, changes in the shunt can be interpreted. Although the
reported experience is small, drugs such as methylprednisolone (Solu-medrol),
tolazoline (Priscoline), and chlorpromazine (Thorazine) have been used to reduce
pulmonary hypertension and thereby reduce shunting across the ductus. Ligation
of the ductus or extra-corporeal membrane oxygenation have also been performed
in desperately ill infants with occasional success.

Long-term studies of adults who had neonatal diaphragmatic hernias have shown
these people living normal lives even though there is pulmonary hypofunction (14).

EVENTRATION

Eventration of the hemidiaphragm, and paralysis of the diaphragm are uncommon.
These entities must be differentiated from the classic hernia because, for the
most part, they can be treated nonoperatively. Paralysis may be diagnosed by
fluoroscopy. Transperitoneal injection (peritoneography) of diatrizoate (Hypaque)
is a very reliable method of demonstrating the presence of an eventration (Fig. 8).
Infants with eventration of the diaphragm, who do not respond to intensive medical
therapy, can succumb as a result of respiratory failure. In these circumstances,
a relatively simple transthoracic plication of the diaphragm will often result in
dramatic improvement in respiratory status.

ESOPHAGEAL ATRESIA AND TRACHEOESOPHAGEAL
FISTULA (TEF)

CLINICAL FEATURES

As a result of accumulated experience, it is now expected that an infant with an
isolated esophageal atresia and tracheoesophageal fistula, who weighs 2000 g or
more, should have a 90% survival. This remarkable improvement in prognosis is
the result of early diagnosis, the control of sepsis, and the availability of both
personnel and equipment specifically geared for the care of sick infants. Despite
all advances, there is still a significant mortality in the premature infant with
esophageal atresia, with or without coexisting major anomalies. About one-third
of these cases have significant associated anomalies and in over half of these,
more than two malformations can be demonstrated (15). In order of frequency,
they involve cardiovascular, gastrointestinal, and musculoskeletal organ systems.
The majority of deaths appear to be related more to the coexistent severe anomaly,
than to the TEF. The term VATER syndrome (16) is the acronym used to describe
the infant with vertebral, vascular (septal defects and a single umbilical artery),
anal, tracheoesophageal fistula, esophageal atresia, renal, and radical anomalies.

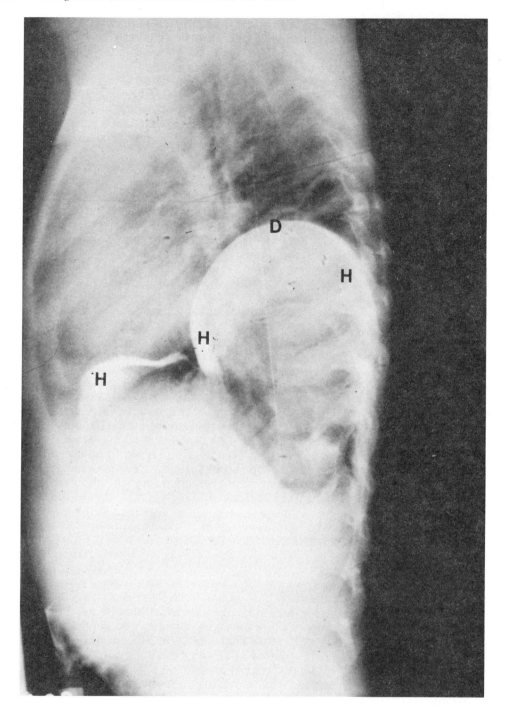

FIGURE 8   Eventration of diaphragm.   Intraperitoneal Hypaque (H) outlining **markedly** elevated diaphragm (D).

The newborn with excessive oral secretions should have an x-ray showing the location of a radiopaque nasogastric tube (Fig. 9a, b). The information available on this x-ray includes coiling of the tube in the air-filled proximal esophageal pouch (usually within 10 cm of the external nares), the presence of pneumonia and atelectasis, the size of the heart, air in the gastrointestinal tract, any abnormal gas patterns, and the skeletal structure. The most common variety of esophageal atresia (85-90%) is one in which there is a blind proximal esophageal pouch and a distal TEF, i. e. , from the level of the tracheal carina to the distal esophageal segment (Fig. 10). This type of esophageal atresia is readily diagnosed by the simple technique described previously. There are, however, uncommon forms of esophageal atresia and TEF, such as the H type (Fig. 11) and the laryngotracheo-esophageal cleft, that may elude detection for a considerable period. The degree of difficulty in both diagnosis and treatment of esophageal atresia is apparent when one reviews a recent atlas of esophageal atresia, in which 95 subtypes are described (17).

TREATMENT

If the newborn with esophageal atresia and TEF is full term, weighs at least 2000 g, and has no aspiration pneumonia, the surgical division of the fistula and primary anastomosis of the esophagus is usually performed within the first day of life. These patients have an excellent prognosis and a smooth recovery. All babies being prepared for surgery have sump suction applied to the blind upper pouch using a Replogle catheter (18). These infants also should be kept at a 30⁰ incline to reduce the likelihood of gastric content refluxing into the tracheobronchial tree. The aspiration of gastric contents produces a severe chemical pneumonitis. If the condition of the patient permits, a gastrostomy under local anesthesia is an important adjunct in the therapy that is aimed at preventing deterioration of pulmonary function. Many pediatric surgeons routinely perform gastrostomy in all their patients regardless of their clinical condition.

Premature infants with aspiration pneumonia may require a staged program of therapy. These patients are first treated with antibiotics, sump suction, and a gastrostomy. If they do not stabilize, it is imperative that the TEF be ligated and divided under local anesthesia. In the very small neonate, an esophageal repair is not done because of the higher morbidity and mortality. If the esophageal separation is considerable, both ends are identified with silver clips to quantitate the effectiveness of any future stretching techniques.

There is a small percentage of patients who undergo primary repair of an esophageal atresia and division of a TEF without a gastrostomy, who never require any further treatment. However, it is not unusual for some patients to develop a small leak at the esophageal anastomosis. Once the leak seals, the resultant esophageal stricture responds readily to dilatation. A reduced incidence of leakage and stricture of the esophagus following an end-to-side, rather than an end-to-end, anastomosis is recommended by some authors (19). Recurrent fistulization does occur in a very small percentage of patients. This complication usually occurs between the fourth and tenth postoperative day and generally requires surgical closure.

There are a number of preoperative solutions to the problem of the wide gap esophageal atresia (Fig. 12a), and these techniques may be used in cases with or without a TEF. One approach is to stretch the proximal esophageal pouch with a 12 F mercury-loaded bougie twice daily (20). The lower esophageal remnant also may be stretched after the construction of a gastrostomy. Although large esophageal defects may be overcome, it may require up to 10 weeks of daily bougienage (21) (Fig. 12b). The incidence of an esophageal anastomotic leak following dilatation is high, but it is an acceptable complication considering the fact that this approach negates the need for a colon interposition.

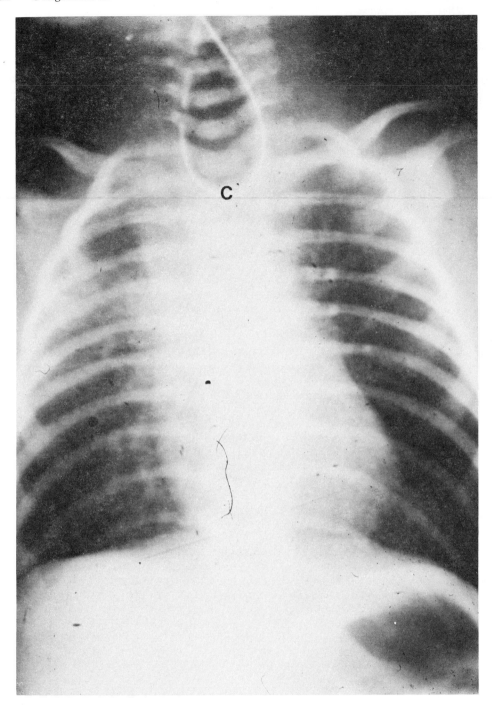

FIGURE 9a   Esophageal atresia with TEF in newborn.   Catheter coiled in blind proximal esophageal pouch (C).

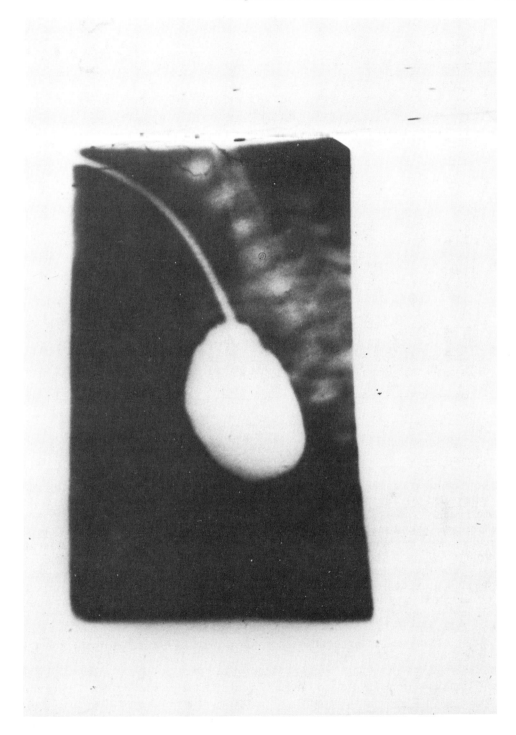

FIGURE 9b   Water-soluble contrast demonstrating proximal esophageal atresia.

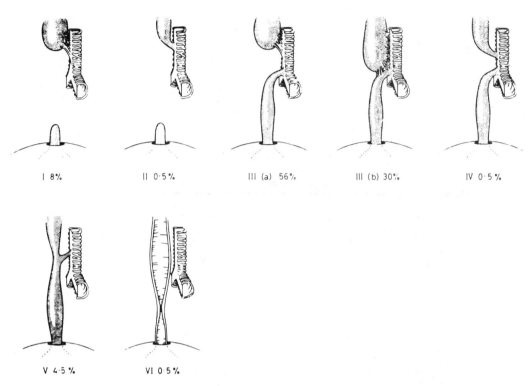

FIGURE 10   Common types of esophageal atresia.   The approximate incidence is given in percentages.

The placing of bougies in both esophageal segments and applying traction sutures threaded through the ends of the pouches is another proven approach (22). The two ends of the esophagus are then slowly pulled together. A circular esophagomyotomy, sometimes performed in a step-wise fashion, of the upper pouch can be made to gain as much as 5 cm of length and to achieve a primary esophageal anastomosis (23). This technique is gaining wide acceptance among pediatric surgeons.   Finally, cases of long-gap esophageal atresia may be treated by a metal bougie placed in each end of the esophagus. The ends of the esophagus are pulled toward each other by intermittently applying an electromagnetic field (24).

In some infants with primary esophageal atresia, the gap between the two ends of the esophagus may be so great as to preclude any hope of an esophageal anastomosis. This form of uncorrectable esophageal atresia is treated by the construction of a substitute esophagus (Fig. 12c).   Esophageal conduits have been fashioned from small bowel, stomach, and colon (25, 26). Over 90% of colon interposition operations, followed for many years, have good results. The recommended approach to the staged repair of esophageal atresia consists of: (1) gastrostomy and division of the tracheoesophageal fistula, (2) bougie dilatation followed by anastomosis, (3) if bougienage is not successful, then a cervical esophagostomy is performed under local anesthesia, and (4) colon interposition.

Long-term follow-up of patients having undergone circular esophagomyotomy has demonstrated that the majority of these patients have satisfactory deglutition. However, some cases have developed ballooning of the esophagus at the site of the myotomy, producing a functional obstruction. These areas lack normal motility and have required resection and reanastomosis with good results.

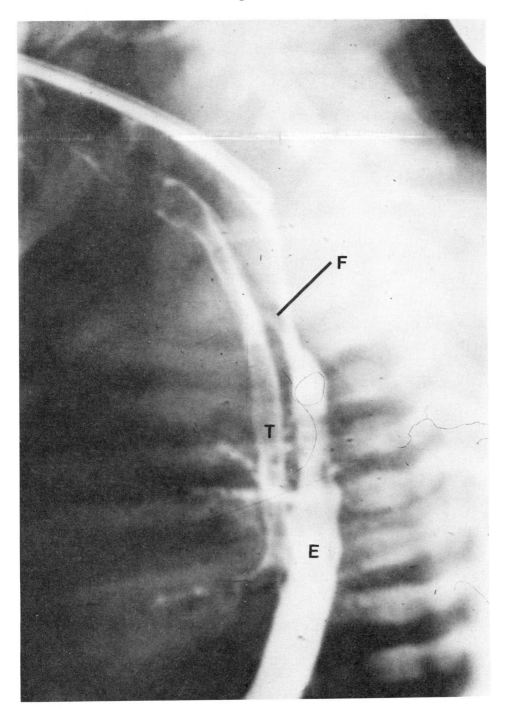

FIGURE 11   Barium swallow demonstrating H-type tracheoesophageal fistula in
infant with aspiration pneumonia; trachea (T), esophagus (E), fistula (F).

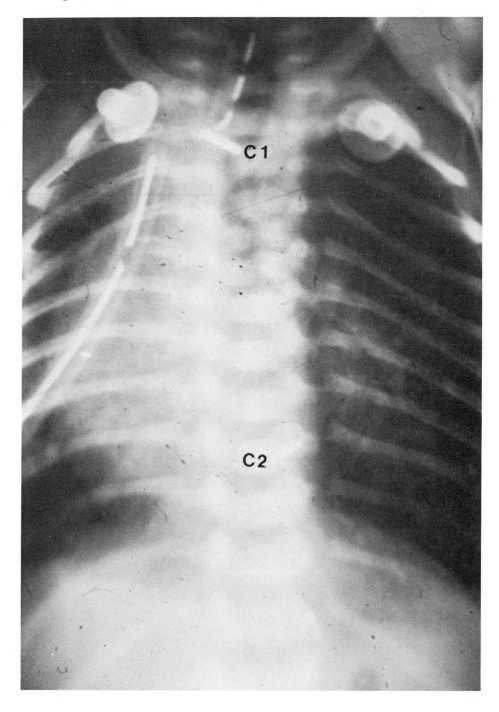

FIGURE 12a   Long-gap esophageal atresia, postoperatively. Metal clip on proximal esophageal pouch (C-1); metal clip on distal esophagus (C-2).

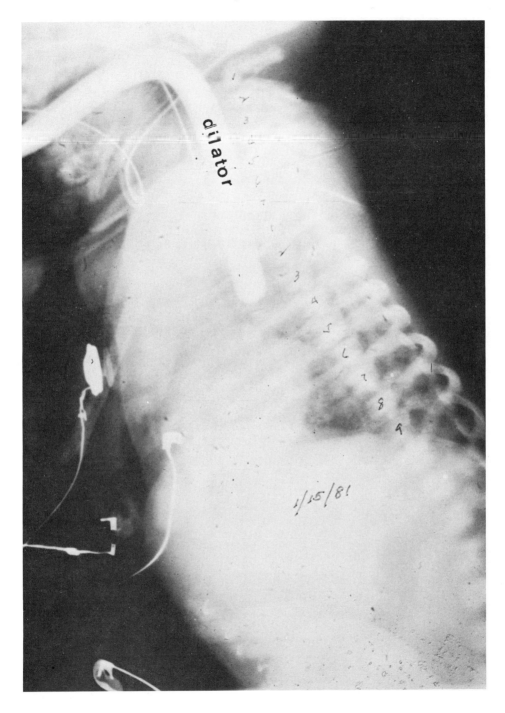

FIGURE 12b   Stretching of proximal esophageal pouch by mercury-weighted bougie in an infant with primary esophageal atresia.

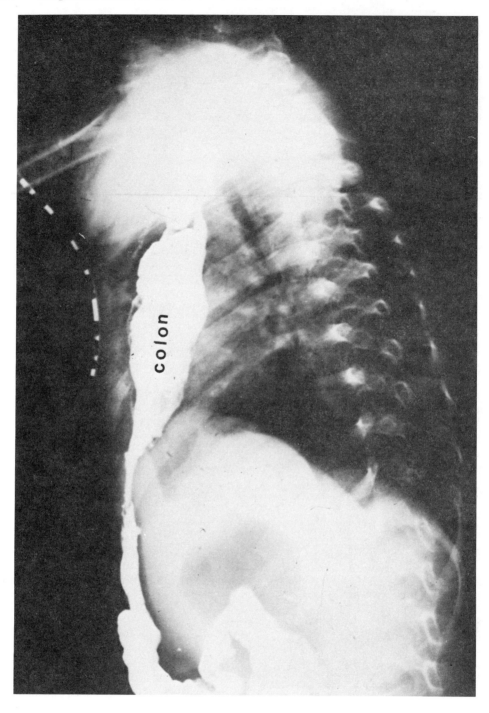

colon

FIGURE 12c   Right colon interposition via substernal tunnel. Cecum anastomosed to proximal esophageal pouch. Distal end of right colon sutured to stomach.

It should be recognized that there are a significant number of newborns with esophageal atresia and TEF whose lives are threatened by other anomalies, especially cardiac defects, i. e. , septal defects, coarctation of the aorta, vascular rings, and patent ductus arteriosus. These infants are often premature, have aspiration pneumonia, and may be on a continuum of treated borderline congestive heart failure. Under these conditions the surgeon must prevent gastric aspiration as soon as the patient is stabilized by performing a gastrostomy under local anesthesia. The timing of any further surgery in these sick infants will depend on their general medical condition. Esophageal pouch stretching in these infants is frequently associated with severe cyanotic spells, and at times, cardiorespiratory arrest.

TRACHEOESOPHAGEAL FISTULA WITH NO ESOPHAGEAL ATRESIA

Approximately 1-2% of tracheoesophageal fistulas are not associated with an atresia of the esophagus (27). These so-called H-type fistulas (see Fig. 11), are usually single, and commonly occur at or above the level of the second thoracic vertebra. The H fistula can be easily repaired through a cervical approach and if necessary, under local anesthesia. On occasion, this variety of fistula may be multiple and can be found anywhere along the tracheobronchial tree. Identifying the fistula(s) in these infants is often the most difficult aspect of their care. Almost all of these cases have choking spells with feeding and about half develop aspiration pneumonia. Excess saliva and abdominal distention are noted in about one-third of the patients. Unlike the other varieties, these cases may present anytime during the first 6 months of life.

The differential diagnosis includes feeding problems, gastroesophageal reflux, aspiration, and palatopharyngeal dyskinesia. Multiple esophagoscopies alone may not identify the fistula, in many cases. Simultaneous bronchoscopy and esophagoscopy along with the instillation of methylene blue near the suspected fistula site has proved to be the most accurate investigative technique.

ESOPHAGEAL WEB AND STENOSIS

Esophageal web is a rare cause of vomiting in the neonate. It is diagnosed by esophagram and esophagoscopy. Occasionally, a patient will present at 6-12 months of age with "dysphagia" and failure to thrive, as a result of an incompletely obstructing esophageal web. It should be recognized that esophageal webs may coexist with other congenital esophageal anomalies such as esophageal atresia and tracheoesophageal fistula. It is good practice to pass a catheter down the distal esophageal segment into the stomach to assure patency of the entire esophagus.

The surgical treatment consists of an esophagotomy, direct exposure of the web, followed by excision of the web, and esophagoplasty. There has been little experience with the use of pediatric fiberoptic resectoscopes in the treatment of esophageal webs.

Esophageal stenosis, usually located within 3 cm of the cardia, can be caused by tracheobronchial remnants (28). In high-grade stenosis, the esophageal wall is circumferentially involved. Histologically, the wall of the esophagus in these patients contains aberrant cartilage, glandular elements, and a stratified ciliated epithelium which act as the obstructing agents. The best treatment is obtained with segmental resection of the esophagus.

PYLORIC STENOSIS

INTRODUCTION AND PATHOGENESIS

Congenital hypertrophic pyloric stenosis causes projectile, nonbilious vomiting in the infant, usually starting at 2-6 weeks of age.   About one case in ten begins to vomit within the first 2 weeks of life, and rare mild cases have not been diagnosed until 6 months of age.   The condition occurs once in every 500 births, with a 4:1 ratio in favor of males.   Familial cases occur in 5%, and offspring of mothers with pyloric stenosis have a four to five times higher incidence than offspring of affected males.   Preterm infants appear to be proportionately less affected.   The obstruction of the pylorus is the result of marked hypertrophy of the circular musculature of the pylorus.   The etiology of pyloric stenosis is obscure, although it has been suggested that the pyloric ganglion cells may be immature.   It also has been hypothesized from experimental studies, that circulating gastrin, whether in normal or excessive amounts, may contribute to pyloric hypertrophy.

CLINICAL FEATURES AND TREATMENT

Palpating the "pyloric tumor," described as an "olive," is diagnostic.   With experience, the pyloric mass is usually palpable to the right of the umbilicus and it is best felt during a feeding or after vomiting.   Visible upper abdominal peristaltic waves can be seen in most cases.   An upper gastrointestinal x-ray is usually unnecessary, but may be obtained in those cases in which the olive is not obvious (Fig. 13).   Unconjugated hyperbilirubinemia occurs in a minority of cases (2%), without a known specific cause.   It has been postulated that the indirect hyperbilirubinemia is the result of a decrease in hepatic glucuronyl transferase, and that this enzyme deficiency is related to starvation.   Preoperatively, the stomach should be decompressed with a nasogastric tube, and corrective measures taken for the everpresent dehydration, metabolic alkalosis, and potassium deficiency. The Fredet-Ramstedt pyloromyotomy is curative and is associated with a mortality of less than 0. 5% (Fig. 14).   Occasionally the duodenum is inadvertently entered; this mucosal penetration must be recognized and repaired to avoid serious complications.   Associated malformations are uncommon, although gastroesophageal reflux has been demonstrated in as high as 10% of the cases.   This may be the explanation for the occasionally reported hematemesis and for those infants who demonstrate persistent postoperative vomiting.

GASTRIC OUTLET OBSTRUCTION

Although bile-free vomitus is a hallmark of pyloric obstruction in the infant, it is not always due to pyloric stenosis.   Congenital pyloric or antral obstruction is rare, and has been reported either as a complete atresia, a fibrous cord, or more commonly a web or diaphragm (30). It is an inherited autosomal-recessive trait in some series.   Siblings with pyloric outlet atresia are well documented.   In patients with incomplete obstruction, clinical manifestations may not appear until adolescence or later. Acquired gastric outlet obstruction occurs in some patients with chronic granulomatous disease, presumably associated with mucosal inflammation.
    Usually there is a history of polyhydramnios during pregnancy, bile-free vomitus, and on x-ray examination, a large distended stomach with no air beyond the gastric antrum.   Surgery entails either resection of the web and pyloroplasty, or an anastomosis between the stomach and duodenum.

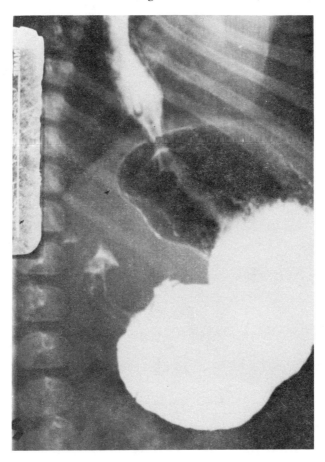

FIGURE 13   Pyloric stenosis.   Six-week-old infant with projectile vomiting and constipation.   Narrowed and flattened pyloric canal with barium trapped at either side producing a double track sign.

DUODENAL ANOMALIES

Duodenal obstruction is the result of atresia, stenosis, a web, an annular pancreas, or peritoneal bands secondary to incomplete intestinal rotation.   Early in fetal life the duodenum goes through a solid phase, and the lack of recanalization produces an atresia or stenosis (29).   Occasionally, the web is stretched out and appears like a "wind sock," with a central aperture.   About 25% of patients with duodenal atresia also have Down syndrome.

An annular pancreas is thought to be the result of failure of the ventral pancreatic anlage to rotate with the duodenum, and as a consequence it becomes wrapped around the second portion of the duodenum.

Bilious vomiting without abdominal distention is the cardinal sign in the patient with a duodenal obstruction.   High-grade duodenal obstruction is easily diagnosed by an upright x-ray of the abdomen showing the typical "double-bubble," with little or no small bowel gas (Fig. 15a).   Uterine sonography of mothers with polyhydramnios can demonstrate a double-bubble in the unborn fetus (Fig. 15b).

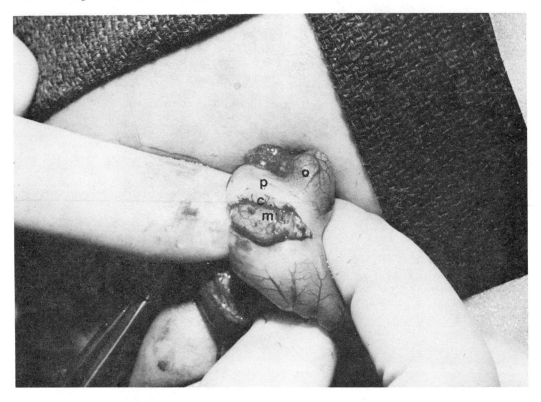

FIGURE 14   Pyloric stenosis. Pyloromyotomy (Fredet-Ramstedt): pyloric muscle (p); cut surface of hypertrophied muscle (c); pyloric mucosa (m); lesser curvature outpouching of antrum, which is usually present (o).

TREATMENT

Except for cases of duodenal web, there is no attempt to resect the obstruction, it
is simply bypassed by either a duodenostomy or a retrocolic side-to-side duodeno-
jejunostomy. In addition to the bypass, a gastrostomy is performed and a feeding
jejunostomy tube is passed through the anastomosis.
    It should be stressed that a partially obstructing annular pancreas or an incom-
plete web may cause symptoms at any time in life. The duodenal web or "wind sock"
obstruction is treated by resection of the web, and not a bypass procedure.

SMALL INTESTINE MALFORMATIONS

Atresia of the small and large bowel is caused by vascular impairment of the intestine (31). The vascular occlusion may be caused by intrauterine volvulus, strangulation, snaring of the intestine by umbilical cord remnants, intussusception, fetal
peritonitis, and primary occlusive lesions in the mesenteric artery. About half of
the cases have an associated major malformation. The major concurrent conditions
are intestinal malrotation, Down syndrome, and cystic fibrosis. Infants with intestinal obstruction beyond the duodenum have bilious vomiting and abdominal

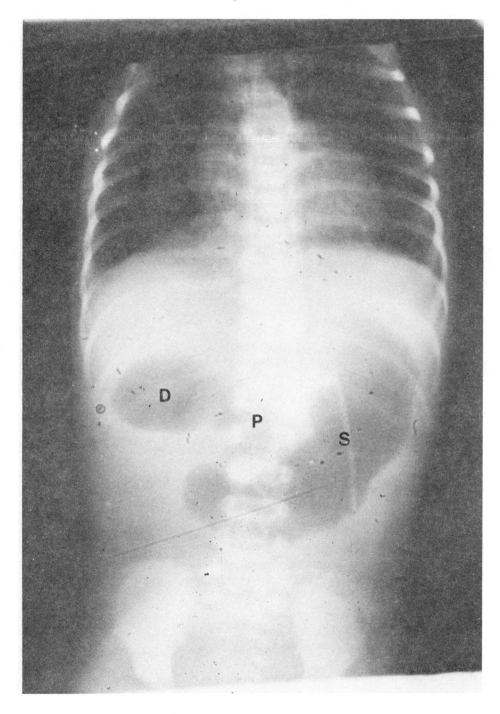

FIGURE 15a   Duodenal atresia in patient with Down syndrome demonstrating "double-bubble": stomach (S); pylorus (P); duodenum (D).

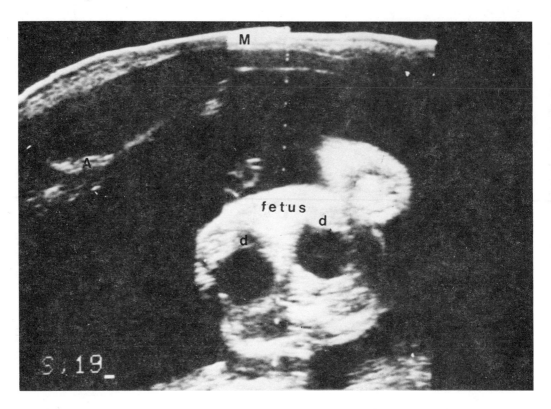

FIGURE 15b   Double-bubble demonstrated by sonogram in utero: double-bubble
(d); mother's abdominal wall (M); amniotic sac (A).

distention. The abdominal x-ray shows dilated loops of bowel, usually with air-
fluid levels (Fig. 16a). These findings pertain to all cases of small-bowel obstruction, whether atresia of the jejunum, ileum (most common) (Fig. 16b), or colon
(rare), and meconium ileus. Multiple skip areas of involvement are reported in
5-25% of the patients. A barium enema may reveal an unused, small colon, often
referred to as a "microcolon," particularly with more distal lesions (Fig. 17).

TREATMENT

At operation, the entire bowel must be inspected so that multiple stenoses and intrinsic webs are not overlooked. An obstructing web may be excised by simple enterotomy, whereas an area of atresia must be resected and intestinal continuity re-
established. The massively distended proximal bowel should be resected in all cases of high-grade small-bowel obstruction in the neonate, since this dilated segment often has neither active peristalsis nor a normal blood supply.

     In a review of 487 cases of congenital duodenal atresia or stenosis, 34% died of
the other associated anomalies seen in about half of these infants (32). In an analysis of 619 patients with congenital atresia and stenosis of the jejunum and ileum,
58% with jejunal and 75% with ileal atresia survived (33). Survival was reduced to
one in seven, when there were multiple bowel atresias.

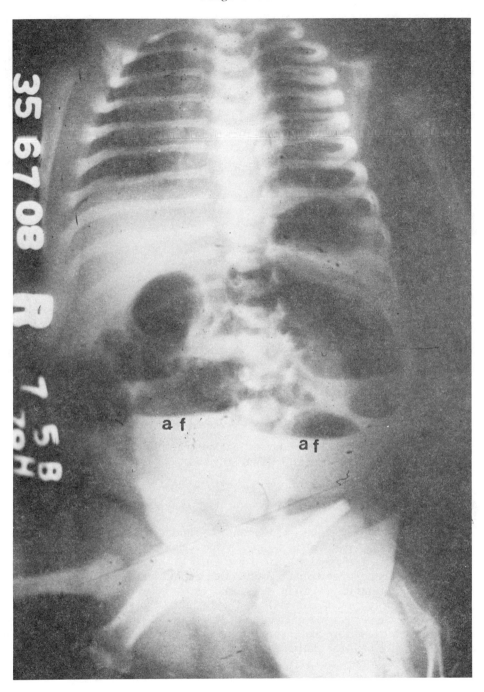

FIGURE 16a   Ileal atresia. Air-fluid levels, (af) and absence of air in distal colon, is suggestive of small-bowel obstruction.

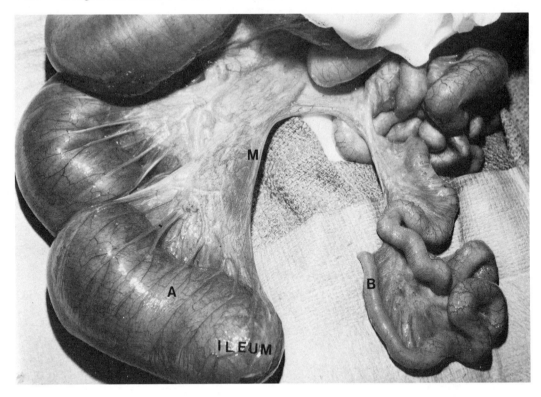

FIGURE 16b   Ileal atresia.   Complete ileal obstruction with dilatation (A), mesenteric defect (M), collapsed distal ileum (B).

LARGE-INTESTINE ANOMALIES

Atresia or stenosis of the colon is uncommon. In most of these cases, there is a complete separation of the atretic segments and a corresponding defect in the mesentery. The defects are usually located proximal to the splenic flexure in either the ascending or transverse colon. Associated anomalies are common with gastroschisis being the most prevalent.

The meconium plug syndrome (34), and its variant the small-left-colon syndrome (35) are unusual causes of low intestinal obstruction. They are relatively benign conditions caused by inspissated meconium which plugs the distal colon and rectum. Up to 40% of these patients subsequently have proved to have Hirschsprung disease. The syndromes can be mimicked by infants who were born to mothers with clinical diabetes which required drug management (Fig. 18).

CLINICAL FEATURES

These are a group of infants with abdominal distention, bile-stained vomiting, and absent spontaneous passage of meconium. The symptoms usually appear on the second day of life. The abdominal x-rays are consistent with small-bowel obstruction and the barium enema shows dilation of the colon proximal to an abrupt cone-shaped transition zone (usually at the splenic flexure), with a colon of

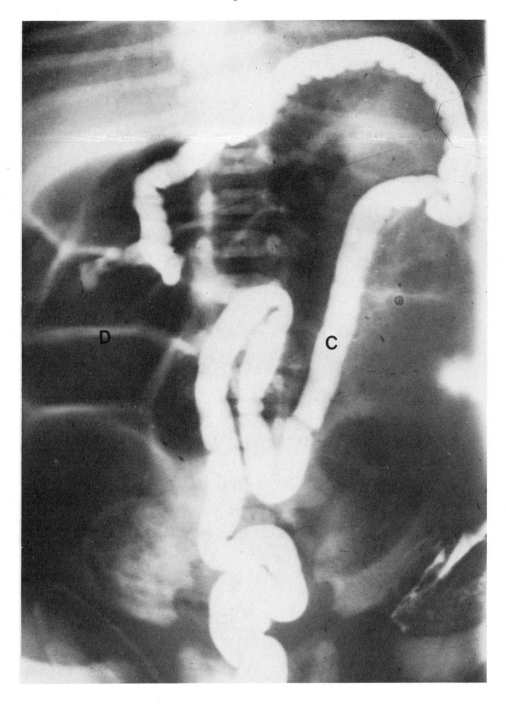

FIGURE 17   Microcolon or unused colon in a newborn with abdominal distention and failure to pass meconium within 56 hours: barium filled microcolon (C); dilated loops of small intestine (D).

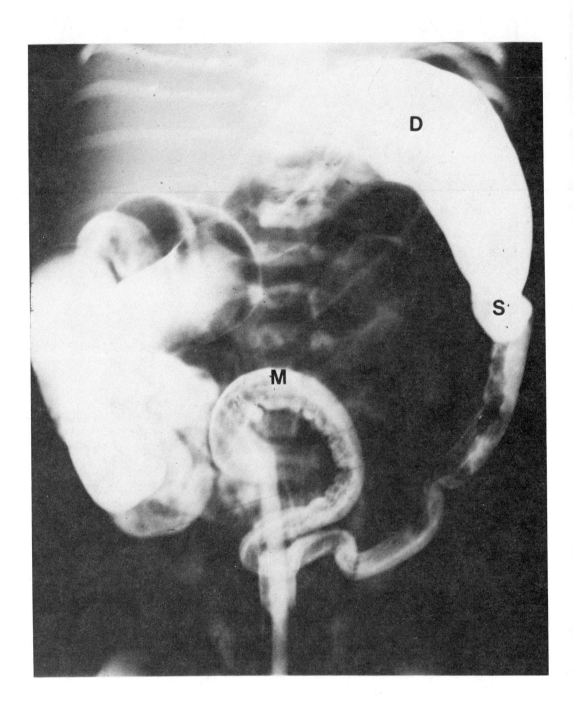

FIGURE 18   Small-left-colon syndrome in newborn of a diabetic mother; dilated proximal colon (D); transition zone at splenic flexure (S); meconium plug in collapsed left colon and sigmoid (M).

reduced caliber distal to the rectum.   The infants have not demonstrated any consistent abnormality of the meconium, nor is there always a meconium plug. Digital examination may be curative in mild cases, and is followed by the explosive expulsion of the meconium plug cast.   In resistant cases, the barium or hypertonic enema will dislodge the plug in most instances.

TREATMENT

Evacuation of the meconium does not always correct the clinical picture of obstruction; in fact, infants can develop late cecal perforations. All these patients have had normal intestinal ganglion cells. Colostomy is indicated in those cases whose functional obstruction does not improve with nonoperative treatment.

HIRSCHSPRUNG DISEASE (See Chap. 8)

MECONIUM ILEUS (Also see Chap. 19)

CLINICAL FEATURES

The differential diagnosis in the newborn with distal small-bowel obstruction consists of ileal atresia or stenosis, meconium ileus, and Hirschsprung disease. Meconium ileus is the earliest manifestation of cystic fibrosis and is present in 10-15% of patients with this disease. The older cystic fibrosis patient also can develop intestinal obstruction, i.e., meconium ileus equivalent, due to inspissation of stool, usually in the terminal ileum.

The neonate with meconium ileus obstruction has a terminal ileum filled with firm, inspissated small concretions. The ileum proximal to this area is dilated, filled with viscid meconium which may give a mass effect, and has ineffective peristalsis. Occasionally, there is a superimposed ileal atresia, presumably the result of a prenatal volvulus of a meconium-filled segment of the distended intestine (Fig. 19).   Radiological examination will demonstrate the many variations of this condition.   The typical x-ray study reveals signs of small-bowel obstruction and a ground-glass or bubbly appearance to intraluminal contents in the right lower quadrant. An abdominal x-ray with diffuse fine spiculated calcifications suggests a meconium ileus with intrauterine bowel perforation and a resultant meconium peritonitis. Meconium peritonitis is associated with a very high mortality. Surgical exploration is indicated as soon as the infant is born.   The abdomen is massively distended.   The abdominal x-ray shows an almost complete absence of intestinal gas, and bulging flanks.   The bowel is often unrecognizable at surgery and fecal contamination is extensive. An intraabdominal pseudocyst covering the bowel is frequently present.   Large portions of the small bowel are commonly gangrenous and require resection.   Sepsis and shock cause the death of most of these patients.   The small percentage of survivors often require very long hospitalizations because of a short-gut syndrome and/or severe intestinal malabsorption.   Almost all infants with meconium peritonitis have cystic fibrosis.

TREATMENT

A few patients respond to nonoperative treatment, consisting of hypertonic acetylcysteine or diatrizoate meglumine (Gastrografin) enemas (36). Those infants who do not respond to this mode of therapy should have surgery. Depending upon the extent of the disease, the surgery may involve just a simple enterotomy with

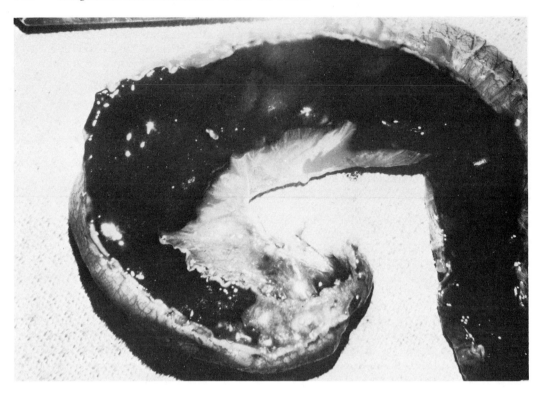

FIGURE 19   Meconium ileus.   Resected ileum filled with inspissated meconium.
Sweat test subsequently diagnostic of cystic fibrosis.

evacuation of the meconium, an exteriorizing Mikulicz bowel resection (37), or a
Bishop-Koop resection (38) and Roux-en-Y anastomosis.   Approximately 75-80%
of the cases will survive the neonatal surgery, but subsequent mortality figures are
closely related to pulmonary complications associated with cystic fibrosis.   Without exception, infants with meconium obstruction in the absence of proven cystic
fibrosis, should be followed until three or four adequate sweat tests (100 mg or
more of sweat, via pilocarpine iontophoresis) are obtained, which may not be
achieved until 3-4 weeks of age (39, 40).   Infants with proven cystic fibrosis require pancreatic enzyme supplement with their feedings.

ABNORMAL INTESTINAL FIXATION

As previously noted, nonrotation of the midgut is a significant finding in all cases
of omphalocele, gastroschisis, and diaphragmatic hernia.   Malrotation or incomplete rotation itself may produce duodenal obstruction, volvulus, internal hernias,
and chronic intermittent obstruction with malabsorption, protein-losing enteropathy, or lactose intolerance in the older patient.   Coincident stenosis or atresias
occurs in 25% of the cases.   Extraintestinal anomalies, particularly of the cardiovascular system, are not infrequent.

Malrotation of the intestine is due to abnormal movement or rotational arrest of the intestine around the superior mesenteric artery. This occurs during the tenth week of embryological development when the midgut returns to the coelomic cavity via a 270° counterclockwise rotation.

CLINICAL FEATURES

There are many variations in the clinical picture, depending upon where the arrest in intestinal rotations occur. High intestinal obstruction in the newborn period is the most common-presenting manifestation. In the classic and most common form, the cecum is in the right hypochondrium. At this level, the cecum lacks its normal attachment to the posterior abdominal wall. Instead, there are abnormal bands extending from the cecum, across the second portion of the duodenum, to the lateral parietal peritoneum. This anatomic variation often causes bilious vomiting in the newborn and the diagnosis is confirmed by barium enema (Fig. 20) which demonstrates the abnormal cecal location. An upper gastrointestinal series also may show that the ligament of Treitz is either in an abnormal location or it may be absent (Fig. 21). The x-ray study may demonstrate that not only the duodenum descends into the right side of the abdomen, but all the small intestine may aggregate on the right side. In these cases of complete nonrotation, the root of the small bowel mesentery is extremely short. This narrow point of fixation is a potential fulcrum about which the entire midgut (duodenum to midtransverse colon) can rotate and produce a volvulus. Very rare paraduodenal and paracecal hernias also have been associated with abnormalities in intestinal fixation.

Obstruction of the duodenum by peritoneal bands from the cecum to the right paravertebral gutter has been described along all portions of the duodenum (Fig. 22). Seventy-five percent of cases with bands require surgery in the neonatal period. These bands may not produce any early symptoms, and are only incidental findings later in life.

TREATMENT

To avoid bowel gangrene and perforation, neonatal midgut volvulus is a high-priority surgical emergency. The most devastating form is the intrauterine midgut volvulus. The newborn with this condition has marked abdominal distention, evidence of peritonitis, and frequently free intraperitoneal air secondary to bowel perforation. Meconium peritonitis is suggested when there are spiculed extraintestinal calcifications on an abdominal x-ray (80% of cases). A midgut volvulus can occur at any age, but is most prevalent in the neonate. The volvulus is usually clockwise. Untwisting of the volvulus and inspection of the bowel for other anomalies is mandatory. At the time of laparotomy it may be obvious that much of the small intestine is gangrenous; however in some patients it is not clear how much bowel is gangrenous. It is crucial to preserve as much bowel as possible and in the circumstance of questionable bowel viability it is best to close the abdomen after untwisting, and reexplore the patient in 24-36 hours. During this interval, antibiotics, fluid and blood replacement, and low-molecular-weight dextran may be administered (41). Any undue delay in making the diagnosis of midgut volvulus frequently results in massive bowel resections and a "short-gut syndrome." A midgut volvulus, progressing to extensive small-bowel gangrene can occur very rapidly. This acute presentation is not limited to the neonate, and may occur at any age. Postoperative recurrent midgut volvulus has been described in those patients who have had a derotational procedure. Postoperative midgut volvulus can occur at any time following the first procedure. This is a rare event. There is a controversy in the literature concerning the need to perform some type of bowel

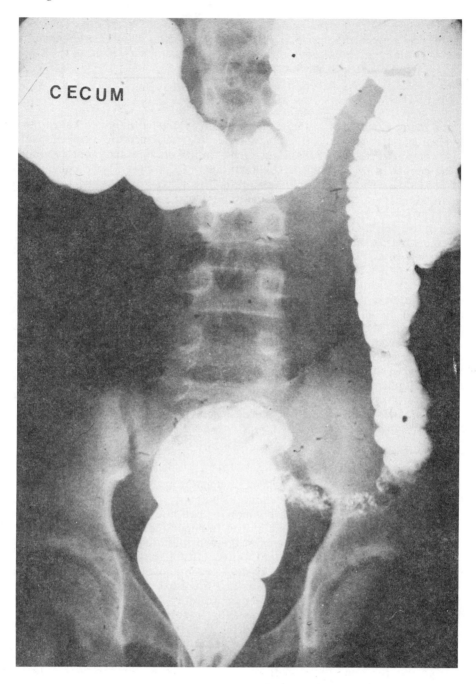

FIGURE 20   Malrotation.   Barium enema demonstrating right upper quadrant location of cecum in malrotation in 14-year-old with recurrent abdominal pain and vomiting.

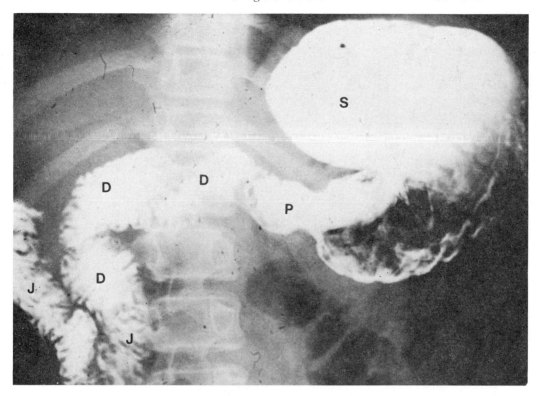

FIGURE 21   Malrotation of duodenal sweep with absent C-loop configuration:
stomach (S); pylorus (P); duodenum (D); jejunum (J).

fixation to prevent a bowel volvulus. Intermittent volvulus occurs mainly in older
children. They are usually small for their age and the history may be vague,
characterized by postprandial pain, associated with nausea and occasional vomiting. Some of these cases have chronic lymphovenous obstruction with a resultant
protein-losing enteropathy and occasional chylous ascites. An upper gastrointestinal series will show evidence of malrotation. At surgery there is often no acute
volvulus, but the findings of chronic venous congestion and serosal congestion
substantiate the intermittent nature of this process. A Ladd procedure results in
dramatic improvement in these individuals.

Paraduodenal (Waldeyere) (42) and paracecal hernias are rare and are related to
errors in rotation and fixation of the midgut. A congenital defect in the mesentery
of the terminal ileum is the most common (Treves field pouch), and it is a potential
site of small bowel incarceration or strangulation. These intestinal hernias are
reported to constitute about 1% of all cases of intestinal obstruction. Rare cases
have both a paraduodenal and paracecal hernia, with a volvulus of the intervening
small bowel (43).

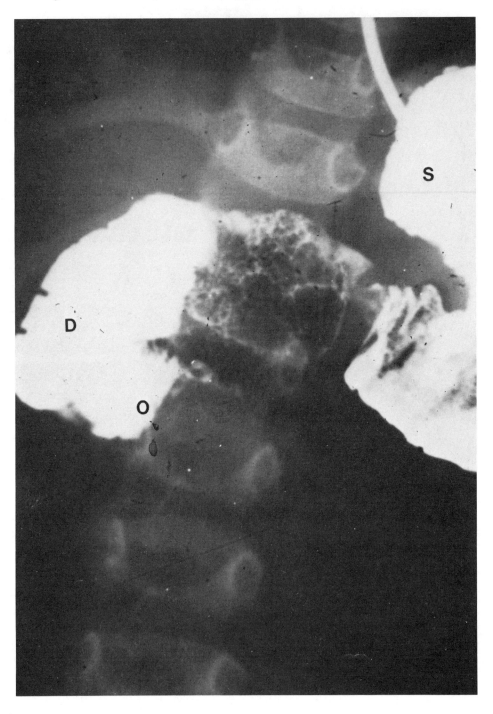

FIGURE 22   Complete obstruction of duodenum by Ladd bands: stomach(S); duodenum (D); obstruction at junction of second and third portions of duodenum (O).

ENTERIC DUPLICATIONS

Alimentary duplications are either cystic or tubular, the former having no communication with the normal intestinal tract, while the latter do communicate. The less common tubular duplication may join the intestine at one or both of its ends. Classically, the diagnostic criteria of a duplication include sharing of a common blood supply, and a common muscular coat between the duplicated segment and the adjacent gut. The duplication must also possess an alimentary epithelium, which need not mimic the mucosa of that portion of the gastrointestinal tract to which it is attached. Small-bowel duplications often contain gastric mucosa and technetium 99m radioimaging may be useful in making the diagnosis.

CLINICAL FEATURES

Enteric duplications occur throughout the gastrointestinal tract. Gastric duplications are the rarest, while ileal duplications are the most common. The complications associated with gastrointestinal duplications include intestinal obstruction, hemorrhage, ulceration, perforation, pancreatitis, jaundice, hematobilia, and cutaneous enteric fistulas. An intrathoracic esophageal duplication may cause respiratory distress, dysphagia, esophagitis, hematemesis, and recurrent pneumonia by erosion into the parenchyma of the lung and/or bronchi. About one-third of the cases have associated congenital anomalies, some of which may be life-threatening.

Gastric duplications are rare, usually found along the greater curvature, and share a common wall, and seem to have a greater propensity to deviate from the classical criteria noted previously. Pedunculated gastric duplications have been described, while other duplications have been found within the pancreas and are free of any attachments to the normal stomach.

Small-bowel duplications are the most common and are usually limited to a small segment of the terminal ileum (Fig. 23). Occasionally, there is a duplication which involves most of the small bowel (45).

Large-bowel duplications, thought to be aborted attempts at total caudal twinning, are frequently combined with complex internal and external genitourinary duplications.

A preoperative diagnosis is often difficult to document by either x-ray contrast or isotope studies. A mass may be palpated or a mass effect on the radiographs of the gastrointestinal tract may be noted. It is essential to delineate any gastric mucosa within the duplication because gastric secretions cause ulceration, bleeding, and perforation at the junction of the duplication and the normal alimentary tract.

TREATMENT

The best surgical treatment is resection of the duplication, followed by an end-to-end anastomosis. Esophageal duplications usually can be separated from the normal esophagus with ease. Gastric duplications are often densely adherent to the stomach and require special measures. The presence of an enteric duplication, even if asymptomatic and an incidental finding, is an indication for its removal. A duplication may be quiescent for many years and present in adulthood with one of the acute complications previously described.

IMPERFORATE ANUS

Anorectal malformations occur in 1:4000-1:5000 births. There is a slight male preponderance, and the more serious types involving a fistula from the colon to the the genitourinary tract are also more common in the male.

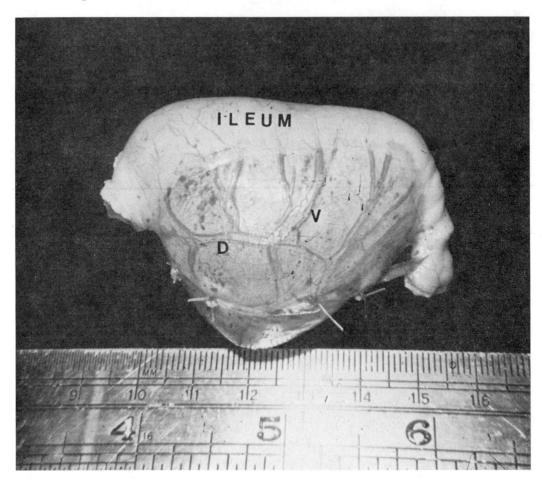

FIGURE 23   Resected segment of ileum with adherent duplication (D) on mesenteric side of normal ileum; common blood supply (V).

CLINICAL FEATURES

Bowel continence depends, in a large part, upon the normal relationship between the rectosigmoid colon and the puborectalis component of the levator ani. Although there are approximately 30 subtypes of anorectal anomalies (46), there are essentially two major groups: the supralevator (high) and translevator (low) imperforate anus. This classification is based upon the location of the blind pouch, i. e. , the high pouches are more common (75%), and are at or above the puborectalis sling (supralevator); the low pouches are below the puborectalis sling (translevator or infralevator). In each group the rectal pouch may end blindly, or communicate by a fistula with a nearby viscus or the perineal surface. The majority of fistulas are present only in cases of high imperforate anus and involve the urinary tract in males (Fig. 24) and the genital tract in females (Fig. 25). In rare cases of proven low imperforate anus, a fistulous tract may be present. The infant with a low pouch may demonstrate a perineal bulge when crying. In the male, the fistula to the urinary tract (usually the prostatic urethra) may produce fecaluria. A

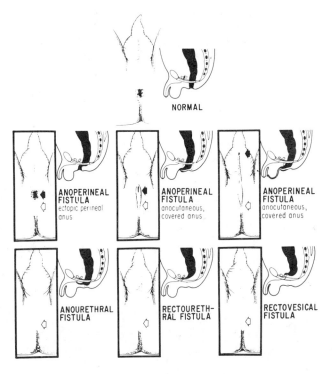

FIGURE 24   Major classes of imperforate anus in the male. (From Ref. 52. Reprinted with permission).

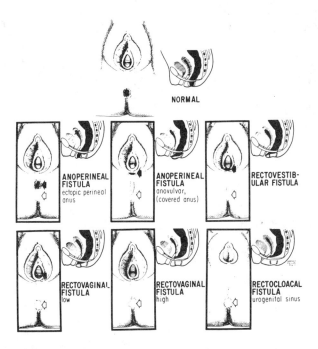

FIGURE 25   Major classes of imperforate anus in the female. (From Ref. 52. Reprinted with permission).

fistulous aperture on the perineum in either sex, is a critical observation, signifying a translevator type of anomaly. The external perineal orifice may be covered by a thickened fold of skin which may contain a minute quantity of meconium (Figs. 26a, b). If the sacrum is normal the anal dimple is always evident, and puckering will occur with stimulation of the overlying thickened skin.

In a female infant, a single perineal orifice suggests the presence of a rectocloacal fistula. This anomaly in the female is the most severe form of imperforate anus. A cloacal deformity is not only difficult to treat, but the long-term results of definitive surgery are disappointing. The female with two perineal openings indicates the presence of a rectovaginal fistula in cases of supralevator imperforate anus. The surgical repair of these cases is not as difficult as the cloacal anomaly, and eventual continence is expected in at least 60% of the cases.

These malformations are associated with other anomalies in two-thirds of the cases. The other systems commonly affected are the vertebral column (28%), the gastrointestinal tract (9%), the heart (9%), and central nervous system (18%). The coexistent anomalies are often severe and lethal in themselves. Additionally, 25% are found in low-birth-weight infants.

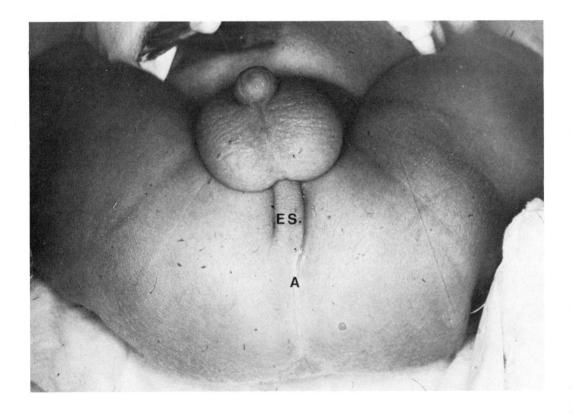

FIGURE 26a   Imperforate anus in the male with excess skin along the median raphe: site of normal anus (A); excess skin along median raphe (ES).

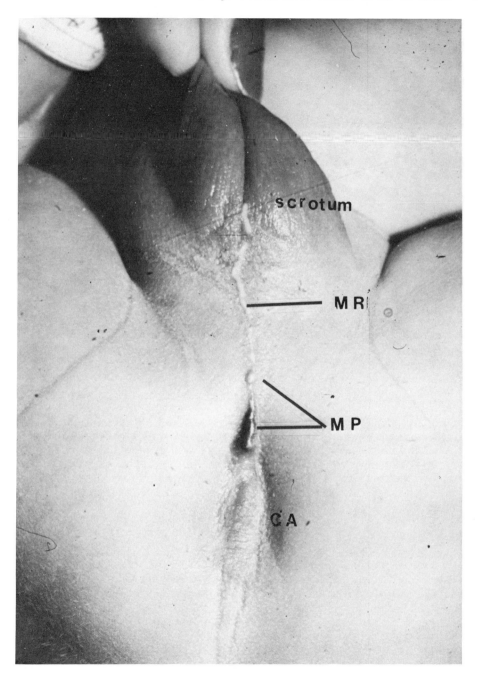

FIGURE 26b   Low imperforate anus in the male. Meconium pearls along median raphe: covered anus (CA); meconium pearls (MP); median raphe (MR) extending to base of scrotum.

DIAGNOSIS

An intravenous pyelogram and a simple x-ray of the spine in all of these babies is imperative. Complete sacral agenesis or the lack of three or more sacral segments is associated with severe pelvic neurological deficits. Sacral deformities are sufficiently common that this anomaly must be identified in every case of imperforate anus. In these circumstances there is no hope of rectal continence, and a pull-through procedure results in a perineal colostomy. A properly performed upside-down lateral pelvic x-ray study (invertograph of Rice-Wangensteen) can aid in the decision as to whether one is dealing with a high or a low pouch (47) (Fig.27). This x-ray study is based upon the fact that gas tends to rise to the apex of the blind bowel within 24 hours of birth. Misinterpretations are due to loss of air through a fistula, or the presence of low, impacted meconium may give a false impression of the level of the blind pouch. More recently, sonography has been used successfully in defining the blind pouch level.

The preoperative workup also may include the injection of a visible fistula. It has been suggested that the perineum be punctured under fluoroscopic control and contrast material introduced into the pouch. A voiding cystourethrogram will demonstrate rectourinary communications, vesicoureteric reflux, and deficiencies in urinary bladder control (Fig. 28). A careful neurological examination should also be performed since the sacral roots that supply the levator ani also innervate the vesical sphincters and the perineal dermatomes. An enlarged expressible bladder indicating bladder atony and perineal anesthesia is a concomitant finding with a paretic levator ani. These observations mandate a permanent colostomy with no attempt at constructing a functioning anus.

It is essential preoperatively, to determine accurately the level of the blind anal or rectal pouch, because this will dictate whether the patient will have a simple sacroperineal repair, or the more complex abdominoperineal or sacroabdominal perineal approach. The pubococcygeal line, drawn on the invertogram, accurately defines the levator ani. Colonic air above the PC line signifies a high imperforate anus and vice versa. The erroneous use of the perineal repair in cases of supralevator anomalies, can severely diminish the chances of ultimately achieving rectal continence. It is generally stated that if one cannot satisfactorily judge the position of the rectal pouch, a decompressing colostomy is the operation of choice.

TREATMENT

Anal deformities associated with an anocutaneous fistula in either sex, may all be treated by a cutback along the fistula to display the "covered anus" (Fig. 29). The prognosis in cases treated adequately by a cutback is excellent. It should be stressed that the female infant with a colovestibular fistula (i. e. , a fistula from the blind rectum to the vaginal fourchette) does not require an urgent colostomy. The fistula is easily dilated and is large enough not only to decompress the large intestine but also to serve as a temporary anus. This "ectopic" anus is then easily transplanted to its normal perineal position at 6 months of age. The outlook in cases of high rectal deformities is problematical because of associated anomalies (e. g. , 10% have tracheoesophageal fistula and esophageal atresia), the magnitude of the corrective surgery, and the existence of neurological deficits. Approximately 70% of the supralevator variety can expect significant fecal incontinence, probably resulting from coexisting absence of both internal and external sphincters and an abnormal levator ani musculature. Regardless of the procedure chosen to repair these cases, the most important feature is the accurate placement of the rectum through the puborectalis sling of the levator ani just behind the urethra.

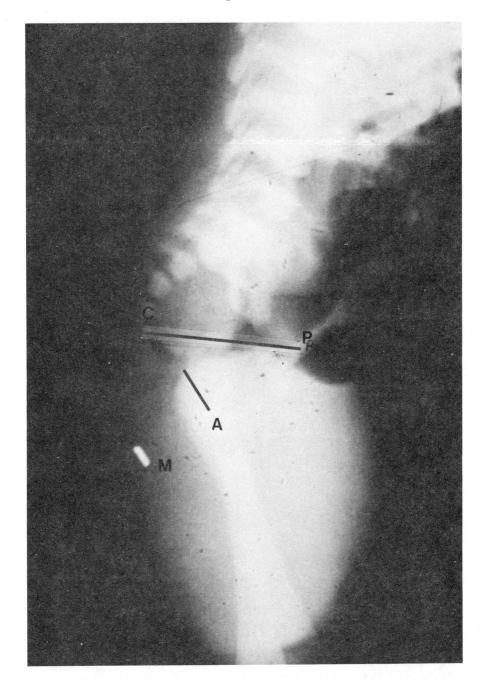

FIGURE 27   Pubococcygeal line (PC), from upper border of pubis to coccyx
(Rice-Wangensteen invertogram): marker on perineum (M); air column (A) below
PC line indicating infralevator (low) imperforate anus. (X-ray photo inverted.)

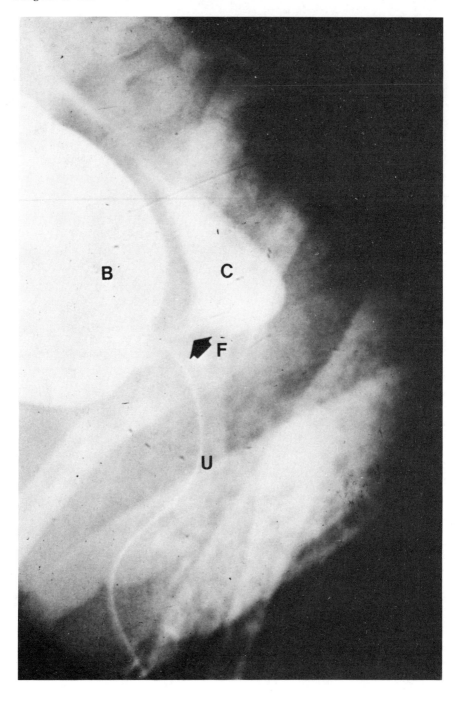

FIGURE 28   Cystogram demonstrating colourethral fistula in newborn with high imperforate anus: urinary bladder filled with Hypaque via urethral catheter (B); imperforate colon (C); urethral catheter (U); colourethral fistula (F) (arrow).

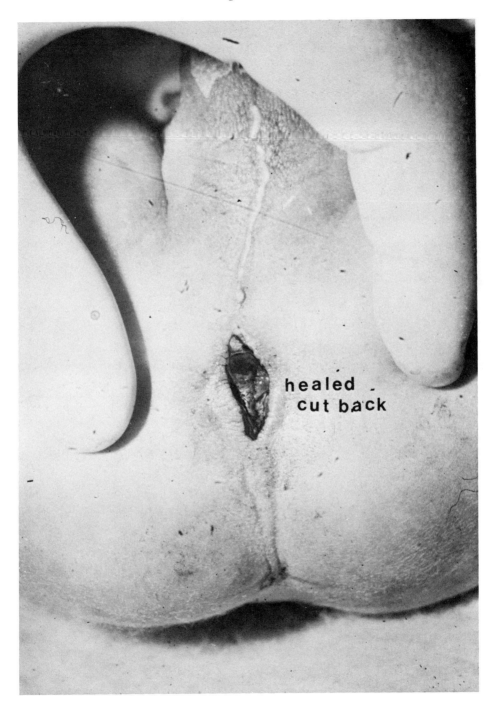

FIGURE 29   Cutback procedure for low imperforate anus along fistula revealing anal canal.

An immediate abdominoperineal pull-through in the newborn with high imperforate anus was initially recommended (48). Early operation yields mixed results, and is generally not considered the optimal time for definitive surgery. Today the approach advocated by most pediatric surgeons is a colostomy in the newborn, followed by construction of a perineal anus at 6-12 months of age. There are several acceptable methods of pulling through the blind rectum, each with its staunch adherents (49-51).

REFERENCES

1. Vassy, L. E. , and T. E. Boles, Jr. : Iatrogenic ileal atresia secondary to clamping of an occult omphalocele. J Pediatr Surg 10: 797-800, 1975.

2. Grob, M. : Lehrbuch Der Kinderchirurgie. Stuttgart, Georg Thieme, 1957, p. 311.

3. Gross, R. E. : A new method for surgical treatment of large omphaloceles. Surgery 24: 277-292, 1948.

4. Schuster, S. R. : A new method for the staged repair of large omphaloceles. Surg Gynecol Obstet 125: 837-850, 1967.

5. Shermata, D. W. , and J. A. Haller, Jr. : A new preformed transparent silo for the management of gastroschisis. J Pediatr Surg 19: 973-975, 1975.

6. Seashore, J. H. , R. J. MacNaughton, and J. L. Talbert: Treatment of gastroschisis and omphalocele with biological dressings. J Pediatr Surg 10:9-17, 1975.

7. Cauty, T. , M. M. Meguid, and A. J. Eraklis: Perforation of Meckel's diverticulum in infancy. J Pediatr Surg 10: 189-194, 1975.

8. Wansbrough, R. M. , S. Thomson, and R. G. Leckey: Meckel's diverticulum: A 42 year review of 273 cases at the Hospital for Sick Children, Toronto. Can J Surg 1: 15, 1957.

9. Simpson, J. S. : Ventral Silon pouch: Method of repairing congenital diaphragmatic hernias in newborns without increasing intra-abdominal pressure. Surgery 66: 798-801, 1969.

10. Geisler, F. , A. Gottlieb, and D. Fried: Agenesis of the right diaphragm repaired with marlex. J Pediatr Surg 12: 587-588, 1977.

11. Berdon, W. B. , D. H. Baker, and R. Amoury: The role of pulmonary hypoplasia in the prognosis of newborn infants with diaphragmatic hernia and eventration. Am J Roentgenol 103: 413, 1968.

12. Raphaely, R. C. , and J. J. Downes: Congenital diaphragmatic hernia: Prediction of survival. J Pediatr Surg 8: 815-823, 1973.

13. Dibbins, A. W. , and E. S. Wiener: Mortality from neonatal diaphragmatic hernia. J Pediatr Surg 9: 653-662, 1974.

14. Reid, I. S. , and R. J. Hutcherson: Long-term follow-up of patients with congenital diaphragmatic hernia. J Pediatr Surg 11:939-942, 1976.

15. German, J. C. , G. H. Mahour, and M. M. Woolley: Esophageal atresia and associated anomalies. J Pediatr Surg 11:299-306, 1976.

16. Quan, L. , and D. W. Smith: The VATER association, Vertebral defects, Anal atresia, T-E fistula with esophageal atresia. Radial and Renal dysplasia: A spectrum of associated defects. J Pediatr 82:104, 1973.

17. Kluth, D.: Atlas of esophageal atresia. J Pediatr Surg 11:901-920, 1976.

18. Replogle, R. L.: Esophageal atresia: Plastic sump catheter for drainage of the proximal pouch. Surgery 54:296-297, 1963.

19. Touloukian, R. J. , L. K. Pickett, T. Sparkman, and P. Biancani: Repair of esophageal atresia by end-to-side anastomosis and ligation of the tracheoesophageal fistula: A critical review of 18 cases. J Pediatr Surg 9:305-310, 1974.

20. Howard, R. , and N. A. Myers: Esophageal atresia: A technique for elongating the upper pouch. Surgery 58:725, 1965.

21. Woolley, M. M. , F. Leix, P. W. Johnston, et al: Esophageal atresia types A and B: Upper pouch elongation and delayed anatomic reconstruction. J Pediatr Surg 4:148-153, 1969.

22. Rehbein, F. , and N. Schweder: Reconstruction of the esophagus without colon transplantation in cases of atresia. J Pediatr Surg 6:746, 1971.

23. Livaditis, A. , L. Radberg, and G. Odensjo: Esophageal end-to-end anastomosis. Reduction of anastomotic tension by circular myotomy. Scand J Thorac Cardiovasc Surg 6:206, 1972.

24. Hendren, W. H. , and J. R. Hale: Esophageal atresia treated by electromagnetic bougienage and subsequent repair. J Pediatr Surg 11:713-722, 1976.

25. Longino, L. A. , M. J. Woolley, and R. E. Gross: Esophageal replacement in infants and children with the use of a segment of colon. JAMA 171:1187-1192, 1959.

26. Azar, H. , A. R. Chrispin, and D. T. Waterston: Esophageal replacement with transverse colon of infants and children. J Pediatr Surg 6:3-9, 1971.

27. Bedard, P. , D. P. Girran, and B. Shandling: Congenital H-type tracheoesophageal fistula. J Pediatr Surg 9:663-668, 1974.

28. Ohkawa, H. , H. Takahashi, Y. Hoshino, and H. Sato: Lower esophageal stenosis in association with tracheobronchial remnants. J Pediatr Surg 10:453-457, 1975.

29. Tandler, J.: Zur entwicklungsgeschichte des mesclilichen duodenum in friiha embryonalstadien. Morphol Jahrb 29:187, 1900.

30.   Szalay, G.C.: Congenital pyloric atresia. Arch Surg 108:248, 1974.

31.   Louw, J.H.: Jejunal atresia and stenosis. J Pediatr Surg 1:8, 1966.

32.   Fonkalsrud, E.W., A.A. deLorimier, and D.M. Hays: Congenital atresia and stenosis of the duodenum. A review compiled from the members of the Surgical Section of the American Academy of Pediatrics. Pediatrics 43:79-83, 1969.

33.   deLorimier, A.A., E.W. Fonkalsrud, and D.M. Hays: Congenital atresia and stenosis of the jejunum and ileum. Surgery 65:819-827, 1969.

34.   Clatworthy, H.W., W.H.R. Howard, and J. Lloyd: The meconium plug syndrome. Surgery 39:131, 1956.

35.   Philippart, A.I., J.O. Reed, and K.E. Georgeson: Neonatal small left colon syndrome: Intramural not intraluminal obstruction. J Pediatr Surg 10:733-740, 1975.

36.   Noblett, H.R.: Treatment of uncomplicated meconium ileus by Gastrografin enema. J Pediatr Surg 4:190-197, 1969.

37.   Donnison, A.B., H. Shwachman, and R.E. Gross: A review of 164 children with meconium ileus seen at the Children's Hospital Medical Center, Boston. Pediatrics 37:833-850, 1966.

38.   Bishop, H.C., and C.E. Koop: Management of meconium ileus: Resection, Roux-en-Y anastomosis and ileostomy irrigation with pancreatic enzymes. Ann Surg 145:410-414, 1957.

39.   Rickham, P.D., and C.R. Boeckman: Neonatal meconium obstruction in the absence of mucoviscidosis. Am J Surg 109:173, 1965.

40.   Dolan, T.F., and R.J. Touloukian: Familial meconium ileus not associated with cystic fibrosis. J Pediatr Surg 9:821-824, 1974.

41.   Krasna, I., J. Becker, K. Schneider, and D. Schwartz: Low molecular weight dextran and re-exploration in management of ischemic midgut-volvulus. J Pediatr Surg 12:615-622, 1978.

42.   Rutherford, H.: Intestinal obstruction in the newborn: Strangulation through a hole in the mesentery. Glasgow Med J 7:87, 1909.

43.   Rubin, S.Z., A. Ayalon, and Y. Berlatzky: The simultaneous occurrence of paraduodenal and paracecal herniae presenting with volvulus of the intervening bowel. J Pediatr Surg 11:205-208, 1976.

44.   Sheppard, M.D., and J.R. Gilmour: Torsion of a pedunculated gastric cyst. Br Med J 1:874, 1945.

45.   Schwartz, D.L., J.M. Becker, K.M. Schneider, and H.B. So: Tubular duplication with autonomous blood supply: Resection with preservation of adjacent bowel. J Pediatr Surg 15:341, 1980.

46.   Stephens, F. D.: Congenital Malformations of the Rectum, Anus, and Genito-Urinary Tract. E and S Livingston, Edinburgh, 1963.

47.   Wangensteen, D. H., and C. O. Rice: Imperforate anus: A method of determining the surgical approach. Ann Surg 92:77-81, 1930.

48.   Rhoads, J. E., R. L. Pipes, and J. P. Randall: A simultaneous abdominal and perineal approach in the operation for imperforate anus with atresia of the rectum and rectosigmoid. Ann Surg 127:552-556, 1948

49.   Rehbein, F.: Imperforate anus: Experiences with abdomino-perineal and abdomino-sacral-perineal pull-through procedures. J Pediatr Surg 2:99-105, 1967.

50.   Kieswetter, W. B.: Imperforate anus II. The rationale and technique of the sacro-abdomino-perineal operation. J Pediatr Surg 2:106-110, 1967.

51.   Hendren, W. H., and R. J. Hale: High-pouch imperforate anus treated by electromagnetic bougienage and subsequent perineal repair. J Pediatr Surg 11:723-732, 1976.

52.   Santulli, T. V.: Malformations of the anus and rectum. in Pediatric Surgery, Vol. 2. 2nd ed. W. T. Mustard et al. (eds.). Year Book Medical Publishers, Chicago, 1969.

6

NORMAL AND ABNORMAL NUTRITION IN CHILDREN

Fima Lifshitz, M. D. and Moshe Berant, M. D.

INTRODUCTION

The study of nutrition in pediatrics concerns the provision of food and its successful intake, as well as the proper absorption and utilization of nutrients. The determination of the quantity and the quality of foodstuffs that are required to meet the
needs of the child, for optimal health, constitutes only a part of the concerns of a
nutritionist. The inadequate availability and intake of food and, especially, deficient environmental conditions, are a major problem and the main cause of malnutrition afflicting a great proportion of the world population (1).

Proper feeding must provide for energy expenditure, normal maintenance, and
repair of body tissues, as well as for the demands for growth and development. A
deficient nutrition will have an adverse impact, especially in the pediatric age
group, because of the special anabolic needs of children. Major efforts have
therefore been invested in the definition of the nutritional requirements and the
dietary policies and practices that may successfully provide proper nourishment.

Deviations from adequate nutrition may cause deviation from good health, or
may be the cause of overt disease, as "single" deficiency or excess states (e. g. ,
rickets or hypervitaminosis D), or "multiple" deficiency or excess states (e. g. ,
protein-energy malnutrition, or obesity). Obesity, as a consequence of excessive
food intake, is receiving increasing attention as the nutritional problem par excel-
lence of an affluent society. However, on the worldwide scale, deficiency diseases still constitute the major problem with overpopulation, poverty, ignorance, war,
and natural catastrophies contributing to the maintenance of nutritional deprivation.

The importance of nutrition for the population as a whole and for the fate of
every individual child, must encourage everyone concerned to be acquainted with
the current concepts of this discipline. In this chapter we review some of these
concepts of normal and abnormal nutrition in pediatrics. We shall not attempt to
review the many factors of an economical, social, political, or cultural nature
which may be most important in determining the nutritional state of a patient or
that of a total population.

ASSESSMENT OF NUTRITIONAL STATUS

Several methods for indexing and quantifying the degree and type of malnutrition have been developed by leaders in the field (2-4). Many of these assessment techniques have proved to be too arduous for most clinicians and are not in widespread use for that reason. However, here we describe a number of clinically necessary evaluations that must be included to assess the nutritional status of patients, although they are often simplified indices. Using some of the measurements described later may uncover nutritional alterations similar to those reported using more detailed and comprehensive methods. While purists may reject this "poor man's" nutritional assessment as being too simplistic, it may be a reasonable way for routinely evaluating adequacy of nutrition on a large-scale, cost-effective basis.

The evaluation of the nutritional status of a patient requires a complete history, a periodic physical examination with accurate body measurements, and a well-focused laboratory profile. These are needed to uncover underlying nutritional alterations in patients who do not necessarily appear to be malnourished (5, 6).

HISTORY

A reliable and complete dietary, nutritional and sociocultural history, in addition to the "conventional" medical history, is important for the evaluation of the patient. Also, the patient's attitudes regarding foods and fads, i.e., vegetarianism or megavitamins, should be disclosed and examined since this may alert the health professional to possible sources of past, present, or future trouble. A single day nutritional survey is an accurate and reproducible estimate of dietary intake and a 24-hour dietary recall should always be obtained as a minimum in clinical situations.

PHYSICAL EXAMINATION

The physical examination should be performed with a specific interest to uncover malnutrition. It should be kept constantly in mind that nutritional alterations may exist, even in communities and neighborhoods where poverty, cultural deprivation, and poor health are not clearly apparent (7, 8). In developed countries, it may be uncommon to find the traditional signs of overt nutritional deficiency, such as angular stomatitis, cheilosis, glossitis, skin lesions, extreme wasting and edema, unless associated with physical or social disease. More commonly, the expression of nutritional deficiency or faulty nutrition will be more subtle, and will therefore become apparent as such only to the minded observer. On the other hand, it may be more common to be faced with nutritional excesses which must be recognized in the early stages, since this is when the individual may be amenable to treatment, as discussed next. The following physical findings are helpful in the assessment of nutritional status:

Weight and Stature (Length or Height)

Weight and stature are traditionally considered to be a convenient, albeit crude, clinical index for nutritional evaluation when correlated with normative values for age (9). Historically, patients may report weight loss or gain and if previous weight is known the percentage deficit or excess weight may be calculated. A better estimate is obtained by assessing weight-for-age with stature-for-age (weight/height index). The child who is underweight for height might then be described as "wasted," whereas the one who is overweight for height may be considered "fat." Similarly, the child who is below the expected height for his weight and his age might be called "stunted" (10).   A weight/height deficit or excess of 10% or less has been considered as being within normal range, with variations beyond that value being abnormal.   A patient with a deficit or an excess of more than 20% in in weight/height is significantly malnourished.   The degree of malnutrition has been classified as "mild" (first-degree), when the weight/height deficit or excess of more than 10% but less than 20%; as "moderate"(second-degree), when there is a digression of more than 20% but less than 40% from normal; and a variation by more than 40% is "severe" (third-degree).   When there is edema in an undernourished child, this classification obviously cannot hold; such a child will be classified automatically as suffering from third-degree malnutrition.

Undernutrition in infants seems to affect mainly weight gain; at a later age, children may have "outgrown" their wasting, and their nutritional deficits may be reflected mainly by decreased stature-for-age (11).   Overnutrition in infancy usually results in accelerated growth both in weight and in length (12).   Therefore, during the first year of life obesity may be difficult to diagnose, as the weight remains proportional to the length; however, as the child grows older the weight/height discrepancies become evident.   Any departure from a child's expected growth pattern or a change in the child's growth velocity characteristics indicates that close investigation is in order, which must include a nutritional evaluation.

Head Circumference

Head circumference and its progress along the curve for age, and correlation with weight and stature, is also contributory to nutritional assessment.   Head circumference may correlate with brain cell number (13) and, according to reported observations (14), serious undernourishment during critical stages of brain development may cause diminished brain growth and consequently, impairment of the normal growth of the head.

Skinfold Thickness

Skinfold thickness and arm circumference measurements provide information on relative body fat content, as subcutaneous tissue is a major depot of body fat (15). Measurements of skinfold thickness have been standardized and are considered to be a reliable index of nutrition (16).   For example, skinfold measurement allows the examiner to distinguish low-birth-weight babies, who are just constitutionally small neonates, from those who are truly undernourished thin-for-dates newborns (17).   The skinfold thickness measurement also helps to interpret weight deviations from normal that are due to alterations in body fat content.   Therefore, skinfold thickness charts should become an integral part of every pediatric chart. Measurements of skinfold thickness with a Lange caliper should be performed on the nondominant midarm, three consecutive times.   The average of the results is then compared with the published standard charts for age and weight (Fig. 1).

The arm/head circumference ratio is a good index of nutritional status (18). This index is obtained by estimating the midportion of the upper arm, measuring the circumference at this location, and measuring the head circumference.   The normal midarm circumference divided by the head circumference is 0.33.   A mild malnutrition exists when the ratio is less than 0.31.   A moderate and a severe malnutrition are present when the ratio is less than 0.27 or 0.25, respectively.

Lean body mass, or for all intents and purposes, skeletal muscle mass, can also be estimated by anthropometric determinations.   The nondominant midarm circumference is measured, and the midarm muscle circumference is subtracted from the value of the triceps skinfold thickness times 0.314 and is then expressed as a percentage deviation from the norm.

Clinical Signs

Clinical signs which contribute to nutritional evaluation, and may give a clue to deviations from normal, include general vitality, muscular development and tone, skeletal structure, and the condition of the gums, teeth, hair, skin, and eyes, and sexual development. Specific clinical signs of nutritional deficiencies will be discussed next.

LABORATORY TESTS

Laboratory investigations should be performed according to the requirements of of the individual clinical situation or as a case-finding method, when certain deficiency states are prevalent in a given population. Laboratory tests which are representative of nutritional state include: hemoglobin concentration and hematocrit values, serum iron, total serum proteins and albumin/globulin ratios, cholesterol, triglycerides, and blood vitamin A (retinol) or carotene levels. Radiological examinations of the bone epiphyses for signs of adequate progression of bone maturation and for evidence of deficiencies such as rickets and scurvy are included. These data have been found to be of value in nutritional screening of pediatric populations (19, 20). For disclosing more subtle, "subclinical" deficiency states, more sophisticated methods are proposed, which include determination of circulating transferrin, ferritin, and diverse vitamins. Lean body mass can be estimated by the level of the urinary excretion of creatine, which is a product of muscle metabolism. The 24-hour urinary excretion is roughly proportional to the skeletal muscle mass. Several methods can be used to assess visceral protein reserve. A serum albumin concentration less than 3.4 g/dl in the absence of liver disease indicates protein malnutrition. The half-life of albumin is approximately 20 days in the normal person, but may be decreased in patients with infection, burns, severe injuries, and protein-losing conditions. The serum transferrin value, directly determined or derived from the total iron binding capacity, also is reduced in conditions of protein deficiency. The half-life of transferrin is 5-7 days. Consequently, a decrease in the transferrin value in starvation can occur before any significant drop in the level of serum albumin. A total lymphocyte count of less than $1500/mm^3$ also is indicative of visceral protein depletion and is commonly associated with cutaneous anergy. Protein requirements can be determined by nitrogen balance, subtracting the nitrogen excretion value from that of nitrogen intake. The 24-hour urinary urea excretion level is a most accurate index of nitrogen excretion that is usable in a clinical setting. A factor of 4 is added to the total urinary urea level to account for other free nitrogen losses (perspiration and feces).

NUTRITIONAL REQUIREMENTS, ALLOWANCES, AND ALTERATIONS

The term "nutritional requirement" is defined as the minimal intake of nutrients that will promote optimal health (21). The recommendations for dietary allowances are not minimum requirements, but will usually exceed the basic needs of "practically all individuals," to provide a margin of safety over the minimal amount of nutrients needed to prevent deficiency states.

The reported Recommended Daily Dietary Allowances (RDA) of the Food and Nutrition Board, National Academy of Sciences—National Research Council (22) are shown in Table 1.

Nutritional needs vary from child to child and are related mainly to the individual body composition, metabolic turnover, and rate of growth. Additional

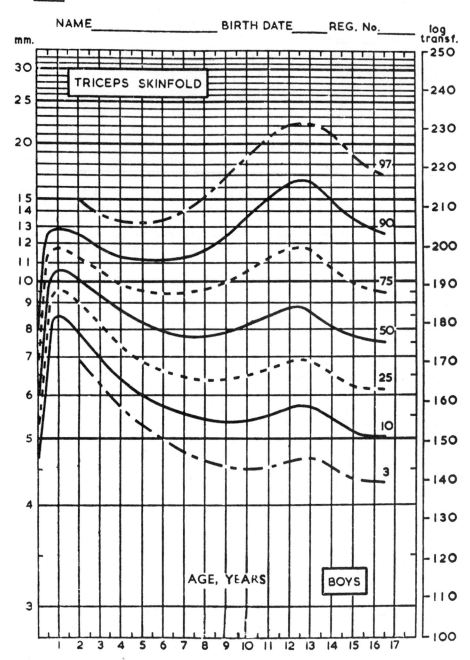

FIGURE 1a   Standards for subcutaneous fat in British boys. (From Lanner, J.M. and R.H. Whitehouse. Br Med J 1:446, 1962. Reprinted with permission.)

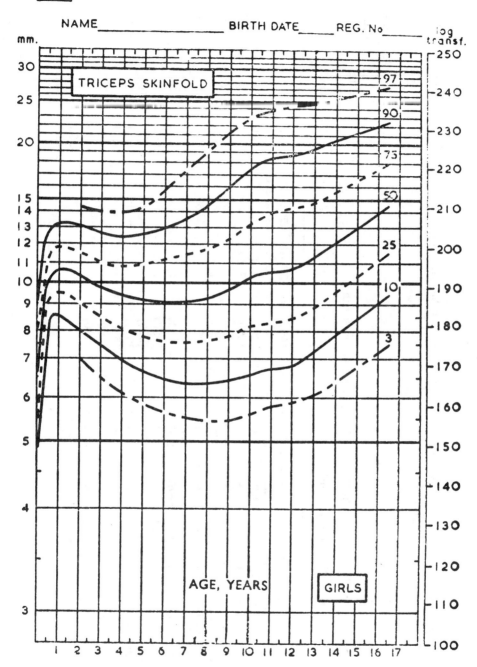

FIGURE 1b   Standards for subcutaneous fat in British girls. (From Lanner, J.M. and R. H. Whitehouse. Br Med J 1:446, 1962. Reprinted with permission.)

TABLE 1   Recommended Daily Dietary Allowances[a], (Designed for the Maintenance of Good Nutrition of Practically All Healthy People in the U.S.A.)

	Age (years)	Weight (kg)	Weight (lb)	Height (cm)	Height (in)	Energy Needs (kcal)	Energy Needs (with range)	Energy Needs (Mj)	Protein (g)	Vitamin A (µg RE)[b]	Vitamin D (µg)[c]	Vitamin E (mg α-TE)[d]
Infants	0.0-0.5	6	13	60	24	kg X 115	(95-145)	kg X 0.48	kg x 2.2	420	10	3
	0.5-1.0	9	20	71	28	kg X 105	(80-135)	kg X 0.44	kg X 2.0	400	10	4
Children	1-3	13	29	90	35	1300	(900-1800)	5.5	23	400	10	5
	4-6	20	44	112	44	1700	(1300-2300)	7.1	30	500	10	6
	7-10	28	62	132	52	2400	(1650-3300)	10.1	34	700	10	7
Males	11-14	45	99	157	62	2700	(2000-3700)	11.3	45	1000	10	8
	15-18	66	145	176	69	2800	(2100-3900)	11.8	56	1000	10	10
	19-22	70	154	177	70	2900	(2500-3300)	12.2	56	1000	7.5	10
	23-50	70	154	178	70	2700	(2300-3100)	11.3	56	1000	5	10
	51+	70	154	178	70	2400	(2000-2800)	10.1	56	1000	5	10
Females	11-14	46	101	157	62	2200	(1500-3000)	9.2	46	800	10	8
	15-18	55	120	163	64	2100	(1200-3000)	8.8	46	800	10	8
	19-22	55	120	163	64	2100	(1700-2500)	8.8	44	800	7.5	8
	23-50	55	120	163	64	2000	(1600-2400)	8.4	44	800	5	8
	51+	55	120	163	64	1800	(1400-2200)	7.6	44	800	5	8
Pregnant						+300			+30	+200	+5	+2
Lactating						+500			+20	+400	+5	+3

Water-Soluble Vitamins

Minerals

Vitamin C (mg)	Thiamin (mg)	Riboflavin (mg)	Niacin (mg NE)[e]	Vitamin B-6 (mg)	Folacin[f] (μg)	Vitamin B-12 (μg)	Calcium (mg)	Phosphorus (mg)	Magnesium (mg)	Iron (mg)	Zinc (mg)	Iodine (μg)
35	0.3	0.4	6	0.3	30	0.5[g]	360	240	50	10	3	40
35	0.5	0.6	8	0.6	45	1.5	540	360	70	15	5	50
45	0.7	0.8	9	0.9	100	2.0	800	800	150	15	10	70
45	0.9	1.0	11	1.3	200	2.5	800	800	200	10	10	90
45	1.2	1.4	16	1.6	300	3.0	800	800	250	10	10	120
50	1.4	1.6	18	1.8	400	3.0	1200	1200	350	18	15	150
60	1.4	1.7	18	2.0	400	3.0	1200	1200	400	18	15	150
60	1.5	1.7	19	2.2	400	3.0	800	800	350	10	15	150
60	1.4	1.6	18	2.2	400	3.0	800	800	350	10	15	150
60	1.2	1.4	16	2.2	400	3.0	800	800	350	10	15	150
50	1.1	1.3	15	1.8	400	3.0	1200	1200	300	18	15	150
60	1.1	1.3	14	2.0	400	3.0	1200	1200	300	18	15	150
60	1.1	1.3	14	2.0	400	3.0	800	800	300	18	15	150
60	1.0	1.2	13	2.0	400	3.0	800	800	300	18	15	150
60	1.0	1.2	13	2.0	400	3.0	800	800	300	10	15	150
+20	+0.4	+0.3	+2	+0.6	+400	+1.0	+400	+400	+150	-[h]	+5	+25
+40	+0.5	+0.5	+5	+0.5	+100	+1.0	+400	+400	+150	-[h]	+10	+50

TABLE 1 (cont'd)

a The data in this table have been assembled from the observed median heights and weights of children together with desirable weights for adults for the mean heights of men (70 in.) and women (64 in.) between ages of 18 and 34 years as surveyed in the U.S. population (HEW/National Child Health Statistics data).

The energy allowances for the young adults are for men and women doing light work. The allowances for the two older age groups present mean energy needs over these age spans, allowing for a 2% decrease in basal (resting) metabolic rate per decade and a reduction in activity of 200 kcal/day for men and women between 51 and 75 years, 500 kcal for men over 75 years, and 400 kcal for women over 75 years. The customary range of daily energy output is shown in parentheses for adults and is based on a variation in energy needs of ± 400 kcal at any one age emphasizing the wide range of energy intakes appropriate for any group of people.

Energy allowances for children through age 18 are based on median energy intakes of children of these ages followed in longitudinal growth studies. The values in parentheses are 10th and 90th percentiles of energy intake, to indicate the range of energy consumption among children of these ages.

The allowances are intended to provide for individual variations among most normal persons as they live in the United States under usual environmental stresses. Diets should be based on a variety of common foods to provide other nutrients for which human requirements have been less well defined.

b Retinol equivalents. 1 retinol equivalent = 1 μg retinol or 6 μg beta carotene.

c As cholecalciferol. 10 μg cholecalciferol = 400 IU of vitamin D.

d α -tocopherol equivalents. 1 mg d-α tocopherol = 1 α -TE.

e 1 NE (niacin equivalent) is equal to 1 mg of niacin or 60 mg of dietary tryptophan.

f The folacin allowances refer to dietary sources as determined by Lactobacillus casei assay after treatment with enzymes (conjugases) to make polyglutamyl forms of the vitamin available to the test organism.

g The recommended dietary allowance for vitamin B-12 in infants is based on average concentrations of the vitamin in human milk. The allowances after weaning are based on energy intake (as recommended by the American Academy of Pediatrics) and consideration of other factors, such as intestinal absorption.

h The increased requirement during pregnancy cannot be met by the iron content of habitual American diets nor by the existing iron stores of many women; therefore the use of 30-60 mg of supplemental iron is recommended. Iron needs during lactation are not substantially different from those of nonpregnant women, but continued supplementation of the mother for 2-3 months after parturition is advisable in order to replenish stores depleted by pregnancy.

Modified from: Food and Nutrition Board, National Academy of Sciences—National Research Council (Revised 1980) (21).

variations are noted in states of exceptional anabolic needs as in the low-birth-weight baby, whose accelerated growth pattern poses higher nutritional demands (23), or in illness, when metabolic needs are always increased (24). Moreover, special nutritional needs have to be considered in children with diarrhea, faulty intestinal absorption, or metabolic disease.

The estimation of requirements for nutrients is based on calculations derived from observations of infant and child populations, and of experimental situations which are brought as close as possible to real life situations. The determination of requirements and the dietary recommendations issued by diverse study groups and committees of experts, are therefore necessarily rough approximations, and may often reflect the philosophy of these experts and also the social, economic, and political setting in which they function.

Nutritional requirements must be met to avoid nutritional alterations. Water, calories, protein, fat, carbohydrates, vitamins, and minerals must be given not only in adequate amounts, but also in properly balanced proportions and combinations, for the efficient digestion, absorption, and utilization of all nutrients. The diet should be presented in a way that will lead to the development of sound eating habits.

WATER

All life processes require water. Water also provides many of the essential minerals. The amount of water needed is proportionally related to the energy expenditure of the individual. The provision of adequate nutrients without adequate amounts of fluid will result in dehydration, an excessive renal solute load, and inefficient utilization and wasting of calories (25). Furthermore, the hyperosmolarity of oral solutions may contribute to other complications, e. g. , enterocolitis in low-birth-weight infants (26). The addition of nutritional supplements, or the increase in calories by providing concentrated formulas to infants who are underweight or have other nutritional alterations is quite popular. This often is done at the expense of water intake and of the proper balance of water to the caloric intake. All diets and formulas must be isocaloric at all times; that is, they must provide anywhere from 1. 25-1. 5 ml of water per kilocalorie (22). In addition, extra fluid should be available to compensate for other alterations which may result in dehydration due to decreased water intake or excessive water losses.

CALORIES

The importance of energy supply is borne out by the observations that even with adequate provision of nutrients, a deficiency in energy will result in deficient growth, whereas an excessive caloric intake will result in obesity. The current expression for energy is kilocalories; however, the joule (J) is the accepted international unit of energy (1 kcal = 4. 184 kJ; 1 kJ = 0. 239 kcal) (22). The energy value of a certain food may be expressed in terms of calories or joules; another practical way is to relate the food's energy value to the equivalent of energy expenditure when performing a certain activity—like walking, running, swimming—during a certain period of time (27). The Food and Nutrition Board (FNB) has recommended a daily calorie intake of 30-120 kcal/kg of body weight, according to the age of the individual (see Table 1). This supply would allow about 50% of those calories for "basal" energy requirements, 30% for growth requirements, and 15-20% for normal variations in activity. Recommendations concerning the relative contributions by protein, fat, and carbohydrate to the supply of calories are in accordance with the medical knowledge and fashion of the day. It has been proposed that the proportions of calories derived from protein, fat, and carbohydrate should be

7-15%, 30-55%, and 35-65%, respectively (20). Currently, the tendency is toward the lower figures of protein and fat and the higher figures of carbohydrate (28, 29).

CARBOHYDRATE

Carbohydrates are an important source of readily available energy for metabolism. An appropriate supply of such energy is imperative for adequate utilization of protein and other nutrients (30). Lack of carbohydrate intake or absorption will result in energy deficiency and this, in turn, will cause a diversion of protein metabolism from its anabolic tasks; thus dietary protein and, subsequently, body proteins will be utilized as a source of energy. The overall result will be a deficiency of energy and a net deficiency of protein—namely, protein-energy malnutrition. An excessive intake of carbohydrates will result in obesity and may expose the infant to the diverse possible consequences of this type of malnutrition (12). Human milk provides about 40% of its calories from carbohydrates, cow's milk provides about 30%, and in most commercial infant formulas, carbohydrates account for 40-50% of the calories. The main carbohydrate in milk is lactose, which yields glucose and galactose by hydrolysis, and thus participates in the synthesis of cerebrosides of myelin and the glycoproteins of collagen (31). Fruits and vegetables in their natural state may contain significant amounts of simple sugars, notably glucose, fructose, and sucrose.

It has been shown that babies tend to consume larger volumes of food when these are sweetened (32). Many commercially prepared baby foods contain added sucrose; also, in many households sucrose is added to the food. An obvious hazard of such practices is that the excessive intake of sucrose will result in obesity, especially if there is also an overall increase of food intake.

The addition of sucrose to the feedings also contributes to the development of dental caries (33), and it has been suggested to play a role in the induction of hyperinsulinism, hyperlipidemia, and diabetes mellitus (34, 35). The present day trend is to advise a restriction in dietary sucrose and to give preference to starches as a source of carbohydrates. Starches are more rapidly evacuated from the stomach than sucrose (36); on the other hand, their digestion is slower and, in consequence, blood glucose will rise more gradually and will evoke a more graded stimulus to insulin production (37).

The feeding of diets high in refined carbohydrates such as sucrose or highly milled flour also has been associated with diverticulosis, artherosclerosis, hiatal hernia, appendicitis, irritable bowel syndrome, hemorrhoids, and malignancies of the colon (38, 39). Although the issue is still highly controversial, there is a current tendency to recommend diets which contain carbohydrates consisting of unprocessed starches and with a high fiber content to provide about 60% of the total caloric intake of the individual.

PROTEIN

Protein intake is necessary for the provision of nitrogen and amino acids for synthesis of tissue and for replacement of nitrogen which is lost from the body. During infancy, protein requirements for growth account for a large percentage of total protein needs. The appropriate expression of protein requirement is per unit of energy (calorie or joule) intake rather than per unit of body weight. The Committee on Nutrition of the American Academy of Pediatrics has recommended (40) that milk formulas for healthy infants must provide a minimum of 1.8 and a maximum of 4.5 g/kcal of protein (the daily allowance by the FNB is around 2.2 g/kg of body weight). The protein which is consumed must offer adequate amounts of essential amino acids. In addition to isoleucine, leucine, methionine, phenylalanine, threonine, tryptophan, and valine, which are the traditional "essential" amino acids for the adult, the full term infant also needs tyrosine, cystine, and histidine (41). Moreover, the proportional amounts of the individual amino acids supplied by protein must be well balanced, since the effects of a relative deficiency of one amino acid may become accentuated by an excess intake of another amino acid (42).

Most infants in developed countries consume an excess of protein. Protein intake in excess of 16% of the caloric supply may not be harmful as long as enough water is ingested, but they are an inefficient and costly source of calories. On the other hand, in the very small, premature infant excessive protein intake can be harmful, although some increased supply of amino acids seems to be very important for survival and better growth in such babies (23).

In developing countries where protein supply may be borderline, the quality, quantity, and variety of the food consumed become of critical importance. The source of dietary protein in these populations is mainly from plant protein, which has a lower biological quality than animal protein because of low levels of one or more essential amino acids. The intake of mixtures of plant proteins, e. g. , cereals and legumes, will make up for the individual amino acid deficiencies and add biological quality to the protein consumed (28). Protein deficiency is likely to occur when protein intake accounts for less than 6% of the total caloric intake. The concomitant intake of adequate amounts of carbohydrate is essential for proper economy in the body, since protein cannot be utilized if an energy source is insufficient. Accordingly, it appears that even in places where marasmus and kwashiorkor are highly prevalent, the role of protein deficiency has been exaggerated. There recently has been a reversal regarding the "protein gap" concept as being the most important single problem causing malnutrition in infants (30, 43).

FAT

The main importance of dietary fat lies in its high caloric value, the feeling of satiety, the supply of essential fatty acids, its role in the absorption of fat-soluble vitamins, and its contribution of products which are necessary for cell membrane stability and function. The Committee of Nutrition of the American Academy of Pediatrics (40) recommends a minimum of 3. 3 g of fat per 100 kcal in infant formulas, and a maximum of 6 g/100 kcal. The recommended minimum for linoleic acid in infant formulas is 300 mg/100 kcal (40), as linoleic acid plays a central role in the prevention of essential fatty acid deficiency (44). A very low fat content in the diet may be associated with an excessive proportion of carbohydrate and protein, while a very high proportion of fat may result in ketosis or acidosis because of the relative reduction in the intake of carbohydrate and protein (40).

Naturally occurring essential fatty acid deficiency is very unusual; however, deficiency states in infants have been induced by the feeding of low-fat diets or a formula that contains mainly saturated fatty acids (45). The prospects of the occurrence of essential fatty acid deficiency has increased because of the greater therapeutic use of fat-restricted diets, oral feeding of medium-chain triglycerides, and especially the widespread application of prolonged fat-free intravenous feeding (46). The linoleic acid group is the most active as a source of essential fatty acids; a linoleic acid content of 3% of the calories in the diet will prevent essential fatty acid deficiency (47). The manifestations of essential fatty acid deficiency include growth retardation, scaly dermatitis, delayed wound healing, capillary fragility, thrombocytopenia, and degenerative changes in the liver and kidneys. There also may be disturbances in the function of the reticuloendothelial system and a greater susceptibility to infection. Laboratory tests show alterations in the fatty acid composition of plasma, platelets, and red blood cells with a decrease in linoleic and arachidonic acid (C-23), and a concurrent increase in 5, 8, 11-eicosatrienoic acid (48). Treatment consists of supplementing oral or parenteral feeding with a soybean oil emulsion containing linoleic acid (49). Prevention and therapy of essential fatty acid deficiency by application of sunflower seed oil to the patient's skin has been reported (50), although more recent studies indicate that this method is not adequate (51).

The recognition that an elevated serum cholesterol concentration in the adult is a reliable risk factor in the prediction of coronary heart disease (52), and the discovery that coronary atherosclerosis may originate in childhood (53), have aroused concern about the cholesterol intake in the pediatric age group. As the serum concentration of cholesterol is related especially to the cholesterol content in the diet (54), demands have arisen for the restriction of cholesterol intake. However, while the cholesterol needed for brain myelinization is synthesized in situ (55), exogenous cholesterol is needed in infancy for the synthesis of bile acids and for the adequate induction of the enzyme system which controls cholesterol metabolism (56). Therefore, reduction in dietary cholesterol intake during infancy has not been recommended. On the other hand, beyond infancy it seems reasonable to moderately restrict the intake of cholesterol. More severe restriction is indicated to families with a high incidence of coronary artery disease at a young age, and especially in cases with familial hyperlipoproteinemia (57).

The popular practice of feeding "low-fat" diets to children has no value since such a diet usually leads to the intake of larger amounts of food containing an increase proportion of carbohydrates. Moreover, feeding skim milk to infants may be dangerous since the intake of essential fats is curtailed and obesity is neither prevented nor effectively treated by this practice (40).

VITAMINS

Vitamin deficiency in normal infants is relatively uncommon in developed countries because the natural supply of vitamins is ample in a varied diet. In addition, public health practices promote adequate vitamin supplementation in instances where their amounts in the food may be borderline (e. g. , vitamins D and K in the exclusively breast-fed infant); or when a relative deficiency is likely (e. g. , vitamin K in the neonate); or when increased needs arise (e. g. , vitamin D and folacin in the premature infant). "Fortification" of foods, like the addition of vitamin D to milk, is also part of an ongoing policy intended to make vitamins available to the population. In addition, many commercially prepared infant foods contain multiple added vitamins. Thus while primary vitamin deficiency should become truly unlikely, vitamin toxicity by excessive intake is being observed with increasing frequency.

When vitamin requirements are estimated, special consideration must be given to the composition of the diet. For example, a higher carbohydrate content demands a higher intake of thiamine; with an increase in dietary protein, the requirements for vitamin B_6 increase and requirements for niacin and pantothenic acid are reduced; an increased intake of polyunsaturated fatty acids increases the requirements for vitamin E (58). The estimated daily requirements and the RDA for vitamins for infants are summarized in Table 1.

A relatively recent development is the response of some inborn errors of metabolism and several aminoacidopathies to treatment with large doses of the vitamin which is involved in the specific metabolic process in question (59). On the other hand, the generally spreading tendency toward indiscriminate and excessive vitamin intake should be condemned.

FAT-SOLUBLE VITAMINS

Vitamin A (Retinol)

Vitamin A is a fat-soluble alcohol found in most animal fats and especially in fish liver oils. In colored vegetables, beta-carotene is the main precursor of vitamin A, and is converted to the active vitamin in the intestinal mucosa (60, 61). The main functions of vitamin A are to participate (1) in the formation of visual pigments in the retina; (2) in the maintenance of the integrity of epithelial structures; and (3) for normal growth of bones and teeth (62).

Vitamin A deficiency is a major nutritional problem and a frequent cause of blindness in many developing countries, especially in southeast Asia. Overt clinical deficiency is very uncommon in developed countries, except as a secondary alteration in intestinal malabsorption, steatorrhea, or "synthetic" feeding. However, subtle effects of mild vitamin A deficiency resulting in impaired visual adaptation to darkness may be encountered with low serum vitamin A levels in apparently healthy individuals in underprivileged communities in industrialized countries. In more advanced stages there is drying, thickening, and wrinkling of the bulbar conjuctiva (xerosis), followed by progressive involvement of the cornea which becomes vascularized and may ultimately liquefy and perforate (keratomalacia). Skin manifestations include follicular hyperkeratosis (63). The diagnosis of vitamin A deficiency can be made by special vision tests, by measurement of serum vitamin A or retinol levels, and by the response to therapy. A retinol serum level below 15 μg/100 ml is considered to reflect vitamin A deficiency. Treatment of clinical vitamin A deficiency should be aggressive—100,000 IU/kg/day orally for 5 days, followed by a 2-week oral course of 25,000 IU/day.

Long-term excessive intake of vitamin A will cause anorexia, irritability, weight loss, hair loss, skin rashes, anemia, jaundice, liver enlargement, hyperostosis, and central nervous system disturbances. Acute poisoning with a massive dose of vitamin A produces transient symptoms of acute intracranial hypertension (63). Discontinuation of vitamin A intake will be followed by the onset of clinical recovery within several days (64).

Vitamin D

Vitamin D is actually a hormone, not a vitamin. This hormone is released into the blood stream by irradiated skin and after a number of metabolic steps, as described later, it becomes active and exerts its action at a site other than where it was produced. Calciferol is thus one of the calcifying hormones which are necessary for calcium homeostasis. Together with parathyroid hormone and calcitonin, as well as other essential minerals, it maintains calcium homeostasis and appropriate bone calcification. Vitamin D plays a major role in the maintenance of extracellular fluid, calcium and phosphorus concentrations, the mineralization of bone, and the maintenance of skeletal integrity (65, 66, 67). The vitamin increases active calcium and phosphorus transport in the duodenum and proximal intestine. Rachitic animals and humans have increased fecal losses of calcium which are reversed by the administration of vitamin D. Furthermore, there is evidence that vitamin D or its metabolites have direct effects upon muscle metabolism and bone cells and upon the mobilization of calcium (65). Finally, the vitamin has pronounced effects upon the maintenance of adequate growth in experimental animals and in man (65, 66).

Man requires exogenous vitamin D only when climatic or sociocultural factors interfere with the exposure to the sun's ultraviolet rays. The natural precursor of endogenous vitamin D, 7-dehydrocholesterol, is stored in the skin (Fig. 2). Ultraviolet light in the spectrum range of 2300-3100Å convert 7-dehydrocholesterol to cholecalciferol. This is a rate-limiting step as vitamin D toxicity cannot ensue as a result of excessive ultraviolet radiation, although vitamin D levels in blood may be higher than those found in patients who are not exposed to excessive sunlight. Cholecalciferol also is derived from the intake of vitamin D in the diet. This source, however, is not a rate-limiting one and there may be vitamin D toxicity occurring when increased quantities of this compound are given. Cholecalciferol is hydroxylated at the 25-position by the liver and the hepatic product 25-hydroxycholecalciferol appears to be the metabolite of vitamin D which accounts for most of the circulating blood level. A further hydroxylation by the kidney to form 1,25-dihydroxycholecalciferol is necessary before vitamin D is transformed into the active compound.

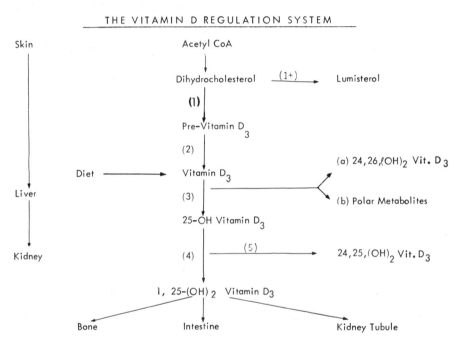

THE VITAMIN D REGULATION SYSTEM

FIGURE 2   Vitamin D requires metabolic activation to exert its action. Sunlight (1) activates 7-dihydrocholesterol and excess sunlight (1[+]) forms other components which are not active, thus avoiding possibility of vitamin D toxicity. However, the skin temperature (2) is the factor responsible for conversion to vitamin D3. This is bound by vitamin D binding protein (3) and transported in the blood into the liver. There, under normal conditions, it is hydroxylated in the microsomes to 25-OH vitamin D3. Under conditions of high calcium (a) 24, 26 $(OH)_2$ vitamin D3 is formed and under the influence of drugs such as steroids or anticonvulsants (b) other polar metabolites which are not active are formed. In the kidney mitochondria, under conditions of low calcium and PO4 (4), 1, 25-$(OH)_2$ vitamin D3 is formed. This is the active compound which exerts action in the bone, intestine, and kidney tubule by enhancing calcium transport. In contrast, under conditions of normal or high Ca and PO4 levels (5) other compounds are formed which do not have the potency or effects of the active metabolite.

The vitamin D content of breast milk remains controversial, since there are difficulties in accurately assaying vitamin D metabolites in human milk. The 25-hydroxycholecalciferol of the lipid fraction of human milk is very low (10-20 IU/L). Whether this vitamin D sulfate, which is assayed in this fraction, is bioavailable, has not been elucidated. On the other hand, the exact amount of vitamin D metabolites in the aqueous fraction is not known at present, although it might be substantial. Alternatively, some factors in breast milk may render the vitamin D more bioavailable than the form present in cow's milk. It is reasonable to speculate that human milk is a complete food when both mother and baby are healthy and are exposed to sunlight irradiation. Recent studies demonstrated that bone calcium content as well as serum 25-hydroxycholecalciferol levels are altered in infants who receive unsupplemented breast milk (68), although other similar studies reported no significant differences (69). In the light of this conflicting data, supplementation of human milk with vitamin D is strongly recommended, since infants may be at an increased risk for rickets even in developed areas of the world where insufficient sunlight exposure could occur because of clothing and other climatic and cultural factors. Vitamin D is found in appreciable amounts in herring, mackerel, salmon, and notably in cod liver oil.

Vitamin D deficiency is customarily listed as a dietary deficiency disease resulting in rickets due to lack of vitamin D. In actual fact, rickets was the earliest air pollution disease, first described in England in the 1600s at the time of the introduction of sulfur coal. Its incidence spread through Europe with the industrial revolution, with the coal smoke and the increasing concentrations of poor people in narrow, sunless, airless, factories in big city slums (70). Now that the new measurements for determining vitamin D and its hydroxylated derivatives are available, the rachitic syndromes have been more precisely classified into two main types: those in which there is a deficiency of active vitamin D metabolite, and those where there is an altered vitamin D responsiveness, usually resulting from an abnormality of the target cell responsible for calcium and phosphate homeostasis (71). In type 1 rickets, lack of active vitamin D compound or lack of action of this compound causes impaired calcium absorption from the intestine, hypocalcemia, and an attempted compensation with secondary hyperparathyroidism which, however, may not be adequate to correct hypocalcemia. In the second group of patients, hypocalcemia and secondary hyperparathyroidism are not present and rickets is primarily a phosphate deficiency phenomenon. In rickets there is an inadequate mineralization of bone matrix and a disproportionate amount of the bone is composed of uncalcified osteoid. Rickets causes disorganization of the chrondro-osseous zone in the growing bones; hence the rachitic rib "rosary" at the costochondral junctions and the enlargement of the epiphyses. Other features of rickets include frontal bossing, bending, and distortion of weight-bearing bones, muscular hypotonia, retarded growth, and a tendency toward pulmonary infection. Laboratory findings show a low or normal serum calcium, low serum phosphorus levels, high alkaline phosphatase, and aminoaciduria. The bony deformities on x-ray are irregularity and widening at the metaphyses, "cupping" and fraying at the ends of the long bones, and loss of radiodensity.

The clinical entity of rickets is seen in growing children. In adults it is called osteomalcia. Today a deficiency in vitamin D is rare in prosperous countries which add this compound to fortify their food. However, numerous recent reports of nutritional rickets in the United States associated with breast-feeding and special dietary practices have occurred (72). Low-birth-weight infants are at particular risk of developing nutritional rickets (73). Calciferol deficiency also may result when intestinal malabsorption impedes the normal absorption of vitamin D from the diet, or by interfering with the enterohepatic circulation of vitamin D metabolites, resulting in great losses of minerals and calciferol.   Any alteration in the metabolic events needed for activation of vitamin D metabolites also may result in rickets, as seen in patients with liver disease or renal disease, or when anticonvulsant drugs are given over a long period (74).   Congenital alteration of vitamin D metabolism due to an inborn error of vitamin D metabolism may result in vitamin D dependency, as the final active compound of vitamin D cannot be manufactured.

Type 2 rickets caused by a target cell abnormality, which interferes with the action of vitamin D, has replaced the term of vitamin D-resistant rickets, applied in the past for some of these patients.   In many instances, evidence of rickets remains despite the presence of vitamin D toxicity, since the primary alteration of the target cell cannot be corrected by vitamin D treatment.   Such alterations also result when there is a calcium and/or phosphate deficiency, either because of low intake, as in premature infants or breast milk feedings or fad diets.   It also may occur in total parenteral nutrition or when there is ingestion of large quantities of phytate in the diet as well as drugs such as aluminum hydroxide.   Disorders of renal tubular reabsorption may also result in type 2 rickets, i. e. , Fanconi syndrome, renal tubular acidosis, and a most prominent example, familial hypophosphatemic rickets.

Routine daily supplementation with vitamin D 400 IU will prevent rickets in normal infants.   Rapidly growing premature infants, convalescent babies, and patients receiving anticonvulsant drugs require approximately 1000 IU/day.   For the treatment of active rickets, 2500-10,000 IU of water-miscible vitamin D is given daily for 1 month, together with adequate supplies of calcium and phosphorus.   Alternatively or when necessary, as in the event of hypocalcemic convulsions, or when there is no assurance that the recommendations for proper vitamin D administration will be followed, a dose of vitamin D, 600,000 IU in oil can be given by oral or intramuscular injection.   If no response to this form of therapy is obtained, type 2 rickets and/or other abnormalities should be sought.

Intake of vitamin D above 2000-4000 IU/day will produce toxicity, eventually manifested by hypercalcemia, with lethargy, nausea, polyuria, diarrhea, and weight loss.   Protracted intoxication may result in irreversible brain damage, nephrocalcinosis, renal failure, and calcifications in soft tissues (75).

Vitamin E (alpha-Tocopherol)

Vitamin E is now recognized to be an essential nutrient (76).   It is present in adequate amounts in breast milk, fish, poultry, plants, and is particularly high in most currently consumed cereals, grain, and vegetable oils.   The main function of vitamin E lies in its properties as an antioxidant, being capable of specifically inhibiting the oxidation of unsaturated fatty acids.   Protection thereby is afforded to cell membranes from oxidation by lipid-free radicals.   Vitamin E may be important in the prevention of retrolental fibroplasia and bronchopulmonary dysplasia in the neonate (77); as a regulator of prostaglandin synthesis and breakdown, this vitamin plays a role in the inhibition of platelet hyperaggregation (78). Vitamin E deficiency can occur in fat malabsorption states, such as cystic fibrosis, cholestatic syndromes, biliary atresia, or celiac disease.   In small premature infants, vitamin E deficiency may result from low stores, diminished absorption, and increased demands due to rapid growth.   The requirements of vitamin E are increased by the intake of polyunsaturated fatty acids and oxidant substances, such as iron.   Indeed, infant formulas containing polyunsaturated fatty acids and fortified with iron can elicit vitamin E deficiency in young premature babies.

The clinical picture of vitamin E deficiency in the premature infant consists of anemia, reticulocytosis, thrombocytosis, and edema.   In children with cystic fibrosis, the hemolysis and edema associated with low levels of vitamin E may be the presenting feature of the disease. Vitamin E deficiency also is associated with creatinuria, ceroid deposition in smooth muscle, and multifocal degeneration in striated muscle.

The diagnosis of vitamin E deficiency can be made indirectly by demonstrating increased in vitro hemolysis of erythrocytes upon exposure to dilute solutions of hydrogen peroxide. Plasma levels of alpha-tocopherol can be measured; the normal range is 0.5-1.3 mg/ml and the ratio of alpha-tocopherol to polyunsaturated fatty acids in the plasma should be above 0.5.

The treatment of vitamin E deficiency consists of supplementation of this vitamin in its water-miscible form (77). Premature infants require the daily administration of 15 mg, and children with cystic fibrosis need 1 mg/kg/day, for the prevention of vitamin E deficiency. In overt deficiency in premature infants the clinical and laboratory abnormalities will revert to normal with four doses of water-miscible vitamin E, 125 mg/kg, given intramuscularly over 1 week. Although the evidence of toxicity is scant, excess vitamin E intake can be harmful by interfering with vitamin K metabolism and thus causing a predisposition to bleeding (78). In addition, excessive vitamin E in man has resulted in gastrointestinal disturbances and creatinuria (79).

Vitamin K

Vitamin K is a napthoquinone that is necessary for the gamma-carboxylation of prothrombin and Factor X, enabling them to bind calcium and to be activated. The chief dietary source of vitamin K is green leafy vegetables (vitamin K_1); an endogenous source is the synthesis of vitamin K (K_2) by intestinal bacteria.

Deficiency of vitamin K will result in a lowering of clotting Factors II, VII, and X, the main finding being a prolonged prothrombin time and partial thromboplastin time. Clinically, there may be bleeding. The newborn baby is in a state of relative vitamin K deficiency. Routine administration of vitamin K is effective for the prevention of "hemorrhagic disease of the newborn." Beyond the neonatal period, vitamin K deficiency can occur in infants with fat malabsorption, as well as in the exclusively breast-fed infant and in those with prolonged total intravenous alimentation. In addition, it may occur in patients in whom prolonged administration of broad-spectrum antibiotics may have suppressed intestinal bacteria (80). In these patients prophylactic supplementation with vitamin K is indicated. In the event of bleeding due to vitamin K deficiency, the intravenous injection of 1-5 mg of vitamin K_1 is indicated. The administration of large doses of vitamin K has resulted in anemia, polycythemia, splenomegaly, renal and hepatic damage, and death (81). It also has been implicated in producing hemolytic anemia, hyperbilirubinemia, and kernicterus in premature infants and in glucose-6-phosphate dehydrogenase deficient patients. In patients with liver disease it may further depress liver function.

WATER-SOLUBLE VITAMINS

Vitamin C (Ascorbic Acid)

Ascorbic acid is an essential nutrient in man. Its main source is from citrus fruits and green vegetables. Breast milk is rich in vitamin C; in contrast, the vitamin C content of unsupplemented cow's milk and strained foods is inadequate. In the strict sense of the word, vitamin C may be said to possess few pharmacological actions. Administration of the compound in amounts greatly in excess of physiological requirements causes few demonstrable effects, except in the patients with scurvy, whose symptoms are rapidly alleviated. However, an extensive literature has accumulated concerning the effect of vitamin C on practically every function of the body. Ascorbic acid affects a number of biochemical reactions mostly involving oxidation. It is also a potent reducing agent and plays an important role in the normal development of fibroblasts, osteoblasts, and osteoclasts. It is active in the conversion of hydroxyproline to proline for collagen synthesis, the formation of hydroxylysine and hydroxytryptophan, and the reduction of folic acid to tetrahydrofolic acid. Vitamin C also participates in the metabolism of tyrosine, and in neonates with a high protein intake, high levels of plasma tyrosine are observed, unless the infant receives vitamin C supplementation. The high content of vitamin C in the adrenal glands may indicate that it also is involved in the formation of adrenal steroids (82).

The manifestation of ascorbic acid deficiency is scurvy (83). Requirements for vitamin C are increased by febrile illness, diarrhea, cold exposure, and iron deficiency; a relative deficiency may then become frank deficiency, giving way to overt disease. The age of occurrence of nutritional scurvy is mainly during the second half of the first year of life. Beyond this age, the main cause of scurvy will be associated with severe feeding problems, as in mental retardation, or with infant neglect. The clinical features of scurvy reflect the biological roles of vitamin C. The onset is usually gradual, with irritability, pallor, diarrhea, and anorexia. Subsequently, there may be spiking fever and the baby will cry whenever handled. Pain and tenderness along the long bones causes "pseudoparalysis" of the limbs, the baby assuming the classic "pithed frog" position. Hemorrhages are common, at the sites of teeth eruption, around hair follicles, into the skin and mucous membranes, and under the periosteum of long bones, probably as a result of disturbed collagen metabolism. In addition, there may be hematuria, melena, and orbital and subdural hemorrhages. A concomitant impaired utilization of iron and folic acid will contribute to the development of severe anemia. Deranged formation of bony matrix leads to epiphyseal fractures and to subluxations, such as the "scorbutic bead" caused by subluxation of the sternal plate at the costochondral junctions. Roentgenograms show the typical appearance of long bones, particularly in the area of the knees. There is a ground-glass appearance of the bone, extreme thinning of the cortex with a "white line" of well-calcified cartilage of the metaphyseal edge (Frankel line), the scorbutic spur reflecting periosteal elevation and detachment (usually by subperiosteal bleeding), and during recovery there is calcification of the elevated periosteum.

Laboratory findings for the diagnosis of scurvy include the absence of vitamin C in the serum and a much-reduced urinary excretion of vitamin C following an intravenous loading dose. A plasma level of 0.6 mg/100 ml rules out vitamin C deficiency.

Scurvy is prevented in the breast-fed infant when the mother takes a daily dose of 150 mg vitamin C. In the artificially fed infant, deficiency will be prevented by a daily intake of 25-50 mg in the diet. Vitamin C is used for treatment of ascorbic acid deficiency, especially "frank" scurvy, which occurs rather infrequently in infants and adults. Treatment by oral or parenteral administration of vitamin C, 100-200 mg or more, will rapidly induce healing. The reducing properties of vitamin C also have been employed to control idiopathic methemoglobinemia, although it is less effective than methylene blue. In addition to this specific use of vitamin C, extensive literature has appeared on the application of this vitamin to a wide variety of diseases. Many such claims are associated with megadose practices, which are stated to prevent or cure viral respiratory infections (84), and to be beneficial in cancer (85, 86) and other diseases (87). However, other studies have not confirmed these claims (87, 88); therefore any benefit that might be derived from such use of ascorbic acid seems small when weighed against the expense and the risks of megadose treatment. The latter include formation of kidney stones, resulting from excessive excretion of oxalate, and rebound scurvy. This phenomenon occurs when subjects who are consuming large amounts of vitamin C suddenly stop; a precipitous reduction in ascorbic acid concentration in plasma follows (89). Rebound scurvy also has been found in the offspring of mothers taking high doses of vitamin C (89, 90). This rebound phenomenon presumably is due to induction pathways of ascorbic acid metabolism as a result of the preceding high dosages, which render the organism vitamin C dependent. Excessive doses of ascorbic acid also can enhance the absorption of iron and interfere with anticoagulant therapy (91, 92).

The Vitamin B Complex

The members of this heterogeneous group of compounds are essential constituents of diverse enzyme systems. They are present in adequate amounts in most of the foods that normally constitute the infant diet. Foods which are deficient in any one factor of the vitamin B complex are often deficient also in other B vitamins. Therefore, there will frequently be considerable overlap in the clinical picture caused by the various vitamin B deficiencies, particularly thiamine, riboflavin, and niacin.

Vitamin B_1 (Thiamine)

Thiamine is a pyrimidine-thiazole compound widely distributed in animal and vegetable foods. Thiamine, as pyrophosphate, is a key participant in the metabolism of carbohydrates and also plays a role in the decarboxylation of pyruvic acid and ketoglutaric acid as they enter the Krebs cycle (93).

Thiamine deficiency is rare in regions where the diet is varied owing to its ubiquity in foods. However, a deficiency can arise due to destruction or extraction of the vitamin in food processing, in dietary faddists, in children with chronic gastrointestinal disease, and in chronic alcoholism. It also may result from consumption of large amounts of raw fish containing thiaminase or large quantities of tea which contain a thiamine antagonist. Beriberi, the disease caused by thiamine deficiency, has a gradual onset beginning with anorexia, apathy, failure to thrive, and progressing to peripheral neurological disturbances, cardiac failure, and edema. Thiamine deficiency has been shown to induce myelin degeneration in the central nervous system and in peripheral nerves, and also degenerative changes in the heart muscle. There may be Wernicke encephalopathy, Korsakoff syndrome, and alcoholic polyneuropathy, depending on the amount of thiamine deprivation. Laboratory tests which will aid in the diagnosis of thiamine deficiency include the demonstration of a low 24-hour urinary excretion of thiamine, an elevated blood pyruvate level, and deviant results in the erythrocyte transketolase stimulation test. Treatment consists of the administration of thiamine hydrochloride, 20-50 mg orally or parenterally, in divided doses for 2 weeks, followed by 10 mg/day orally.

Large doses of thiamine may also be helpful in the treatment of subacute necrotizing encephalomyelopathy, inducing temporary improvement (94). Other inborn errors of metabolism that are sensitive to the administration of thiamine have also been described (95).

Vitamin B_2 (Riboflavin)

Riboflavin is a component of many respiratory enzymes and is essential in the energy metabolism of all body cells. Various foods, such as milk, eggs, leafy vegetables, and whole grain have a high riboflavin content.

Riboflavin deficiency may result from inadequate dietary intake and chronic digestive disease. The characteristic symptoms include cheilosis, angular stomatitis, spreading seborrheic dermatitis, conjunctivitis, weight loss, weakness, and photophobia. Severe manifestations are edema, anemia, corneal vascularization, and cataract formation. The urinary 24-hour excretion of riboflavin is a fairly accurate index of riboflavin nutritional status.

The only established therapeutic application of riboflavin is to treat or prevent disease caused by deficiency.   Ariboflavinosis seldom occurs in the United States as a discrete deficiency, but usually accompanies other nutritional diseases, particularly pellagra.   Therefore, therapy of ariboflavinosis should include other members of the B complex in addition to riboflavin. Specific therapy with riboflavin usually consists of the oral administration of 5-10 mg/daily.

Niacin (Nicotinic Acid)

Niacin is a component of coenzyme I and coenzyme II, which, among others, participate in glycolysis, protein, amino acid and lipid metabolism, pentose biosynthesis, and in the formation of high-energy phosphate bonds. Dietary tryptophan can be converted into niacin and niacin deficiency can result from low niacin and tryptophan intake, as in the case of indigent maize-consuming peoples.

Niacin deficiency also is observed in chronic alcoholism, chronic gastrointestinal disease, malignant carcinoid tumors, diabetes mellitus, and in liver cirrhosis. Pellagra also occurs in Hartnup disease in which there is a defect in the absorption of tryptophan (96), and in patients with carcinoid tumor. The disease resulting from niacin deficiency is pellagra, which is classically characterized by four "ds": dermatitis, diarrhea, dementia, and death. Early or mild symptoms include soreness of the skin and tongue, burning and itching on the back of the hands, and subsequently symmetric dermatitis appearing on the backs of the hands, wrists, forearms, and neck, worsened by exposure to sunlight, heat, or mild trauma. The skin lesions progress to cracks and fissures with hemorrhagic crust formation and secondary infection. The buccal mocosa, the tongue, the rectum, and the anus become severely inflamed and stubborn diarrhea sets in. Neurological involvement causes weakness, psychiatric disturbances, peripheral nerve lesions, and pyramidal signs.   The outcome of pellagra can be fatal.

A laboratory aid in the diagnosis is the urinary excretion of N-methyl-nicotinamide and 2-pyridone, expressed in terms of creatinine excretion and their ratio. Nicotinic acid, nicotinamide, and their derivatives are used for prophylaxis and treatment of pellagra. In the acute stages of the disease, therapy must be intensive. The recommended oral dose is 50 mg, given up to ten times daily. If oral medication is impossible, intravenous injection of 25 mg is given two or more times daily. Pellagra is now quite uncommon in the United States, probably as a direct result of supplementation of food with nicotinic acid since 1939. When observed, it is usually secondary to chronic gastrointestinal disease or to alcoholism, and in these cases multiple nutritional deficiencies often exist. Large doses of niacin are recommended, especially when there is psychosis associated with encephalopathy.

Vitamin B$_6$ (Pyridoxine, Pyridoxal, and Pyridoxamine)

Vitamin B$_6$, particularly as pyridoxal-5-phosphate, serves as a coenzyme in well over 60 different enzyme systems, mainly associated with protein and amino acid metabolism, but also with metabolism of carbohydrates and fats. Vitamin B$_6$ is widely distributed among foods, but deficiency may arise because of its ease of depletion, marked losses by food processing, antagonism by certain drugs and hormones (e.g. isoniazid, hydralazine, oral contraceptives), participation in numerous metabolic functions, and its association with brain metabolism and development.   A high protein intake will increase the requirements of vitamin B$_6$.

Deficiency of vitamin B$_6$ can occur in malabsorption syndromes, or when the intake is low either by nutritional deprivation or by destruction of the vitamin by food processing.   The clinical picture consists of cheilosis, dermatitis, glossitis, peripheral neuritis, anemia, and convulsions.   The differential diagnosis of convulsive disorder in infants must include the possibility of vitamin B$_6$ deficiency, which causes a decrease of gamma-aminobutyric acid in the brain, thereby lowering the threshold of central nervous system irritability. Vitamin B_6-responsive convulsions may occur in infants in whom an inborn error of metabolism causes a 100- to 500-fold increase in vitamin B_6 requirement. This condition has been termed "vitamin B6 dependency" as opposed to true deficiency. In vitamin B6 deficiency there is an impairment of hemoglobin synthesis which results in a hypochromic, microcytic anemia with normal levels of serum iron (97).

A satisfactory laboratory test for assessing the vitamin B6 status is the tryptophan loading test and measurement of abnormal urinary excretion of tryptophan metabolites. In vitamin B_6 deficiency there will be an excretion of xanthurenic acid greater than 25 mg in 6 hours, following a dose of 50 mg/kg tryptophan. Treatment of vitamin B6 deficiency with pyridoxine 10-50 mg/day will induce recovery from all the symptoms. The convulsions and the severe electroencephalographic disturbances will disappear almost immediately upon an intravenous 10 mg dose of pyridoxine. For vitamin B_6 "dependency," a daily dose of over 300 mg pyridoxine may be required. For patients who take drugs which antagonize vitamine B_6, a supplementation with 10-25 mg/day of the vitamin is suggested.

Folic Acid (Folacin)

The physiologically active derivative of folic acid is folinic acid, or citrovorum factor. The requirement of folic acid is in part supplied by intestinal bacteria, and meats and leafy green vegetables are rich dietary sources of this vitamin. The most important role of folacin is its participation in the synthesis of the purine and pyrimidine compounds used for the formation of nucleoproteins. Every cell, in every tissue, needs a proper supply of folacin, particularly where cell turnover is high. Therefore, folacin requirements will be greatly increased in pregnancy, hemolytic disorders, inflammatory conditions of the gastrointestinal tract, in rapidly growing premature infants and in convalescent patients. Oral contraceptives can increase the requirements, and anticonvulsant drugs may interfere with the intestinal absorption of folacin. Vitamin C deficiency impairs the conversion of folic acid into tetrahydrofolic acid, which is the precursor of the active compound, folinic acid. Folacin deficiency is frequently observed in malabsorption syndromes, notably in celiac disease (98). Folacin deficiency causes an impairment in cellular multiplication and growth. Antenatal folacin deficiency, as in Rh-hemolytic disease, may result in the birth of a small-for-date infant, who will show a slower growth pattern during the first year of life unless timely supplementation of folacin is given (99). Diminished cell turnover becomes manifest as bone marrow insufficiency, ranging from megaloblastic anemia to pancytopenia, and atrophy of the intestinal epithelium which results in digestive and absorbtive disturbances (100). Folacin deficiency can be demonstrated by finding a serum folate level less than 3 ng/ml, or a red cell folate concentration of less than 140 ng/ml. For the management of folacin deficiency the suggested threatment is supplementation with folic acid 1-5 mg/day, although smaller doses may also be effective.

Vitamin B_{12} (Cyanocobalamin)

Vitamin B_{12} is essential for the normal functioning of all cells. It serves as a coenzyme in multiple enzyme systems and its metabolism is in many ways interrelated with folacin metabolism (101). Vitamin B_{12} is found almost exclusively in animal products (meat, milk, eggs, cheese), and true dietary deficiency of vitamin B_{12} is rare, although it may occur in vegans who subsist exclusively on vegetables (102). Specific malabsorption of vitamin B12 has been described in several familial congenital conditions. The main manifestations of vitamin B_{12} deficiency include a megaloblastic anemia, peripheral neuropathy, and subacute combined degeneration of the spinal cord. Other features are glossitis, diarrhea, and jaundice.

While the megaloblastic anemia responds to administration of folic acid, such treatment may worsen the neurological disturbances caused by vitamin B_{12} deficiency. For the treatment of vitamin B_{12} deficiency, the administration of 15-25 mg/day of the vitamin will result in complete recovery. In conditions where there is vitamin B_{12} malabsorption a periodic loading dose of the vitamin must be given parenterally.

Pantothenic Acid

Pantothenic acid is a component of coenzyme A and thus participates in numerous enzymatic reactions. It is widely distributed in foods and a clearly defined deficiency of the vitamin has not been described in the human. Nevertheless, in the severely malnourished patient, a deficiency of pantothenic acid may be an unrecognized part of the total clinical picture (103).

Biotin

Biotin is an essential nutrient which serves as a cofactor in numerous enzyme functions; however, a deficiency state has been reported only very rarely. Children suffering from extensive seborrheic dermatitis have been found to have a reduced urinary excretion of biotin, and the parenteral administration of biotin has been recently reported to induce dramatic improvement in such children (104).

MINERALS

Minerals, both "major" and "trace" elements, are well established as having definite nutritional importance in humans and are essential for life. Minerals play an essential role in the maintenance or body homeostasis and the constancy of the cellular milieu. A growing number of minerals is found to be linked with enzyme structure and function, and to play a part in the synthesis of proteins and nucleic acids. They also participate in the organization of mitochondrial function, membrane transport, nerve conduction, and muscle contraction, as well as in many other vital functions (105).

The nutritional requirement for minerals is relatively low, but their availability in many diets is correspondingly small. Growth alone may enhance mineral requirements. This process increases the requirements of these elements and an insufficient positive balance may result in mineral deficiencies which would not occur in nongrowing organisms (106). When allowances for minerals are recommended (see Table 1), an important factor to consider is that their absorption is influenced by their chemical form, by the amount and the nature of other nutrients in the diet, and by the presence or absence of substances which interfere with absorption. For example, iron in human milk is absorbed to a much greater extent than iron in cow's milk (107); or, dietary iron absorption is enhanced by ascorbic acid and reduced by a high protein content (91). Indeed, a recent publication reviews the many interactions among minerals and other dietary foodstuffs that may modify the absorption of specific elements (108).

Thus, the normal daily requirements may not be met under a variety of conditions. For example, the typical American breakfast, consisting as it does of a high proportion of milk, sugar, and refined cereal, may well provide insufficient quantities of absorbable manganese and zinc. To make matters worse, this type of breakfast may actually reduce absorption of such trace minerals owing to the presence of either metal-binding compounds or excessive concentrations of less essential minerals that display competitive kinetics with respect to the trace metal transport sites in the intestinal mucosa. In contrast, these same foods would appropriately meet the normal daily requirements, if they were given alone.   In addition, potential problems arising from deficiencies of these minerals may result from the increased use of elemental diets or total parenteral nutrition (TPN). Further research will be necessary before any such deficiences can be detected and prevented and their role in the growth and well being of children evaluated.

MINERAL DEFICIENCIES

Mineral deficiencies in children may result from two basic mechanisms: (1) increased losses which lead to a negative mineral balance, and (2) an insufficient positive mineral balance in which available minerals do not meet the requirements of a growing organism, but are not associated with abnormal losses of endogenous mineral.   Both mechanisms have a different physiological significance.   The losses of endogenous minerals may affect cellular function in a different form from that seen during a state of insufficient positive balance where cellular function may be able to proceed without loss of the mineral already present.   Moreover, the manifestations of mineral deficiencies in a growing organism may be more severe and may have little in common with the clinical picture seen in an adult (106).

The causes of mineral deficiencies are listed in Table 2.   This classification includes a variety of diseases that may not share much in common except for "mineral deficiencies."   Often, the only evidence of disease may be poor growth. For example, in familial hypophosphatemia, the failure to grow might be the most prominent sign of the disease (109).   Similarly, poor growth may precede, for years, the development of any other sign or symptom that indicates the type of disease, e. g. , chronic inflammatory bowel disease (110).   Mineral deficiencies also could be the consequence of iatrogenic manipulations such as steroids or other drugs (111, 112), or the result of specific inborn errors of metabolism, which could affect the absorption or excretion of specific minerals (113, 114). There may be different pathogenic processes leading to mineral deficiencies in each or any-one of these groups of patients; similarly, there may be one or several minerals involved.

Specific deficiency syndromes in children for Ca, P, Mg, Na, K, iron, zinc, copper, fluoride, and chromium have been identified. It is quite likely that deficiencies of other trace elements necessary for normal growth will be recognized in the future.   Trace elements of established importance which have not yet made an impact on clinical problems include manganese, cobalt, molybdenum, selenium, nickel, vanadium, tin, cadmium, silicon, lead, and even arsenic. In some instances considerable information is already available on the biochemistry, the physiological role, and the effects of these elemental deficiencies in animals (Table 3).

TABLE 2   Causes of Mineral Deficiency States

---

1.   Increased losses with negative mineral balance –
     Primary disorders of mineral metabolism:
        Isolated defects: Familial hypophosphatemia, hypomagnesemia, etc.
     Secondary disorders of mineral metabolism:
        Gastrointestinal (e.g. , diarrhea, CIBD), renal, diabetes mellitus, drugs, etc.

2.   Insufficient positive mineral balance –
     Increased requirements during growth
     Decreased intake: fad diets, primary malnutrition, failure to thrive, anorexia
                    nervosa
     Decreased absorption:
        Intestinal malabsorption, phytate in diet, etc.

TABLE 3   Classification and Actions of Essential Trace Elements

| Element | Function | Deficiency signs | | Occurrence of imbalances in humans |
		Animals	Humans	
Fluorine	Structure of teeth, possibly of bones; possibly growth effect	Caries; possibly growth depression	Increased incidence of caries; possibly risk factor for osteoporosis	Deficiency and excess known
Silicon	Calcification; possibly function in connective tissue	Growth depression; bone deformities	Not known	Not known
Vanadium	Not known	Growth depression, change of lipid metabolism, impairment of reproduction	Not known	Not known
Chromium	Potentiation of insulin	Relative insulin resistance	Relative insulin resistance, impaired glucose tolerance, elevated serum lipids	Deficiency known in malnutrition, aging, total parenteral alimentation
Manganese	Mucopolysaccharides metabolism, superoxide dismutase	Growth depression, bone deformities, β-cell degeneration	Not known	Deficiency not known; toxicity by inhalation
Iron	Oxygen, electron transport	Anemia, growth retardation	Anemia	Deficiencies widespread; excesses dangerous in hemochromatosis; acute poisoning
Cobalt	As part of vitamin B_{12}	Anemia; growth retardation in ruminant species	Only as vitamin B_{12} deficiency	Inability to absorb vitamin B_{12}; low B_{12} intake from vegetarian diets

Element	Function	Deficiency signs in animals	Deficiency signs in humans	Occurrence in humans
Nickel	Interaction with iron absorption	Growth depression, anemia, ultrastructural changes in liver; impaired reproduction	Not known	Not known
Copper	Oxidative enzymes; interaction with iron; cross-linking of elastin	Anemia, rupture of large vessels, disturbances of ossification	Anemia, changes of ossification; possibly elevated serum cholesterol	Deficiencies in malnutrition, total parenteral alimentation
Zinc	Numerous enzymes involved in energy metabolism and in transcription and translation	Failure to eat, severe growth depression, skin lesions, sexual immaturity	Growth depression, sexual immaturity, skin lesions, depression of immunocompetence, change of taste acuity	Deficiencies in Iran, Egypt, in total parenteral nutrition, genetic diseases, traumatic stress
Arsenic	Not known	Impairment of growth, reproduction; sudden heart death in third generation lactating goats	Not known	Not known
Selenium	Glutathione peroxidase; interaction with heavy metals	Different, depending on species; muscle degeneration (ruminants), pancreas atrophy (chicken)	Endemic cardiomyopathy (Keshan disease) conditioned by selenium deficiency	Deficiency and excess in areas of China; one case resulting from total parenteral alimentation
Molybdenum	Xanthine, aldehyde, sulfide oxidases	Difficult to produce; growth depression	Not known	Excessive exposure in parts of Soviet Union associated with goutlike syndrome
Iodine	Constituent of thyroid hormones	Goiter, depression of thyroid function	Goiter, depression of thyroid function, cretinism	Deficiencies widespread; excessive intakes may lead to thyrotoxicosis

(From: Mertz, W: The essential trace elements. Science 213:1332, 1981. Copyright 1981 by the American Association for the Advancement of Science. Reprinted with permission.)

For example, manganese has an essential role in mucopolysaccharide synthesis and its deficiency in young birds causes, among other effects, a variety of skeletal abnormalities with stunted growth (115). There is data on the effects of selenium deficiency in animals (116). Though only suggestions of possible deficiencies in malnourished infants exist (117), in the case of other minerals, data are even more limited at this time, although all these elements appear to be necessary for normal growth.

A frequent problem is confusion in the diagnosis of mineral deficiencies. Only a few minerals have definitive markers to make the diagnosis in clinical medicine, such as iron deficiency. Most other minerals are intracellular ions which are not readily accessible for measurement by clinical means. In addition, the criteria for diagnosis is not well established. Thus when we talk about a deficiency state, it may be confused with the term applied to a low serum level. For example, potassium deficiency may be present even when there are normal serum potassium levels and vice versa. A high serum potassium level may not represent an increased bodily content of this ion. Similarly, a decreased ion level in hair cannot be taken as prima facie evidence of deficiency, particularly since this measurement is so unreliable in the majority of instances. Mineral deficiencies can only be established with certainty when the total body content of the mineral is diminished. Since this measurement is not practical for clinical purposes, the clinician must establish the diagnosis by a variety of measurements, all of which are indirect. Therefore, only a series of measurements may ensure an appropriate diagnosis. For example, several tissues may have to be analyzed including RBCs, hair, and muscle. Bone biopsies also are not accessible under ordinary clinical circumstances. The urinary excretion of these minerals almost always will be diminished if a body deficiency exists, since the organisms will attempt to conserve these ions unless the primary defect involves excessive urinary losses. Finally, the serum levels, which are easily obtained, have to be interpreted with caution since they may be high, normal, or low without necessarily indicating a deficiency or normalcy of those elements. For example, magnesium deficiency may occur with or without hypomagnesemia (118), and the same may be said of all other ions. Therefore, it is important to document both a negative balance which would explain the suspected deficit and the possible cause, as well as a positive balance once the mineral is given, in other words, a therapeutic diagnostic trial (106, 118).

SODIUM

It is worth mentioning that the amount of salt in the diet of infants has aroused concern. Present intakes of salt provide more sodium than is required by the infant and a relationship has been suggested between increased salt intake early in life and the future development of essential hypertension (119). Such an association has been demonstrated in rats, especially in a genetically hypertension prone strain (120). There is no conclusive evidence that this holds true in the human; however, excess salt intake is considered to be one possible contributory factor to hypertension. In the opinion of the Committee on Nutrition of the American Academy of Pediatrics (121), there is no reason to restrict the intake of salt in the general infant population, but reduced salt consumption may be advisable for infants with a strong family history of essential hypertension. Diets of cow's milk and proprietary solid foods which generally have added salt, have been estimated to provide 2 g or more of sodium chloride daily to the 5-month-old infant—a definitely excessive intake.

CALCIUM

Calcium is important in the formation of bones and teeth, in blood coagulation, in the maintenance of proper muscle and nerve function, and it is also an activator of multiple enzymes. Calcium also participates in the maintenance of the acid-base balance of body fluids. A deficiency of calcium may arise in the rapidly growing premature baby who is usually born with a low calcium endowment. Lack of vitamin D and parathyroid insufficiency result in defective calcium transport in the intestine; malabsorptive conditions, such as celiac disease, impair the intestinal absorption of calcium. An adequate intake of dairy products along with the required vitamin D—by exposure to ultraviolet radiation or by supplementation—will prevent a nutritional calcium deficiency (122).

MAGNESIUM

Magnesium is a constituent of several enzymes and also catalyzes diverse enzymatic reactions. The metabolism of magnesium is interrelated with the metabolism of calcium and phosphorus, and the serum level of magnesium is partly influenced by parathyroid hormone. Low levels of magnesium are found in protein-energy malnutrition, malabsorption syndromes, liver disease, hyperthyroidism, hyperaldosteronism, hyperphosphatemia, diabetes, and following intensive diuretic therapy. Hypomagnesemia in the neonate can be observed in infants of diabetic mothers and in babies born to mothers with hyperparathyroidism. In addition, a specific magnesium malabsorption has been described in male newborns (123).

Hypomagnesemia is frequently accompanied by a mild to moderate hypocalcemia that will not respond to the administration of calcium. The clinical features are those of neuromuscular hyperirritability and manifested by twitching, eye-rolling, and convulsions (123). Hypermagnesemia can happen in neonates of mothers who are treated with parenteral magnesium sulfate for preeclampsia (124). Neonatal toxicity will manifest as respiratory depression and muscular paralysis.

PHOSPHORUS

Most body phosphorus is found in the skeleton. The organic moiety of body phosphorus is an important component of nucleoproteins, phospholipids, and of the compounds related to cellular respiration and energy transformation. The requirements of phosphorus are increased in periods of rapid growth; however, with an adequate intake of dairy products dietary phosphorus deficiency is not likely to occur. Phosphate deficiency may occur in the premature baby fed human milk (125).

SULFUR

Sulfur is a constituent of all body proteins and it functions predominantly as an integral part of an organic molecule. The main provision of dietary sulfur must come from sulfur-containing amino acids. Specific sulfur deficiency has not been described, but it is most likely to play a role in the disturbances caused by general nutritional deprivation.

IRON

Iron is required as a constituent of hemoglobin, of myoglobin, and as part of, or a cofactor to, numerous enzyme systems, and plays a key role in oxygen transport and cellular respiration. Iron deficiency seems to be the most common specific nutritional deficiency, anywhere. Iron deficiency can be caused by inadequate intake, while contributory factors are low iron stores at birth, prematurity, rapid growth, protracted illness, and blood loss. The ultimate result of iron deficiency is classically a hypochromic, microcytic anemia, with a low level of serum iron and a low saturation of transferrin. On the other hand, even before the appearance of anemia, the depletion of iron stores can become clinically manifested as poor appetite, poor weight gain, lassitude, susceptibility to infection, and perhaps, behavior disturbances. Severe iron deficiency contributes to an impairment in the intestinal absorption of nutrients and is also a cause of bleeding into the gastrointestinal tract. All these abnormalities are reversed by appropriate therapy with iron (126). Iron deficiency stands out as a common finding and constitutes an important public health problem, which has led to the "fortification" of milk and many types of infant foods with added iron—often to contain more than ten times its concentration in human milk (127). The fortification of foods with iron is probably beneficial for the prevention of iron deficiency in the general infant population, but should be applied with caution in small premature infants, in whom vitamin E levels are low and the addition of iron may cause hemolysis (128).

IODINE

Iodine is needed for the synthesis of the thyroid hormones. Iodine deficiency can occur in regions where the iodine content in the soil and its produce is poor. The clinical picture consists of hyperplasia of the thyroid gland (goiter), and hypothyroidism. Because of almost universal use of iodized salt, iodine-deficiency goiter is now rare. An excess intake of iodine also will result in goiter, which may be observed in long-term users of iodine-containing drugs, such as cough medicines (129).

ZINC

Zinc is the metallic component in a variety of enzyme systems and is important for the mobilization of vitamin A from the liver. A high dietary content of phytate and fiber greatly inhibits the intestinal absorption of zinc, and thus may be instrumental in producing zinc depletion in populations where such a diet is consumed. There is a high correlation of zinc intake with protein intake; consequently, zinc deficiency is often seen concomitantly with protein deficiency (130). The clinical syndrome caused by zinc deficiency includes retarded growth, delayed sexual maturation, impaired taste acuity, delayed wound healing, a roughened skin with hyperpigmentation, anemia, and pica. The glucose tolerance curve may be abnormal. The full-blown picture of zinc depletion is frequently seen in Middle Eastern countries. In Western countries, nutritional surveys of children have disclosed zinc deficiency in patients with inadequate growth and altered taste acuity. Hypozincemia and zinc depletion also may be involved in the growth retardation of malnutrition, malabsorption syndromes, and inflammatory bowel disease (106, 110). Recently, it has been demonstrated that acrodermatitis enteropathica can be completely cured by supplementation with zinc. An inborn error of zinc absorption or zinc metabolism seems to be implicated (131). Congenital anomalies may be produced in the offspring of animals which have been rendered zinc deficient during pregnancy (132). Zinc also may play an important role in liver disease and myocardial infarction, as well as in acute stress of many causes. In addition, it may be of importance in wound healing and in sickle cell anemia.

COPPER

All mammalian cells contain copper, mainly as a constituent of tissue oxidases and respiratory pigments. Copper is so widely distributed in foods that severe deficiency is rarely seen. Hypocupremia can occur in severe malnutrition, and malabsorption, and in protracted parenteral or oral synthetic feeding. The clinical features of copper deficiency are relatively dramatic and acute (133). Early manifestations are neutropenia and anemia which does not respond to iron, since copper is involved in iron release from stores and in iron transport within the normoblast. Additional features are progressive osteoporosis, cupping and flaring of long bone metaphyses, periosteal reactions, and spontaneous fractures of ribs. The pathogenesis of the bone lesions is ascribed to the lack of copper which is required for the cross-linking of bone collagen. There is a decrease in the pigmentation of the skin and hair, dilatation of superficial veins, seborrheic dermatitis, anorexia, diarrhea, and hepatosplenomegaly. Neurological disturbances include hypotonia, apneic episodes, and possible psychomotor retardation. Copper deficiency with severe central nervous system involvement is seen in Menkes "kinky hair" syndrome (134), in which the profound copper deficiency results from an X-linked genetic defect in intestinal copper absorption. The recognition of nutritional copper deficiency has enabled the successful prevention of this condition in the population at risk. The administration of copper will correct the clinical and biochemical abnormalities of copper depletion. Copper deficiency has not been found in full-term or premature infants of more than 1500 g. However, in smaller infants, the small liver may also have reduced concentration of copper and thus they are unable to keep up with the demands for the mineral, particularly when given unmodified cow's milk formula, which is significantly lower in concentrations of copper than human milk. Copper deficiency also is found in patients with proximal renal tubular acidosis, as a result of alkali therapy that binds the mineral in the intestinal tract (135), and in a baby fed cow's milk (136).

CHROMIUM

The main physiological role of this element is as a cofactor for insulin at the insulin-responsive cell membrane. Chromium deficiency has been shown to be one of the factors responsible for the impairment in glucose tolerance associated with protein-energy malnutrition and also for growth retardation. Chromium supplementation in these cases of chromium deficiency will promote growth and the glucose intolerance will revert to normal (137, 138). Chromium deficiency is likely to occur in man because the Western diet contains only small quantities of this ion, and it becomes even less by food processing. This problem is magnified by the decreased absorption of chromium in the presence of a high carbohydrate intake. Chromium is an important factor in glucose tolerance and diabetes mellitus (137, 138).

MANGANESE

Manganese is the metallic component of a number of enzymes and is, among other minerals, involved in bone metabolism and in the urea cycle. Manganese deficiency has not been described in the human, but in the experimental animal it has been shown to impair growth and reproduction and to cause damage to the bony skeleton (115, 139). In mice carrying a mutant gene for spontaneous congenital ataxia, prenatal administration of manganese prevented the appearance of the ataxia, whereas manganese deficiency in normal pregnant mice could cause congenital ataxia in their offspring (140).

SELENIUM

Selenium has been found to be a component of the enzyme glutathione peroxidase and has a protective function against lipid peroxide-induced damage. In this way it appears that selenium is involved in vitamin E metabolism. In addition, supplementation with selenium has been found to promote growth in some children with protein-energy malnutrition. The mechanism involved is poorly understood (141). Selenium deficiency may be induced in animals and may have occurred in men with endemic cardiomyopathy (142), and in a 2-year-old girl (143). However, selenium in the sulfite form is frequently incorporated into shampoos and ointments and although of low toxicity it has been shown that high urinary excretion of this mineral is associated with its use, especially when open skin lesions are present. Symptoms included tremors and loss of appetite, as well as poor growth.

COBALT

The main known biological function of cobalt is as a component of vitamin B_{12}. Cobalt also has been shown to activate a number of enzymes, such as phosphotransferases. The administration of pharmacological amounts of cobalt will produce polycythemia, probably by stimulating the synthesis of erythropoietin or by inhibiting its breakdown. Excessive intake of cobalt may cause cardiomyopathy with heart failure and eventually a fatal outcome (144). Clinically, therapy with cobalt has been effectively used as a hematinic in some patients with uremia, but it may result in toxicity with production of goiter.

MOLYBDENUM

Molybdenum is a component of flavoprotein enzymes which participate in the uptake and release of iron from ferritin in the intestinal mucosa, and the release of iron from ferritin in the liver and in the bone marrow. Deficiency of molybdenum may thus adversely affect iron utilization (145).

FLUORIDE

The role of fluoride in dental caries in humans has been studied (146). The adjustment of this element to 1 ppm in drinking water appears to be optimal for the prevention of caries. Continual use of drinking water with 4-6 ppm of fluoride causes mottled and pitted teeth, and if higher concentrations exist there may be skeletal fluorosis. Administration and supplementation of fluoride has been recommended at times when the tooth is erupting or has recently erupted. Administration of supplemental fluoride at other times may not be of value or may be even detrimental, especially when given in conjunction with other trace minerals. The local administration of frequent doses of fluoride to the erupted teeth seems to be a good approach for the maximum effectiveness of this highly beneficial element to oral health.

BREAST-FEEDING

Human milk is the preferable and the best food for human consumption in the first year of life. Breast-feeding alone suffices for the nutritional needs of babies during the first few months of life. The need for other food supplements or formulas arises only when the mother's milk production diminishes or when it cannot suffice for the caloric needs of the child. This does not occur as frequently as thought (147). In developing countries and in areas where sanitation is unsatisfactory, breast-feeding plays an important role in reducing infant morbidity and, especially, infant mortality. A reduced morbidity and mortality of breast-fed infants also has been observed in industrialized countries (148). The association of breast-feeding with decreased incidence of disease and malnutrition in less-developed countries has become apparent (149). Indeed, decreased rates of breast-feeding and increased usage of commercial formulas have been blamed for many of the problems of malnutrition and diarrhea throughout the world (147-149), becoming more important than protein-energy deficits (150, 151). Whereas, when breast-feeding prevails, malnutrition is rare even in the most primitive conditions (152).

The demands and cultural trends that modern society impose on women and the convenience and availability of modified cow's milk formulas for infant feeding (153) have led to a marked decline, until recently, in the prevalence of breast-feeding, up to the extent of breast-feeding being regarded as a custom fitting only to "primitive" mothers. As a result, mothers—especially from underdeveloped areas and low socioeconomic status—had abandoned breast-feeding in an effort to appear "progressive." Infants are thus arbitrarily denied the advantages of breast milk and are being unnecessarily exposed to the disadvantages of cow's milk and formula-feeding (154, 155).

In addition to the previously mentioned problems of increased morbidity and mortality, "artificial" feeding may be associated with a variety of hazards. These include the possibility of allergy to cow's milk; mistakes or negligence in the preparation of the feeding where underdilution will result in hyperosmolar solutions and overdilution will cause an insufficient calorie supply; neonatal hypocalcemia, which is related to the high phosphate concentration of cow's milk; and metabolic derangements in the premature infant by his limited ability to metabolize certain of the amino acids which are found in a high concentration in cow's milk.

Breast milk is bacteriologically safe, and also is beneficial by fostering an intestinal flora characterized by the prevalence of Lactobacillus bifidus. Bacterial colonization of the intestine in bottle-fed infants is predominantly by a gram-negative flora. Furthermore, it appears that human milk has a protective role against enteric infections in the young infant (156). Breast milk contains immunoglobulins (notably IgA) with antibody activity against several microorganisms, including Escherichia coli (149). Breast milk also contains lymphoid cells that produce IgA, lymphocytes capable of participating in processes of cellular immunity, phagocytizing neutrophils and macrophages, complement components, lactoperoxidase, lysozyme, and lactoferrin—an iron-binding protein with a strong bacteriostatic effect on E. coli (Table 4). Clinical and experimental observations suggest that breast

TABLE 4   Anti-Infective Factors in Human Milk

Factor	Capacity
Secretory IgA	Specific activity against microorganisms
IgM, IgG, IgD	Specific activity against allergens
Lactoferrin	Bacteriostasis
Lysozyme	Bacterial lysis
Complement (C3, C4)	Opsonization
Lactoperoxidase	Bacterial lysis
Anti-Staphylococcal factor	Inhibits systemic staphylococcal infections
Bifidus factor	Promotes growth of bifidus bacteria
Antiviral RNA-ase	Inhibits viral activity
Interferon	Inhibits viral infection
Lymphocyte	Synthesis of immunoglobulins
Macrophage and neutrophils	Bacterial killing and phagocytosis

(From Ref. 149. Reprinted with permission.)

milk provides protection from necrotizing enterocolitis (157). The composition of breast milk is favorable in terms of the protein quality and content, its mineral content with a low potential renal solute load, and also its nutrient interactions. For example, the lower protein content improves iron absorption, and breast-feeding is thus associated with a lower incidence of iron deficiency than the use of unfortified cow's milk formulas (158). The curd which is formed in the stomach from human milk is soft and flocculent, enabling further good transit and digestion.

Another advantage of breast-feeding over bottle-feeding is that the breast-fed infant may self-determine the volume of milk that will be consumed at each feeding, while the bottle-fed infant is usually being persuaded to "finishing the bottle to the last drop," in amounts set by others. The tendency will be to offer amounts that are larger than those actually needed by the infant. Indeed, during the first months of life bottle-fed infants gain more in weight than breast-fed infants; this implies overfeeding and setting a feeding pattern that may lead to obesity. In recent years these nutritional advantages of human milk feeding are beginning to be appreciated and in some instances being rediscovered as reviewed elsewhere (159). In addition to the immunological benefits of decreased infection rates, there is also a reduction in the incidence of allergic disorders (159). It also may be of benefit in the eventual development of atherosclerosis and possible obesity.   Breast-feeding may protect the baby from the intellectual impairment that would result in infants with undiagnosed congenital hypothyroidism. Maternal benefits from breast-feeding include a reduction in the incidence of breast cancer and a reduction in the incidence of early repeat pregnancy. The early and intimate physical contact between mother and infant that is associated with breast-feeding has been observed to create better mother-child interaction (160), resulting in less problems and setting the stage for a better family integration. Child abandonment rates also seem to be reversed by breast-feeding (161).

Breast-feeding should thus be encouraged by adequate information and propaganda, educational programs for adolescents and parents (or parents-to-be), and by the creation of employment policies and working conditions that will enable mothers to breast-feed. The hypothesis has been advanced that infant-mother separation after delivery is an important cause of decreased breast-feeding (161). This, however, can be reversed by increasing rooming-in policies and postpartum stimulation by health personnel contacting the mother after delivery and counteracting some of the commercial promotions of formula-feeding and weaning foods.

FOOD FADS

Good nutrition requires no single food pattern; man requires specific nutrients, not specific food items. Therefore, it is possible to obtain satisfactory nutrition by the proper selection of indigenous foods throughout the world. As simple as this concept may be, individuals are still susceptible to the lure of faddism. Food fads or cults are considered when popular pursuit, diversions, or fashions in food consumption prevail for a period of time. These trends are certainly not new and have been part of our culture for several generations (162). However, because of many sociocultural factors, food faddism has created a new public nutritional health problem. A new industry has been created, that of "health foods." In general, there are three basic types of food fads: (1) those in which special virtues of a particular food are exaggerated and purported to cure specific diseases; (2) those in which certain foods are eliminated from the diet because of a belief that harmful constituents are present; and (3) those in which emphasis is placed on a "natural" food. The appeal of food fads and cultism to a significant segment of the population may undermine the teaching and implementation of sound nutrition principles. Moreover, more serious hazards of food faddism include the false promises of superior health and freedom from diseases that are believed to accrue from use of health foods, delaying individuals from obtaining the necessary competent medical attention.   Economic extravagance is another consequence of food faddism since foodstuffs which attach the word "health," implying health-giving, curative properties, are more expensive than their natural counterparts.

The number of people involved in food faddism is difficult to assess but it is estimated to be in the millions (163-165).   The use of organically grown foods is an important aspect of the health food movement.   The term "organic" describes "all living things," therefore, it is more accurate to speak of organically grown foods which are those grown without the use of food chemicals or additives.   However, there is no way of monitoring such claims, nor are there laws which define and certify these labels.   Claims have been made that organically grown foods are nutritiously superior to foods grown under standard agricultural conditions using chemical fertilizers (165-167).   There is no scientific basis for this claim. Plants use only inorganic food and there are no organic forms of plant food. Therefore, it is relatively immaterial whether traditional agricultural methods using chemical fertilizers or organic farming practices are followed.   Moreover, the use of organic farming techniques have added the disadvantage of possible contamination with Salmonella, which can result in food poisoning (166-168).   As far as taste is concerned, there are no objective tests to support or disclaim the beneficial taste of organically grown foods.

Claims are made also that our food supply is being poisoned with pesticides and food additives.   The use of additives and pesticides is regulated by law.   The Federal Drug Administration regularly conducts "market-basket" studies in several regions of the United States and although many of our common foods may contain unknown substances, some of which are toxic (169, 170), these are usually present in amounts which do not cause any difficulty.   There is a document which lists over 250 toxic compounds normally present in many common foods and food additives (165).   Accidental contamination of food sources also have been reported. However, this large amount of knowledge contrasts sharply with the lack of knowledge about naturally occurring toxicants in foods which may be present in the so-called organically grown type (166).

The third issue is the cost of these foodstuffs which is usually 30-100% higher as compared with nonorganic counterparts.

Natural foods are considered to be those foods which are in their original state or have minimal refinement and minimal processing.   Some examples of such foods are fresh fruits and vegetables or milk, unrefined sugar, honey, and whole grain flour and cereals.   It has been found that labels of natural or organic products can be misleading.   For instance, vitamin preparations of the so-called natural type are prepared similarly to those of the other types whose synthetic chemicals are added to natural bases.

Part of the movement toward natural foods is expressed by the increased demand for certified, unpasteurized milk.   Raw milk, because of its excellent nutrient composition, is a favored medium for bacterial growth; therefore, pasteurization of all market milk has been encouraged.   Raw certified milk is basically pure, fresh, nutritious milk, in its natural state, not having been heated, and without the addition of caloric matter or preservatives, "nothing having been added or taken away." Unfortunately, this type of milk is costly and does not ensure absolute safety from pathogenic organisms (171).   The requirements and checking systems to enforce "health food" standards may not be optimal, whereas, pasteurization of milk as performed by the dairy industry, which has developed excellent pasteurization equipment, offers fine control of all the above factors.

The Zen macrobiotic diet is the most dangerous current fad and represents an extreme example of the trend toward natural foods (172-174); Zen means medication, and macrobiotic suggests longevity.   The purpose of this fanatical adherence to rigid nutritional principles is to create a spiritual awakening.   There are many stages of this diet in which natural foods have been advocated, and emphasis is placed on whole grain cereals and avoidance of sugar and fluids. The philosophy behind this diet is to prevent and cure every disease from dandruff, psychosis, arthritis, and heart disease, to cancer, thus, a panacea. In the advanced degrees of this diet, seven cereals constitute 100% of the daily intake. Therefore, scurvy and death can result from adherence to such diets for only a few months. Followers of such diets are those with a strong system of philosophical and religious beliefs and have generally been found to be of middle and upper economic classes, fairly intelligent, and seeking a new belief being totally unconcerned with the data and teaching of established nutrition (175).

Frequently, it is difficult to separate fact from fiction. Nutrition misinformation can arise from many sources, some accidental and some intentional. Many prominent nutritionists have noted that some information published by nutritional gurus is not in accord with established scientific knowledge. In those publications (176, 177), although research studies are quoted, the interpretation and conclusion of such studies are often unjustified, and in many cases are speculative and at variance with the accepted medical practice. One of the themes promoted is the need for increased protein, implying that we as a nation are protein deficient. Another one is a recommendation for extra dietary supplements, namely 5000 units of vitamin D and 25,000 units of vitamin A. These dosages are at least five times those of the human recommended dietary allowances.

Only by effective nutritional education is it possible to counteract the false propaganda of food fads. However, there are many self-appointed "advisors" and the public does not adequately recognize glaring differences between fact and fancy. In many cases where nutritional knowledge exists, it is not applied. A positive aspect of food faddism is that it has brought nutrition to the forefront, and as the general educational level of the public has increased, individuals are seeking nutrition facts beyond the four basic concepts. Nutrition education should stress that knowledge increases as research continues and that it is important to evaluate the validity of claims of food faddists.

TOTAL PARENTERAL NUTRITION

Parenteral nutrition can provide the essential nutrients necessary to maintain positive nitrogen balance and to achieve weight stability or gain in adults and normal growth and development in infants under a variety of conditions usually associated with a catabolic state. Total parenteral nutrition (TPN) is indicated for the support and management of patients who cannot eat, who will not eat, who should not eat, or who cannot eat enough. The technique of parenteral nutrition is relatively safe when performed in specific centers where specialized care is available. There, the benefits from its application outweigh reported potential risks which can be prevented or treated. However, TPN should not be used without proper consideration for available nutritional support, which may be provided orally by administering food or specialized enteral feedings, without the risks of intravenous infusion, particularly in places where no such specialized care is available.

For patients with a functional gastrointestinal tract, the best route for satisfying nutritional requirements is through oral nutrition. When oral or enteral feedings become inadequate, or impossible to provide essential nutrients, parenteral nutritional support is indicated. This technique is often referred to as intravenous hyperalimentation because in all cases extra calories are provided to prevent negative energy and nitrogen balance from occurring during or following illness. Following its first successful use in 1968 (178), the decade that followed was marked by a tremendous surge of interest and progress in the field, as evidenced by the creation of the American Society of Parenteral and Enteral Nutrition. Enteral nutrition with elemental diets and nutrient formulations are reviewed elsewhere (179-181).

NUTRITIONAL ASPECTS OF TPN

A patient requiring TPN usually is suffering from malnutrition and other complications. Ideally, TPN solutions must, therefore, alleviate these conditions and provide nutrients in amounts sufficient to achieve tissue synthesis and an anabolic state. The energy must cover resting metabolism, physical activity and specific dynamic action. The patient's condition and particular disease state also must be regarded as significant factors dictating the amount of energy required (182). Recommendations of energy value in clinical situations range from 150-250 kcal/g of utilizable nitrogen supplied, or more when other alterations exist. This should be adjusted downward as the weight increases after therapy is started.

The two most important sources of energy are carbohydrates and fats. A minimum of 100 g of carbohydrates per day will prevent ketosis and decrease protein catabolism in adults. Hypertonic glucose solutions have been the major parenteral energy source of TPN in the United States (182). Until definitive evidence is gathered through using randomized control studies for other sources of energy supplementation from nonglucose carbohydrates in TPN, glucose should remain the carbohydrate of choice for this type of feeding. A great demand for energy can be supplied with available intravenous fat emulsions, in combination with no less than 20% of the total calories derived from carbohydrates. The advantage of fat emulsions is that a large amount of energy (9 kcal/g) can be given in a small volume of isotonic fluid. Because of the isotonicity of fat emulsions, these may be administered via peripheral veins. This contrasts with the irritating hypertonic TPN glucose solutions which usually have to be administered through catheters in central veins. Fat emulsions will also both prevent and correct essential fatty acid deficiency. However, it should be remembered that contraindications to the use of fat emulsion are pathological hyperlipidemia, advanced hepatocellular injury, coagulation disturbances, and allergy (182-185). The fat emulsion which has gained wide acceptance in the United States is a 10% soybean and oil emulsion with egg yolk, phospholipids, and glycerol (185).

Several nitrogen sources for TPN are available and are basically of two types: protein hydrolysates and mixtures of crystalline amino acids. The requirements for amino acids depend upon the metabolic and physiologic conditions, the need increasing accordingly as protein catabolism is increased. The following amounts are recommended for TPN: 0.4-0.6 g of protein per kilogram body weight per day for patients with renal insufficiency; 0.8-1.6 g/kg for adults; 2-3 g/kg for infants, pregnant women, and postoperative patients, and 2-4 g/kg for premature babies and postoperative neonates (186).

Several guidelines for the amino acid composition of solutions for long-term parenteral infusion of seriously ill or injured patients appear reasonable. The indispensable, or essential amino acids should be patterned to the needs of the growing child. They should be maintained at a ratio of a 1:1.5 with the dispensable amino acids and they should contain alanine, proline, arginine, glutamic acid, and histidine, with tyrosine, and cystine also added (187). For optimal utilization of the amino acids, even parenterally, energy requirements must be made simultaneously by infusion of both protein and glucose sources. TPN solutions must also contain vitamins in sufficient quantities to reverse prior deficiencies as well as to meet increased metabolic demands associated with the disease and other anabolic processes. It should also contain sufficient quantities to compensate for excessive urinary losses, particularly water-soluble vitamins administered via the venous catheter (188). Consideration should be given for replenishing essential minerals and electrolytes as well as trace elements (185, 189).

A large number of factors influence fluid losses and fluid requirements in TPN. Metabolic water formed by the conversion of protein, carbohydrate and fat must be considered when calculating fluid balance. Care must be taken not to provide excessive fluid and electrolytes in patients who are older, critically ill, or those with an organ failure, i. e. , kidney or liver. However, sufficient water to provide for the energy that is being administered must be provided (185).

INDICATIONS FOR TPN

There are many specific conditions in which the use of the alimentary tract for nourishing patients optimally may be impossible. These include mechanical obstruction, postoperative illness, short-gut syndrome, inflammatory and malabsorptive processes. There are also instances when attempting adequate enteral intake may be inadvisable, e.g., in patients with very severe diarrhea and chronic inflammatory bowel disease, or in patients with acute renal failure, hepatic dysfunction, etc.

TPN also may be indicated for a diverse group of patients with disease states in which maintenance of an adequate enteral dietary regimen is improbable, even though the alimentary tract may be potentially or partially functional. A combination of oral supplements and TPN may be effective adjuncts in patients with several types of cancer and those undergoing chemotherapy or irradiation, as well as those with severe malnutrition of other types. In some low-birth-weight infants there are difficulties in establishing a successful enteral feeding schedule. Utilization of TPN and infusion of feedings into the stomach or jejunum may allow the nutritional delivery which will insure survival and growth of these patients. TPN can also be a valuable means for restoring nutritional status when use of the gastrointestinal tract is avoided for other reasons as in patients with anorexia nervosa. However, other modalities of feedings must be first exhausted in these patients.

Finally, there are rare conditions during which adequate enteral intake is hazardous and often associated with an unacceptable high incidence of aspiration pneumonia. Examples are cerebrovascular accidents, coma, tetanus, laryngeal incompetence, tracheoesophageal fistulas, etc. In these patients TPN may be indicated.

COMPLICATIONS OF TPN

Potential complications and hazards of TPN have been identified, including: (1) metabolic, (2) technical, (3) sepsis, and (4) incompatibilities.

Metabolic Complications

Glucose intolerance is the most common metabolic complication that results because of an inability to utilize the high concentration of glucose in TPN (190). Two opposite and extreme manifestations of this problem may occur: (1) hyperosmolar nonketotic hyperglycemia, resulting from reduced glucose tolerance or excessive total dose or rate of infusion with production of osmotic diuresis and dehydration; (2) severe hypoglycemia resulting from persistence of endogenous insulin production, secondary to prolonged stimulation of islet cells by high carbohydrate infusion or from sudden cessation of the concentrated glucose infusion (190). Complications relative to amino acid metabolism alterations, i. e. , imbalance, may also occur (176). Hyperchloremic metabolic acidosis may result from excessive chloride in the crystalline amino acid solution delivered (191). Hyperammonemia also may occur especially in premature infants and in patients with hepatic disorders. Prerenal azotemia may complicate excessive total dose or rate of protein infusion (183). Abnormal plasma aminograms often are found. Essential fatty acid metabolism may be impaired by inadequate essential fatty acid and vitamin E administration (184).   Similarly, mineral and vitamin deficiencies are known to occur with particular emphasis on hypophosphatemia, hypocalcemia, hypomagnesemia, etc. , although other more unusual deficiencies, i. e. , chromium, also have been reported (192).

Technical Complications

Technical complications of TPN include problems which may result from hyperosmolar solutions leading to infiltration or thrombophlebitis.   Thrombosis of great veins may occur, but may not become a clinical problem until they prevent catheterization, cause emboli or become septic. When these occur, thrombosis can become a major threat to survival (193). Mechanical malfunction of catheters has posed potential hazards to TPN recipients.   Air emboli may occur during the process of insertion when the syringe is removed, or if the intravenous line becomes inadvertently detached from the intravenous catheter.   Other complications related to catheters include malposition, pneumothorax, dislodgment, leaks, and liver disease with progressive cholestasis and abnormal elevations of liver enzymes also have been reported (194). Some authors consider the hepatic dysfunction as a metabolic disorder.

Septic Complications

Septic complications are frequent because of the deficient immune mechanisms of patients who are recipients of TPN.   Catheter-related sepsis is also a frequent problem.   Although TPN solutions are able to sustain growth of many pathogens, solution contamination is rare as a cause of sepsis.   The most frequent cause is growth of organisms along the course of the cutaneous vascular prosthesis and through the catheter due to contamination of a closed system.   These occur despite implementing certain procedures and techniques which are aimed at reducing the incidence of sepsis and are essential whenever TPN is used.

Incompatibilities

Patient versus solution incompatibilities have also been described (190).   There are two types: fever and typical allergy.   These reactions are usually seen with protein hydrolysate solutions and disappear when replaced by crystalline amino acid solutions.

Finally, death resulting from overzealous TPN has been reported (195).   This is of particular importance, as it may occur whenever there is an overzealous refeeding of a malnourished population.   It is known as the refeeding syndrome, which may be worse than the malnourished state.   Cachectic patients are relatively well adapted to their calorically deprived state, and thus they are prone to acute metabolic imbalances and other incompatibilities when infused with TPN.

HOME TPN

Home parenteral nutrition is now the treatment of choice for chronically ill patients who have little hope of restoring and maintaining nutrition by oral means. It has radically altered our attitude and treatment endeavors toward patients after massive small-bowel resection, or other abnormalities which were previously not compatible with life.   Such patients who heretofore died may now maintain excellent nutrition at home and resume a nearly normal life (196).

REFERENCES

1. Mata, L. J. , R. A. Kromal, J. J. Urrutia, and B. Garcia: Effect of infection on food intake and the nutritional state: Perspectives as viewed from the village. Am J Clin Nutr 30:1215, 1977.

2. McGovern, G. : Address to the American Society for Parenteral and Enteral Nutrition for the Third Clinical Congress. J Parent Ent Nutr 3:137-138, 1979.

3. Kaminski, M. V. , and A. L. Winborn: Nutritional Assessment Guide. Monograph, Midwest Nutrition Education and Research Foundation, Inc. 1978.

4. Seltzer, M. H. , J. A. Bastidas, D. M. Cooper, et al. : Instant nutritional assessment. J Parent Ent Nutr 3:157-159, 1979.

5. Bistrian, B. R. , G. L. Blackburn, J. Vitale, et al. : Prevalence of malnutrition in general medical patients, JAMA 235:1567-1570, 1976.

6. Butterworth, C. E. : The skeleton in the hospital closet. Nutr Today 9:4-8, 1974.

7. Baker, H. , O. Frank, S. Feingold, G. Christakos, and H. Ziffer: Vitamins, total cholesterol, and triglycerides in 642 New York City school children. Am J Clin Nutr 20:850, 1967.

8. Ten-State Nutrition Survey. 1968-1970. DHEW Publication No. (HSM) 72:8132, July, 1972.

9. Jelliffe, D. B. : Assessment of Nutritional Status of the Community. WHO Monograph Vol. 53, Geneva, 1966.

10. Waterlow, J. C. : Note on the assessment and classification of protein-energy malnutrition in children. Lancet 2:87, 1973.

11. Waterlow, J. C. , and I. H. E. Rutishauser: Malnutrition in man. in Symposia of Swedish Nutrition Foundation, XII. Almqvist and Wiksell, Stockholm, 1974.

12. Weil, W. B. , Jr. : Current controversies in childhood obesity. J Pediatr 91:175, 1977.

13. Winick, M. , and P. Rosso: Head circumference and cellular growth of the brain in normal and marasmic children. J Pediatr 74:774, 1969.

14. Dobbing, J. : Later growth of the brain: Its vulnerability. Pediatrics 53:2, 1974.

15. Dauncey, M. J. , G. Gandy, and D. Gairdner: Assessment of total body fat from skinfold thickness measurements. Arch Dis Child 52:223, 1977.

16. Tanner, J. M. , and R. H. Whitehouse: Revised standards for forceps and subscapular skinfolds for British children. Arch Dis Child 50:142, 1975.

17. Ounsted, M., and C. Ounsted: On fetal growth rate. Clinics in Developmental Medicine, No. 46, Heinemann, London, 1971.

18. Kanawati, A.A., and D.S. McLaren: Assessment of marginal malnutrition. Nature 228:573, 1970.

19. U.S. Dept. of HEW: Screening children for nutritional status: suggestions for child health programs. U.S. Government Protocol Office, Washington, 1971.

20. Fomon, S.J.: Infant Nutrition, 2nd ed. W.B. Saunders Co., Philadelphia, 1074.

21. Food and Agriculture Organization: Energy and Protein Requirements. FAO Nutrition Meeting Report Series, No. 52, Rome, 1973.

22. Recommended Dietary Allowances. Food and Nutrition Board, National Academy of Sciences—National Research Council, 9th ed. Publ. No. 2216, Washington, 1980.

23. American Academy of Pediatrics. Committee on Nutrition: Nutritional needs of low-birth-weight infants. Pediatrics 60:519, 1977.

24. Beisel, W.R.: Magnitude of the host nutritional response to infection. Am J Clin Nutr 30:100, 1976.

25. Davies, D.P., and R. Saunders: Blood urea: Normal values in early infancy relating to feeding practice. Arch Dis Child 48:563, 1973.

26. Willis, D.M., J. Chabot, I. Radde, and G.W. Chance: Unsuspected hyperosmolality of oral solutions contributing to necrotizing enterocolitis on very low birth weight infants. Pediatrics 60:535, 1977.

27. Komishi, E.: Food energy equivalents of various activities. J Am Diet Assoc 46:3, 1965.

28. Payne, P.R.: Safe protein calorie ratios on diets. The relative importance of protein and energy intake as causal factors of malnutrition. Am J Clin Nutr 28:281, 1975.

29. Select Committee on Nutrition and Human Needs, U.S. Senate: Dietary goals for the United States. U.S. Gov't Printing Office, Washington, 1977.

30. Waterlow, J.C., and P.R. Payne: The protein gap. Nature 258:113, 1975.

31. Baum, J.D.: Nutritional value of human milk. Obstet Gynecol 37:126, 1971.

32. Desor, J.A., O. Maller, and R.E. Turner: Taste in acceptance of sugars by human infants. J Comp Physiol Psychol 84:496, 1973.

33. Makinen, K.K.: The role of sucrose and other sugars in the development of dental caries: A review. Int Dent J 22:363, 1973.

34. Yudkin, J.: Sucrose, insulin and coronary heart disease. Am Heart J 80: 444, 1970.

35.   Antar, M. A. , J. A. Little, C. Lucas, G. C. Buckely, and A. Csima: Inter-relationship between the kind of dietary carbohydrate and fat in hyperlipo-proteinemic patients.   Part 3. Synergistic effect of sucrose and animal fat on serum lipids. Atherosclerosis 11:191, 1970.

36.   Husband, J. , P. Husband, and C. N. Mallonson: Gastric emptying of starch meals in the newborn. Lancet 2:290, 1970.

37.   Anderson, T. A. , S. J. Forson, and L. J. Filer, Jr. : Carbohydrate toler-ance studies with 3-day-old infants. J Lab Clin Med 79:31, 1972.

38.   Burkitt, D. P. : Some diseases characteristic of modern Western civilization. Br Med J 1:274, 1973.

39.   Trowell, H. C. : Ischemic heart disease and dietary fiber. Am J Clin Nutr 25:926, 1972.

40.   American Academy of Pediatrics.   Committee on Nutrition: Commentary on breast feeding and infant formulas, including proposed standards for formu-las.   Pediatrics 57:278, 1976.

41.   Snyderman, S. E. , A. Boyer, E. Roitman, L. E. Holt, Jr. , and P. H. Prose: The histidine requirement of the infant. Pediatrics 31:786, 1963.

42.   Harper, A. E. , N. J. Benevenga, and R. M. Wahlhueter: Effects of ingestion of disproportionate amounts of amino acids. Physiol Rev 50:428, 1970.

43.   McLaren, D. S. : The great protein fiasco. Lancet 2:93, 1974.

44.   Schlenk, H. : Odd numbered and new essential fatty acids. Fed Proc 31:1430, 1972.

45.   Holman, R. T. : Essential fatty acid deficiency. in Progress in the Chemistry of Fats and Other Lipids, Vol. 10. Pergamon, Oxford, 1971.

46.   Caldwell, M. D. , H. T. Jonsson, and H. B. Othersen, Jr. : Essential fatty acid deficiency in an infant receiving prolonged parenteral alimentation. J Pediatr 81:894, 1972.

47.   Holman, R. T. : Function and biologic activities of essential fatty acids in man. in Fat Emulsions in Parenteral Nutrition. American Medical Associ-ation, Chicago, 1976.

48.   Pikaar, N. A. , and J. Fernandes: Influence of different types of dietary fat on the fatty acid composition of serum lipid fractions in infants and children. Am J Clin Nutr 19:194, 1966.

49.   Forget, P. P. , J. Fernandes, and P. H. Begemann: Utilization of fat emulsion during total parenteral nutrition in children. Acta Paediatr Scand 64:377, 1975.

50. Friedman, Z. , S. J. Shochat, and J. Maisels, et al. : Correction of essential fatty acid deficiency in newborn infants by cutaneous application of sunflower seed oil. Pediatrics 58:650, 1976.

51. Hunt, C. E. , R. R. Engel, S. Modler, W. Hamilton, S. Bissen, and R. T. Homan: Essential fatty acid deficiency in neonates: Inability to reverse deficiency by topical application of EFA-rich oil. J Pediatr 92: 603, 1978.

52. Kannel, W. D. , W. P. Castelli, 1. Gordon, and P. M. McNamara: Serum cholesterol, lipoproteins and the risk of coronary heart disease. Ann Int Med 74:1, 1971.

53. Kannel, W. B. , and T. R. Dauber: Atherosclerosis as a pediatric problem. J Pediatr 80:544, 1972.

54. Council on Foods and Nutrition: Diet and coronary heart disease. JAMA 222:1697, 1972.

55. Plotz, E. J. , J. J. Kabara, M. E. Davis, G. V. LeRoy, and R. G. Gould: Studies on the synthesis of cholesterol in the brain of the human fetus. Am J Obstet Gynecol 101:534, 1968.

56. Hahn, P. , and L. Kirby: Immediate and late effects of premature weaning and of feeding a high fat or high carbohydrate diet to weanling rats. J Nutr 103:690, 1973.

57. American Academy of Pediatrics. Committee on Nutrition: Childhood diet and coronary heart disease. Pediatrics 49:305, 1972.

58. Gershoff, S. N. : Effects of dietary levels of macronutrients on vitamin requirements. Fed Proc 23:1077, 1964.

59. Rosenberg, L. E. : Inherited aminoacidopathies demonstrating vitamin dependency. N Engl J Med 281:145, 1969.

60. Olson, J. A. : The metabolism of vitamin A. Pharmacol Rev 19:559, 1967.

61. Roels, O. A. : Vitamin A physiology. JAMA 214:1097, 1970.

62. Hayes, K. C. : On the pathophysiology of vitamin A deficiency. Nutr Rev 29:3, 1971.

63. Morrice, G. , Jr. , W. H. Havener, and F. Kapetansky: Vitamin A intoxication as a cause of pseudotumor cerebri. JAMA 173:1802, 1960.

64. Persson, B. , R. Tunell, and K. Ekengren: Chronic vitamin A intoxication during the first half year of life: Description of 5 cases. Acta Paediatr Scand 54:49, 1965.

65. DeLuca, H. F. : The vitamin D system in the regulation of calcium and phosphorus metabolism. Nutr Rev 37:161, 1979.

66. Haussler, M. R. and T. A. McCain: Basic and clinical concepts related to vitamin D metabolism and action. N Engl J Med 297:974, 1977.

67. Omdahl, J. L. and H. F. DeLuca: Regulation of vitamin D metabolism and function. Physiol Rev 53:327, 1973.

68. Greer, F. R. , V. E. Sency, R. S. Levin, J. J. Steider, P. S. Asche, and R. C. Tsang: Bone mineral content in breast fed infants with and without supplemental vitamin D. Pediatr Res 14:500, 1980.

69. Roberts, C. C. , G. M. Chon, D. Folland, and R. Jackson : Adequate bone mineralization and serum vitamin D in breast fed term infants not supplemented with vitamin D. Pediatr Res 14:509, 1980.

70. Loomis, W. F.: Rickets. Scien Amer 222:77, 1970.

71. Harrison, H. E. and H. C. Harrison: Rickets then and now. J. Pediatr 87:1144, 1975.

72. Edidin, D. V. , L. L. Levitsky, W. Schey, N. Dinboiac, and A. Compos: Resurgence of nutritional rickets associated with breast feeding and special dietary procedures. Pediatrics 65:232, 1980.

73. Hoff, N. , J. Haddad, S. Teitelbaum, W. McAlister, and L. S. Hilmon: Serum concentrations of 25-hydroxyvitamin D in rickets of extremely premature infants. J Pediatr 94:460, 1979.

74. Lifshitz, F. and N. Maclaren: Vitamin D dependency rickets in institutionalized mentally retarded children on long-term anticonvulsant therapy. I. A survey of 288 patients. J Pediatr 83:612, 1973.

75. National Research Council, Food and Nutrition Board: Hazards of overuse of vitamin D. Am J Clin Nutr 28:512, 1975.

76. Oski, F.A.: Nutritional anemias of infancy. in Pediatric Nutrition: Infant Feedings – Deficiencies – Diseases. F. Lifshitz (ed.). Marcel Dekker, New York, 1982, pp. 123-138.

77. Johnson, L. H. , D. B. Schaffer, D. E. Goldstein, and T. R. Boggs: Influence of vitamin E treatment and blood transfusions on mean severity of retrolental fibroplasia in premature infants. Pediatr Res 11:983, 1977.

78. Hypervitaminosis E and coagulation. Nutr Rev 33:269, 1975.

79. Hillman, R. W.: Tocopherol excess in man: Creatinuria associated with prolonged ingestion. Am J Clin Nutr 5:597, 1957.

80. Ansell, J. E. , R. Kumar, and D. Deykin: The spectrum of vitamin K deficiency. JAMA 238:40, 1977.

81. Finkel, M. J.: Vitamin K and vitamin K analogues. Clin Pharmacol Ther 2:794, 1961.

82. King, C. G.: Present knowledge of ascorbic acid (vitamin C). Nutr Rev 26:33, 1968.

83. Hodges, R. E. , J. Hood, J. E. Canham, H. E. Samberlich, and E. M. Baker: Clinical manifestations of ascorbic acid deficiency in man. Am J Clin Nutr 24:432, 1971.

84. Pauling, L. : Evolution and the need for ascorbic acid. Proc Natl Acad Sci 67:1643, 1970.

85. Cameron, E. and L. Pauling: Supplemental ascorbate in the supportive treatment of cancer: Prolongation of survival times in terminal human cancer. Proc Natl Acad Sci 73:3685, 1978.

86. Creagan, E. T. , C. C. Moertel, J. R. O'Fallon, A. J. Schutt, M. J. O'Connell, J. Rubin, and S. Frytak: Failure of high dose vitamin C to benefit patients with advanced cancer. N Engl J Med 301:687, 1979.

87. Goodman, A. , and L. S. Gilman: The Pharmacological Basis of Therapeutics, 6th ed. Macmillan Co. , New York, 1980, p. 1576.

88. Pitt, H. A. and Costrini, A. M. : Vitamin C prophylaxis in marine recruits. JAMA 241:908, 1979.

89. Herbert, V. : The rationale of massive-dose vitamin therapy. in Proceedings, Western Hemisphere Nutrition Congress IV. Publishing Sciences Group, Inc. , Acton, MA, 1975, p. 84.

90. Anderson, T. W. : Large scale studies with vitamin C. Acta Vitaminol Enzymol (Milano), 31:43-50, 1977.

91. Cook, J. D. , and E. R. Monsen: Vitamin C, the common cold and iron absorption. Am J Clin Nutr 30:235, 1977.

92. Rosenthal, G. : Interaction of ascorbic acid and warfarin. JAMA 215:1671, 1971.

93. Ariaey-Nejad, M. R. , M. Balaghi, E. M. Baker, and H. E. Sauberlich: Thiamine metabolism in man. Am J Clin Nutr 23:764, 1970.

94. Pincus, J. H. , J. R. Cooper, J. V. Murphy, E. F. Rabe, D. Lonsdale and H. G. Dunn: Thiamine derivatives in subacute necrotizing encephalomyelopathy: A preliminary report. Pediatrics 51:716-721, 1973.

95. Scriver, C. R. : Vitamin-responsive inborn errors of metabolism. Metabolism 22:1319-1344, 1973.

96. Darby, W. J. , K. W. McNutt, and E. N. Todhunter: Niacin. in Present Knowledge in Nutrition. D. M. Hegsted, C. O. Chichester, W. J. Darby, K. W. McNutt, R. M. Stalvey, and E. H. Stotz (eds.). The Nutrition Foundation, Washington, 1976, p. 162.

97. Hines, J. D. and J. W. Harris: Pyridoxine-responsive anemia. Am J Clin Nutr 14:137, 1964.

98. Bernstein, L. H. , S. Jutstein, S. Weiner, and G. Efron:The absorption and malabsorption of folic acid and its polyglutamates. Am J Med 48:570, 1970.

99. Sandy, G. and W. Jacobson: Influence of folic acid on birth weight and growth of the erythroblastotic infant. I, II and III. Arch Dis Child 52:1, 1977.

100. Herbert, V.: The five possible causes of all nutrient deficiency: Illustrated by deficiencies of vitamin B_{12} and folic acid. Am J Clin Nutr 26:77, 1973.

101. Nixon, P. F. and J. R. Bertrino: Interrelationships of vitamin B_{12} and folate in man. Am J Med 48:555, 1970.

102. Baker, S. J.: Human vitamin B_{12} deficiency. World Rev Nutr Diet 8:62, 1967.

103. Kerrey, E., S. Crispin, H. M. Fox, and C. Kies: Nutritional status of preschool children. I. Dietary and biochemical findings. Am J Clin Nutr 21:1274, 1968.

104. Messaritakis, J., C. Kattamis, C. Karabula, and N. Matsnitis: Generalized seborrhoeic dermatitis. Clinical and therapeutic data of 25 patients. Arch Dis Child 50:871, 1975.

105. Ulmer, D. D.: Trace elements. N Engl J Med 297:318-321, 1977.

106. Lifshitz, F., and Y. Nishi: Mineral deficiencies during growth in pediatric diseases related to calcium. in Pediatric Diseases Related to Calcium. H. DeLuca and C. Anast (eds.). Elsevier, New York, 1980, pp. 305-321.

107. American Academy of Pediatrics. Committee on Nutrition. Iron supplements for infants. Pediatrics 58:686-691, 1976.

108. Levander, D. A. and C. Lorraine: Micronutrient interactions: Vitamins, minerals and hazardous elements. Ann NY Acad Sci, Vol. 355, Dec. 1, 1980.

109. Harrison, H. E., H. C. Harrison, F. Lifshitz, and A. D. Johnson: Observations on the growth disturbance of hereditary hypophosphatemia. Am J Dis Child 112:290-297, 1966.

110. Nishi, Y., F. Lifshitz, M. A. Bayne, F. Daum, M. Silverberg, and H. Aiges: Zinc status and its relation to growth retardation in children with chronic inflammatory bowel disease. Am J Clin Nutr 33:2613-2621, 1980.

111. Henkin, R. I.: On the role of adrenocorticosteroids in the control of zinc and copper metabolism. in Trace Elements in Animals, Vol. 2. W. G. Hoekstra, J. W. Suttie, H. E. Ganther, and W. E. Mertz (eds.). University Park Press, Baltimore, 1974, pp. 647-651.

112. Wester, P. O.: Zinc during diuretic treatment. Lancet I: 578, 1975.

113. Booth, B. and A. Johanson: Hypomagnesemia due to renal tubular defect in reabsorption of magnesium. J Pediatr 84:350-354, 1974.

114. Skyberg, D., J. H. Stromme, R. Nesbakken, et al.: Neonatal hypomagnesemia with selective malabsorption of magnesium - a clinical entity. Scand J Clin Lab Invest 21:355-363, 1968.

115. Leach, R. M. , Jr. , A. M. Muenster, and E. M. Wein: Studies on the role of manganese in bone formation: Effect upon chrondroitin sulfate synthesis in chick epiphyseal cartilage. Arch Biochem Biophys 133:22-28, 1969.

116. Scott, M. D.: The selenium dilemma. J Nutr 103:803-810, 1973.

117. Simkin, P. A.: Zinc sulphate in rheumatoid arthritis. in Zinc Metabolism: Current Aspects in Health and Diseases. G. J. Brewer, and A. S. Prasad (eds.) Alan R. Liss, Inc., New York, 1977, pp. 343-351.

118. Fort, P.: Magnesium and diabetes mellitus. in Pediatric Nutrition. Infant Feedings - Deficiencies - Diseases. F. Lifshitz (ed.). Marcel Dekker, Inc., New York, 1982, p. 223.

119. Dahl, L. K. and R. A. Love: Etiological role of sodium chloride intake in essential hypertension in humans. JAMA 164:397-400, 1957.

120. Dahl, L. K.: Effects of chronic excess salt feeding: Induction of salt-sensitive hypertension in rats. J Exp Med 114:231-236, 1961.

121. American Academy of Pediatrics. Committee on Nutrition: Salt intake and eating patterns of infants and children in relation to blood pressure. Pediatrics 53:115-121, 1974.

122. Irwin, M. I. and E. W. Kienholz: A conspectus of research on calcium requirements of man. J Nutr 103:1019-1095, 1973.

123. Cockburn, F. , J. K. Brown, N. R. Belton, and J.O. Forfar: Neonatal convulsions associated with primary disturbance of calcium, phosphorous, and magnesium metabolism. Arch Dis Child 48:99-108, 1973.

124. Lipsitz, P.J.: The clinical and biochemical effects of excess magnesium in the newborn. Pediatrics 47:501-509, 1971.

125. Greer, F.R. , J.J. Steichen, and R.C. Tsang: Calcium and phosphate supplements in breast milk - related rickets. Am J Dis Child 136:581-585, 1982.

126. Woodruff, C.W.: Iron deficiency in infancy and childhood. Pediatr Clin N Amer 24:85-94, 1977.

127. Nelson Textbook of Pediatrics. 10th ed. V.C. Vaughn, III and R.J. McKay (eds.). W. B. Saunders Co. , Philadelphia, 1975, p. 174.

128. Williams, M. L. , R. J. Shott, P. L. O'Nela, and F. A. Oski: Role of dietary iron and fats on vitamin E deficiency anemia of infancy. N Engl J Med 292: 887-890, 1975.

129. Rall, J. E.: Recent advances in the diagnosis of the disease of the thyroid. Clin Chim Acta 25:339-344, 1969.

130. Hambridge, K. M.: The role of zinc and other trace metals in pediatric nutrition. Pediatr Clin N Am 24:95-106, 1977.

131. Kelly, R. , G. P. Davidson, R. R. W. Townley, and P. E. Campbell: Reversible intestinal mucosa abnormality in acrodermatitis enteropathica. Arch Dis Child 51:219-222, 1976.

132. Hurley, L. S. and P. B. Mutch: Prenatal and postnatal development after transitory zinc deficiency in rats. J Nutr 103:649-656, 1973.

133. Ashkenazi, A., S. Cevon, M. Djaldeffi, E. Fishel, and D. Benvensti: The syndrome of neonatal copper deficiency. Pediatrics 52:525-533, 1973.

134. Holtzman, N. A.: Menkes' kinky hair syndrome: A genetic disease involving copper. Fed Proc 35:2276-2280, 1976.

135. Nishi, Y., E. Kittaka, K. Fukuda, S. Hatano, and T. Usui: Copper deficiency associated with alkali therapy in a patient with renal tubular acidosis. J. Pediatr 98:81-83, 1981.

136. Navech, Y., A. Hazani, and M. Berant: Copper deficiency with cow's milk diet. Pediatrics 68:397, 1981.

137. Levine, R. A., D. H. P. Streeten, and R. J. Doisy: Effects of oral chromium supplementation on the glucose tolerance of elderly human subjects. Metab Clin Exp 17:114-125, 1968.

138. Mertz, W.: Biological role of chromium. Fed Proc 26:186-193, 1967.

139. Shrader, R. E., L. C. Erway, and L. S. Hurley: Mucopolysaccharide synthesis in the developing inner ear of manganese-deficient and pallid mutant mice. Teratology 8:257-266, 1973.

140. Erway, L. C., L. S. Hurley, and A. Frazer: Neurological defect: Manganese in phenocopy and prevention of a genetic abnormality of inner ear. Science 152:1766-1768, 1966.

141. Rotruck, J. T., A. L. Pope, H. E. Janther, A. B. Swanson, D. G. Haferman, and W. G. Hoekstra: Selenium: Biochemical role as a component of glutathione peroxidase. Science 179:558, 1973.

142. Keshan Disease Research Group of Chinese Acad Med Sci, Beijing. Observations on the effect of sodium selenite in prevention of keshan disease. Chin Med J 92:471-6, 1979.

143. Collipp, P. J. and S. Y. Chen: Cardiomyopathy and selenium deficiency in a 2-yr-old girl. N Engl J Med 81:1304, 1981.

144. Underwood, E. J.: Trace Elements in Human and Animal Nutrition. 3rd ed. Academic Press, New York, 1971.

145. Seelig, M. S.: Review: Relationships of copper and molybdenum to iron metabolism. Am J Clin Nutr 25:1022, 1972.

146. Newbrun, E.: Dietary fluoride supplementation for the prevention of caries. Pediatrics 62:733-737, 1978.

147. Jelliffe, D. B., and E. P. T. Jeffiffe: Human Milk in the Modern World. Oxford University Press, London, 1976.

148. Robinson, M.: Infant morbidity and mortality. Lancet 1:788, 1951.

149. Mata, L.: Breast feeding, neonatal disease and malnutrition in less developed countries. in Pediatric Nutrition. Infant Feedings - Deficiencies - Diseases. F. Lifshitz (ed.). Marcel Dekker, Inc., New York, 1982, pp. 355-372.

150. Lifshitz, F.: The effects of diarrhea on infant nutrition. in Textbook of Gastroenterology and Nutrition in Infancy. Vol. II. E. Lebenthal (ed.). Raven Press, New York, 1981, p. 1003.

151. Lifshitz, F., S. Teichberg, and R. Wapnir: Malnutrition and the intestine. in Nutrition and Child Health. R. Tsang and B. Nichols (eds.). Alan R. Liss, New York, 1981, p. 1.

152. Fagundes-Neto, U.: Malnutrition and the intestine. in Clinical Disorders in Pediatric Gastroenterology and Nutrition. F. Lifshitz (ed.). Marcel Dekker, Inc., New York, 1980, pp. 249-263.

153. Sloper, K., L. McKean, J.D. Baum: Factors influencing breast feeding. Arch Dis Child 50:165, 1975.

154. Hambraeus, L.: Proprietary milk versus human breast milk in infant feeding. Pediatr Clin N Am 24:17, 1977.

155. Jelliffe, E.F.P.: Infant feeding practices: Associated iatrogenic and commerciogenic diseases. Pediatr Clin N Am 24:49, 1977.

156. Goldman, S.A. and C. Wayne Smith: Host resistance factors in breast milk. J Pediatr 82:1082, 1973.

157. Barlow, B., T.V. Santulli, W.C. Heird, et al.: An experimental study of acute necrotizing enterocolitis. The importance of breast milk. J Pediatr Surg 9:587, 1974.

158. McMillan, J.A., S.A. Landaw, F.A. Oski: Iron sufficiency in breast fed infants and the availability of iron from human milk. Pediatrics 58:686, 1976.

159. Oski, F.A.: The non-nutritional benefits of human milk. in Pediatric Nutrition. Infant Feedings - Deficiencies - Diseases. F. Lifshitz (ed.). Marcel Dekker, Inc., New York, 1982, pp. 55-69.

160. Lozoff, N., G.M. Brittenham, M.A. Trause, et al.: The mother-newborn relationship: Limits of adaptability. J Pediatr 91:1, 1977.

161. Mata, L., S. Murillo, P. Jimewez, M.A. Allen, and B. Garcia: Child feedings in less developed countries. Induced breast feeding in a transitional society. in Pediatric Nutrition. Infant Feedings - Deficiencies - Diseases. F. Lifshitz (ed.). Marcel Dekker, Inc., New York, 1982, pp. 35-53

162. Deutsch, R.M.: The Nuts Among the Berries. An Exposé of America's Food Fads. Ballantine Books, New York, 1961.

163. Sipple, H.L. and C.G. King: Food fads and fancies. J Agr Food Chem 2: 352-354, 1954.

164. Wagner, M. G. : The irony of affluence: Adult nutrition problems and programs. J Am Diet Assoc 57:311-315, 1970.

165. Von Elbe, J. H. : Organic food—another consumer hoax? J Milk Food Tech 35:669-671, 1972.

166. White, H. S. : The organic food movement. Food Tech 26:29-30, 32-33, 1972.

167. Deutsch, R. : If you dare to look: A nutrition guide to favorite foreign delectables. French, Chinese, Italian. Today's Health 50:44-47, 1972.

168. Jukes, T. H. : Fact and fancy in nutrition and food science. Chemical residues in food. J Am Diet Assoc 59:203-211, 1971.

169. Wolnak, B. : Health foods: Natural, basic and organic. Food Drug Cosmet Law J 27:453-459, 1972.

170. Kermode, G. O. : Food additives. Sci Am 226:15-21, 1972.

171. Lampert, L. M. : Modern Dairy Products. Chemical Publ. Co. , Inc. , New York, 1970.

172. Sherlock, P. and E. O. Rothschild: Scurvy produced by a Zen macrobiotic diet. JAMA 199:794-798, 1967.

173. Council on Foods and Nutrition: Zen macrobiotic diets. JAMA 218-397, 1971.

174. Wohl, M. G. and R. S. Goodhart: Modern Nutrition in Health and Disease, 4th ed. Lea & Febiger, Philadelphia, 1968.

175. Prout, C. : Dietary restriction: The new nirvana. Trans Am Clin Climatol 83:219-225, 1972.

176. Davis, A. : Let's Get Well. Harcourt, Brace and World, Inc. , New York, 1965.

177. Davis, A. : Let's Eat Right to Keep Fit. The New American Library, Inc. , New York, 1970.

178. Dudrick, S. J. , D. W. Wilmore, H. M. Vars, and J. E. Rhoads: Long-term total parenteral nutrition with growth development and positive nitrogen balance. Surgery 64:134-142, 1968.

179. Bury, K. D. : Elemental diets. in Total Parenteral Nutrition. J. E. Fischer, (ed.). Little, Brown and Co. , Boston, 1976, pp. 395-411.

180. Shils, M. D. (ed.): Defined-Formula Diets for Medical Purposes. American Medical Association, Chicago, 1977.

181. Mitty, W. F. , T. F. Nealon, and C. Grossi: Use of elemental diets in surgical cases. Am J Gastroenterol 65:297-304, 1976.

182. Giovanni, R.: The manufacturing pharmacy: Solutions and incompatibilties. in Total Parenteral Nutrition, J. E. Fischer (ed.). Little, Brown and Co., Boston, 1976, p. 27-53, WB, 410, F52.

183. Law, D. H.: Current concepts in nutrition: Total parenteral nutrition. N Engl J Med 297:1104-1107, 1977.

184. Grotte, G., S. Jacobson and A. Wretlind: in Total Parenteral Nutrition. Proceedings of International Symposium on Intensive Therapy, Rome, May 30-June 2, 1975. C. Manni, S. I. Magalini and E. Scrasla (eds.). Elsevier, New York, 1976, pp. 47-73.

185. Shenkin, A., and A. Wretlind: Parenteral nutrition. World Rev Nutr Diet, 28:1-111, 1978.

186. Silberman, H., M. Freehauf, G. Fong, and N. Rosenblatt: Parenteral nutrition with lipids. JAMA 238:1380-1382, 1977.

187. Munro, H. M.: Basic concepts for parenteral nutrition. in Total Parenteral Nutrition. Symposium on Total Parenteral Nutrition, Nashville, Tenn., 1972. P. L. White, M. E. Nagy, and D. C. Fletcher (eds.). Publishing Sciences Group, Inc., Acton, MA, 1974, pp. 7-34.

188. Greene, H. L.: Vitamins. in Total Parenteral Nutrition. Symposium on Total Parenteral Nutrition, Nashville, Tenn., 1972. P. L. White, M. E. Nagy, and D. C. Fletcher (eds.). Publishing Sciences Group, Inc., Acton, MA, 1974, pp. 78-91.

189. Shils, M. E.: Minerals. in Total Parenteral Nutrition. Symposium on Total Parenteral Nutrition, Nashville, Tenn., 1972. P. L. White, M. E. Nagy, and D. C. Fletcher (eds.). Publishing Sciences Group, Inc., Acton, MA, 1974, pp. 92-113.

190. Cahill, G.: Carbohydrates. in Total Parenteral Nutrition. Symposium on Total Parenteral Nutrition, Nashville, Tenn., 1972. P. L. White, M. E. Nagy, and D. C. Fletcher (eds.). Publishing Sciences Group, Inc., Acton, MA, 1974, pp. 45-51.

191. Dudrick, S. J., B. U. MacFadyen, C. T. VanBuren, R. L. Roberg, and A. J. Maynard: Parenteral hyperalimentation, metabolic problems and solutions. Ann Surg 176:259-264, 1972.

192. Freund, H., S. Atamian and J. E. Fischer: Chromium deficiency during total parenteral nutrition. JAMA 241:496-498, 1979.

193. Ryan, J. A., Jr.: Complications of total parenteral nutrition. in Total Parenteral Nutrition. J. E. Fischer (ed.). Little, Brown and Co., Boston, 1976, pp. 50-100.

194. Postuma, R. and C. L. Trevenen: Liver disease in infants receiving total parenteral nutrition. Pediatrics 63:110-115, 1979.

195. Weinsier, R. L. and C. L. Krumdieck: Death resulting from overzealous to-
      tal parenteral nutrition: The refeeding syndrome revisited.   Am J Clin Nutr
      34:393-399, 1980.

196. Richard, F.C., R.W. Beart, Jr., S. Berkner, D.B. McGill, and R. Gaf-
      fron: Home parenteral nutrition for management of the severely malnour-
      ished adult patient. Gastroenterology 79:11, 1980.

7

IMMUNOLOGICAL ASPECTS OF THE
GASTROINTESTINAL TRACT

Mervin Silverberg, M.D.

The intestinal tract is one of the main interfaces between the external and internal body environments. Therefore, a vital discriminatory function is necessary to develop mechanisms for handling the large variety of potential penetrating substances, which include bacteria, viruses, toxins, and food antigens.

IMMUNOLOGICAL DEFENSES

Throughout the gut in a subepithelial location, there are abundant lymphoid and plasma cells both in isolated and in aggregate forms, e.g., lymph follicles, Peyer patches (Fig. 1), and the appendix, i.e., gut-associated lymphoid tissues (GALT). Peyer patches and isolated lymph nodules can be identified in the lamina propria throughout the small intestine along the antimesenteric border, the former being most abundant in the terminal ileum. Peyer patches usually contain at least five lymph follicles and increase in number of follicles and number of patches with age, up to puberty, when the reverse process sets in. The surface epithelium overlying the nodules and patches differs from that found on adjacent villi and crypts, i.e., nuclei are not basal, goblet cells are sparse, and intraepithelial lymphocytes are common (Figs. 2, 3). The appendix in man seems to function immunologically as a large Peyer patch. All of these tissues presumably act as a peripheral lymphoid organ, since attempts to relate them to the avian bursa of Fabricius have been unsuccessful.

Additionally, the mesenteric lymph nodes receive and process antigenic material from the bowel, and large numbers of free cells mainly in the lamina propria throughout the intestine, are engaged in the body's immune responses. These include lymphocytes, plasma cells, macrophages, mast cells, eosinophils, and polymorphonuclear leukocytes.

Two main processes represent the major defense mechanisms uniquely adapted to the gastrointestinal tract.

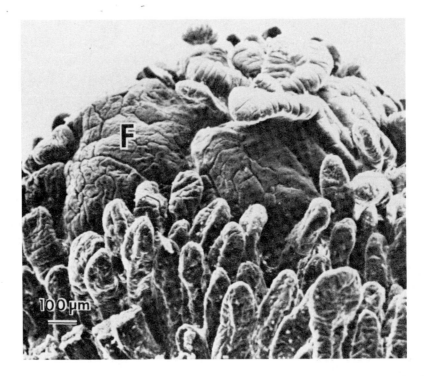

FIGURE 1   Scanning electron micrograph revealing a single Peyer patch, lymphoid follicle which protrudes among finger-shaped villi in the human ileum. (From Ref. 40. Reprinted with permission.)

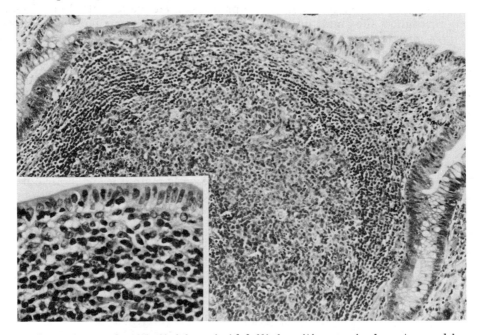

FIGURE 2   Ileum-subepithelial lymphoid follicle with germinal center and lymphoid mantle. Insert—surface epithelium above lymphoid follicle without goblet cells and irregular nuclei. Hematoxylin-eosin stain. Original magnification x306. (Courtesy of Dr. Ellen Kahn.)

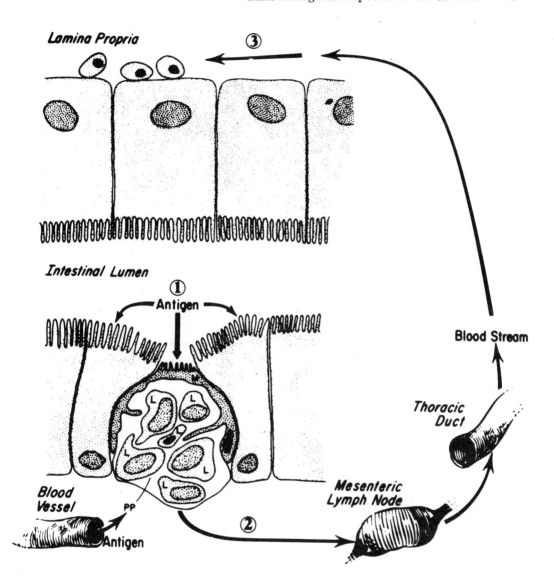

FIGURE 3   Schematic representation of the cell cycle for IgA-producing plasma cells populating the intestinal mucosa. Lymphocytes (L) within gut-associated lymphoid tissues (GALT), particularly Peyer's patches (PP) of the ileum, are stimulated by antigens entering from the intestinal lumen ① via specialized membrane like cells (M), across conventional absorptive cells or from the systemic circulation. Lymphoblasts migrate to mesenteric nodes for further maturation ② and then enter the systemic circulation as plasmablasts to redistribute along intestinal mucosal surfaces ③ and produce secretory IgA antibodies in response to intestinally absorbed antigens. Homing of committed IgA-producing lymphoblasts to the mammary gland provides the breast-fed baby with mucosal protection against many antigens and bacteria. (Reprinted with permission, Ref. 40.)

TABLE 1   Immunoglobulins

Class	Heavy Chain	Mol. Wt. (Daltons)	Placental Transfer	Comments	Probable Mechanism of Action
IgA	α	160,000	–	2 Subclasses, IgA$_1$ predominant; 1-3 monomers	Coating foreign antigens
S-IgA	α	395,000	–	Dimeric form; secretory component-60,000 daltons; joining piece-15,000 daltons	Sequestration of foreign antigens
IgD	δ	180,000	–	Monomeric form, no subclasses	? Important in newborns
IgE	ε	180,000	–	Monomeric form, no subclasses	Antibody-dependent cell-mediated cytotoxicity
IgG	γ	150,000	+	Monomeric form, 4 sub-classes, IgG$_1$ predominant	Complement activation, opsonization, antibody-dependent cell-mediated cytotoxicity
IgM	μ	900,000	–	Pentameric form with joining and secretory component	Same as IgG + coating antigens

IMMUNOGLOBULINS OR
LOCAL IMMUNITY (TABLE 1)

The predominant immunoglobulin in all intestinal secretions is immunoglobulin A (IgA) with immunoglobulin M (IgM) a distant second. This corresponds to immunofluorescent studies of immunoglobulin-bearing cells in the subepithelial layers that show a ratio of IgA/IgM/IgG/IgE of 20:3: 1:0.5.

Most of the IgA in secretions is in the secretory dimeric form, i.e., consists of two monomeric IgA molecules linked by a J chain of polypeptides, also produced by mucosal cells, and coupled with a glycoprotein carrier, the secretory component (Fig. 4). The dimeric IgA and J piece are produced in local plasma cells and then released into the interstitial tissues of the lamina propria near the crypts of Lieberkuhn. Here they diffuse into the epithelial cell where they link up with locally produced secretory component. The secretory-IgA (S-IgA) is released into the lumen by reverse pinocytosis and in this form is capable of complexing with antigens and is resistant to proteolysis. Additionally, S-IgA has been shown to interfere with the adherence of toxins and bacteria (1, 2) to microvillar receptor sites, and to prevent the uptake of inert antigenic macromolecules into the enterocyte (Fig. 5). S-IgA, found in bile, probably plays an important role in the local gut immunity, as well.

Immunoglobulin M in secretions is also in polymeric form linked to a secretory component, with a similar secretory process. Immunoglobulin D, IgE, and IgG normally appear in much smaller concentrations in secretions in monomeric forms.

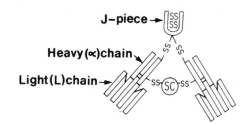

SECRETORY IgA

FIGURE 4   Structural mode of dimeric secretory IgA. The U-shaped chain is the joining piece common to all polymeric immunoglobulins. SC is the secretory component and the disulfide bonds (-S-S-) of the monomeric units are indicated by lines between the chains.

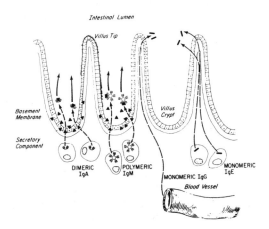

FIGURE 5   Schematic representation of local immunoglobulin defense processes.

Immunoglobulin D, IgE and IgG, like other intraluminal proteins, are secreted at the villous tips, and reach protective levels only with inflammation or hypersensitivity.

The newborn infant has an underdeveloped secretory immunoglobulin system. With antigenic stimulation by food and microorganisms, the S-IgA response develops rapidly. At 1 month of age almost all infants have demonstrable S-IgA. The preterm infant is even more compromised and is transiently more vulnerable to intestinal penetration.

CELL-MEDIATED IMMUNITY

Special lymphocytes from the thymus, called T cells, are responsible for cell-mediated immunity, and they migrate to peripheral lymphoid tissue everywhere in the body, including the gut. The T cells have a variety of functions, including (1) interaction with B lymphocytes by either helping or suppressing the antibody responses, (2) differentiation into and interaction with cells that are able to kill host cells that have changes on their surface, i. e. , "killer" or K cells, (3) becoming long-term memory cells and (4) production of lymphokines, which can mediate a number of biological activities.

Other factors that are important in cell-mediated immunity include monocytes, macrophages, "null" lymphocytes, and eosinophils.

The exact role all these agents play in protecting the bowel or causing disease is only now being studied. They probably will be found to participate in disorders such as food allergies, gluten-induced enteropathy, and various infectious diseases, particularly of parasitic origin.

NONIMMUNOLOGICAL DEFENSES

A number of nonspecific factors play an important role in controlling the intraluminal antigenic challenge during normal and disease states.

NORMAL INTESTINAL FLORA

The normal intraluminal microorganisms act to keep the balance and prevent overgrowth within relatively narrow limits. For example, short-chain fatty acids produced by colonic bacteria prevent colonization by Salmonella and Shigella species. The newborn gut is rapidly colonized by various organisms depending on dietary and sanitary factors. The proximal gastrointestinal tract, by the age of 1 month, contains facultative gram-positive organisms of less than 10^5/ml of intestinal aspirate. The distal ileum and colon have aerobic coliforms and anaerobic bacteroids in concentrations in excess of 10^9/ml of intestinal fluid.

INTESTINAL SECRETIONS

Numerous factors in saliva, gastric juice, bile, and succus entericus interfere with microorganisms or antigen penetration of the mucosal barrier. Glycoproteins (3) in saliva and in the glycocalix coating the epithelial surfaces of the absorptive cells, inhibit bacterial adherence to receptor sites. The same substances may interact with other antigens preventing them from moving across the mucosal epithelium. Lysozyme combined with complement and specific S-IgA, can control bacterial proliferation. Gastric secretions, particularly hydrochloric acid, appear to play a major defense role, since in achlorhydria there is an increased absorption of macromolecules and an excessive number of gastrointestinal infections (4).

PERISTALTIC MOVEMENT

Peristalsis plays an important role in moving intestinal contents forward and thus reducing the time for the "antigenic mass" to challenge the mucosa. This is particularly important when receptor sites have been made unavailable by various competitive inhibitors, e.g., mucins and secretory antibodies. In the presence of bowel stasis syndromes, bacterial overgrowth is common with considerable disruption of local defense barriers.

GASTROINTESTINAL ALLERGIC DISORDERS

Sensitization of the gastrointestinal tract to dietary proteins is relatively infrequent, despite the fact that up to late infancy the child absorbs intact macromolecules and is therefore at risk for subsequent challenges (5). Predisposing circumstances such as a familial atopic background, other protein intolerance, gastroenteritis, and malnutrition presumably play some role. The exact mechanisms of action of these disorders are not completely understood.

COW'S MILK PROTEIN-SENSITIVE
ENTEROPATHY (CMPSE) (Also see Chap. 15)

Clinical reactions following the ingestion of bovine proteins, i.e., milk, other dairy products, beef, and veal, have been described for about a century. Most of the examples have been anecdotal and often were unproven guilt-by-association. The major clinical reaction involves: (1) the respiratory tract—upper respiratory infections, asthma, pneumonia; (2) skin eczema and hives; (3) the intestinal tract (see later). Unproven causal relationships have been claimed for colic, irritability, hyperkinesis, tension-fatigue, and learning disabilities. Less critical estimates claim an incidence of these disorders up to 7% in the pediatric population, although values around 2% are probably more accurate. The risk is highest for infants with previous atopic disease, with IgA deficiency, or with a family history of milk allergy. Infants who have been breast-fed since birth appear to be less susceptible, however, this is still controversial.

Of the more than 22 different proteins in cow's milk, beta-lactoglobulin appears to be most antigenic, followed in order by alpha- and beta-casein, alpha-lactalbumin, and bovine serum albumin (6). Only the latter is heat labile and reactions to it do not appear until after the infant stops drinking proprietary formulas. Immune complexes have been implicated as the presumed, but not proven, mechanism of the underlying reaction for many of the gastrointestinal complaints.

CLINICAL FEATURES

Various alleged clinical syndromes have been described, although many are unproved. Most of the patients develop signs within the first 6 months of life, the majority affecting extraintestinal systems (Table 2).

A variety of gastrointestinal disturbances have been attributed to CMPSE.

Diarrhea

Diarrhea with or without gross blood has been noted in 25-75% of these cases (7). It is usually found in younger infants, and the stools may vary from soft to very watery with gross or occult blood and often containing mucus. The latter colitislike picture is occasionally associated with shock and prostration, and the rectal mucosa is grossly and histologically indistinguishable from the nonspecific ulcerative colitis

TABLE 2   Alleged Association Between Cow's Milk Protein-Sensitive Enteropathy and Clinical Manifestations

Gastrointestinal Manifestations	Respiratory Manifestations
Vomiting	Rhinitis
Abdominal pain	Chronic cough
Diarrhea	Bronchitis
Steatorrhea	Asthma
Malabsorption	Recurrent pneumonia
Intestinal bleeding	Pulmonary hemosiderosis
gross	Upper airway obstruction
occult	Serous otitis media
Protein-losing enteropathy	
Enterocolitis	Dermatologic Manifestations
Ulcerative colitis	
Constipation	Atopic dermatitis
Proctalgia	Urticaria
Refusal of milk	Angioedema
Stomatitis	Seborrheic rashes
	Contact rash
Hematologic Manifestations	Perianal rash
	Purpura
Anemia	Dermatitis herpetiformis
Hypoproteinemia	
Thrombocytopenia	Cardiovascular Manifestations
Eosinophilia	
	Anaphylactic shock
Central Nervous System Manifestations	Coronary heart disease
Allergic Tension-Fatigue Syndrome	Cor pulmonale
	Cardiac arrhythmias
Urinary Manifestations	
	Miscellaneous Manifestations
Enuresis	
Cystitis	Failure to thrive
Orthostatic albuminuria	Sudden infant death syndrome
Nephrotic syndrome	Infantile cortical hyperostosis
	Ocular allergy

seen in older children. Diarrhea may be intermittent or sufficiently prolonged to be associated with failure to thrive, dehydration, or malnutrition.

Vomiting

Vomiting is relatively common, and may be the presenting complaint, particularly when associated with an anaphylactoid reaction. It usually occurs within an hour after ingestion, and not infrequently it is reported to be projectile in nature (8).

Abdominal Pain

Abdominal pain may be noted in one-third of the patients (9, 10). The pains vary from mild and vague to severe colic, usually occurring during or shortly after the feeding. The location is variable. Occasionally, the clinical picture may be confused with an intussusception.

Iron Deficiency Anemia (Wilson-Lahey Syndrome) (11, 12)

Iron deficiency anemia involves prolonged occult blood loss, usually with minimum alteration of bowel habits, and may lead to iron deficiency anemia. Some of these patients have hypoproteinemia as well, including the copper and iron-carrying serum proteins ceruloplasmin and transferrin, respectively. It occurs most commonly from 6-12 months of life. Many of these infants improved on boiled or evaporated milk. Fecal losses may reach 5-10 ml/day, determined by infusing ^{51}Cr-labeled autologous red blood cells and measuring the radioactivity appearing in the stools.

Allergic Gastroenteropathy (13)

Allergic gastroenteropathy is a rare hypersensitivity syndrome with the intestinal tract as the "shock organ" presenting with edema, usually periorbital at first, iron deficiency anemia, failure to thrive, and minimal to mild diarrhea. An atopic history will be uncovered in the family or in the patient, although many will not develop atopic features until they are older. Hematocrits as low as 10% have been recorded in association with the chronic loss of iron into the gastrointestinal tract, both as blood and bound to transferrin. Peripheral eosinophilia may be as high as 50% of blood leukocytes with extensive infiltration of eosinophils into the mucosa throughout the gastrointestinal tract. Extrusion of sufficient eosinophils into the lumen may be demonstrated by a Hansel stain. Charcot-Leyden crystals may be seen in fresh stool smears. There is usually a panhypoproteinemia and the low serum albumin and anemia may combine to cause cardiac decompensation. In one report, the putative protein was proved to be beta-lactoglobulin.

Celiac-Sprue Syndrome

Celiac-sprue syndrome is both a transient and typical long-standing intolerance to gluten and has been reported to be etiologically related to "milk allergy." Patients with this syndrome usually are affected more severely by diarrhea and poor weight gain and may not manifest spruelike signs until 2 years after the onset of the milk protein sensitivity (14).

Nutriment Malabsorption

Both steatorrhea and lactose intolerance have been reported after the administration of whole milk. Steatorrhea was noted following as little as 8 mg of beta-lactoglobulin (15). The role of rapid transit is unclear; however, rapid passage through the small intestine has been documented in these patients following milk ingestion.

DIAGNOSIS

Although presumed to have an immunological basis, there are no reproducible tests of immunological dysfunction that have been of diagnostic value. The demonstration of circulating antibodies of various types (5) has not been helpful, since up to 95% of controls have similar findings within the first 2 years of life. The use of the more specific radioallergosorbent test (RAST) to demonstrate IgE-related antibodies has not improved the value of circulating antibody studies. A drop in C_3 complement following a milk challenge involved only five patients, and has never been corroborated by other investigators (16). IgA antibodies to milk protein are found in the stool of these patients; however, these coproantibodies also have been shown in normal nonsensitized children (17).

    The problem was first critically appraised by the establishment of clinical "Goldman criteria " (18). The clinical impression is confirmed, following the development of similar adverse reactions repeated on three separate occasions, within 48 hours of challenge with up to 100 ml of reconstituted powdered skim milk. Lactose intolerance should be excluded before the initial challenge. A recent modification of the challenge test accepts a reaction to single administration, after a 1-month period on a hypoallergenic diet. If diarrhea ensues, a Wright stain of the stool should reveal both erythrocytes and leukocytes (19). In patients who are thought to be very sensitive, the initial challenge should involve no more than 5 ml milk with hourly increments up to 120 ml in 6 hours, to avoid an anaphylactoid reaction.

Histological changes can be demonstrated with a milk challenge. Within 12 hours, the lamina propria will be irregularly infiltrated by eosinophils, neutrophils, plasma cells, and mast cells. The plasma cells have been shown to stain for IgE, and mast cells may be degranulated (20).

TREATMENT

The elimination of milk and dairy products from the diet will correct the clinical abnormalities in almost all patients within 72 hours. In rare cases of allergic gastroenteropathy, the peripheral eosinophilia persists until beef and veal are likewise withdrawn. If the response is poor after 1 week of dietary manipulations, other factors or diagnoses should be sought, e.g., sensitization to other proteins such as soy and gluten. Soy-based formulas are usually ideal milk substitutes, except with combined sensitivities. Goat's milk is not appropriate since there is cross-reactivity between human and goat lactoglobulin. Most of these children can tolerate the reintroduction of bovine products within 2 years of the onset of the hypersensitivity. The remainder react normally by the time they enter school. Predigested formulas, e.g., Pregestamil, or elemental formulas, e.g., Vivonex, may be necessary under special circumstances, although their high osmolarity may aggravate diarrhea and cause abdominal discomfort. Those patients with iron deficiency will not respond to iron therapy without dietary restrictions, as well. If iron administration alone successfully treats the anemia, the patient probably has a primary iron deficiency with secondary involvement of the intestinal mucosa, which allegedly may simulate allergic gastroenteropathy.

SOY PROTEIN-SENSITIVE ENTEROPATHY

Soy protein-sensitive enteropathy has been well documented in children with a clinical picture indistinguishable from the more common, and occasionally coincident bovine protein allergy. The presence of gross or occult blood in the stools is relatively common (21).

EOSINOPHILIC GASTROENTERITIS (22)

Eosinophilic gastroenteritis is an unusual clinical syndrome found mainly in older children and adults. An allergic diathesis, particularly food allergy, has been considered as the most likely cause. Unfortunately, there is weak evidence to support this theory, although many patients have been atopic.

CLINICAL FEATURES

Most patients present with abdominal pain, intermittent diarrhea, and vomiting. Protein-losing enteropathy, iron deficiency anemia, and steatorrhea are common.

Radiographic studies reveal narrowing of the lumen involving the gastric antrum, proximal small intestine, esophagus, and colon, in order of frequency (23). There is usually significant elevation of eosinophils and occasionally IgE, in the peripheral blood, and intestinal biopsies reveal eosinophilic infiltrations of one or more of the bowel layers—particularly in the narrowed segments. In the rare case, when the serosal surface is involved, eosinophilic ascites may develop.

TREATMENT

If an offending food is implicated, this should be avoided. Usually, even a meticulous elimination diet is not successful, and corticosteroids are required, in either a 2-week or prolonged course, with alternate day therapy.

PRIMARY IMMUNODEFICIENCY SYNDROMES AFFECTING THE GASTROINTESTINAL TRACT

Although respiratory infections represent the most serious clinical problems in primary immunodeficiency syndromes (PIDS), gastrointestinal disorders are very common. Indeed, in children, intestinal dysfunction may be the presenting complaint. The list of PIDS and the putative defects are noted in Table 3. The diseases are heterogeneous and affect B and T lymphocytes. Frequent and/or severe infections by bacteria, viruses, and fungi are not unusual. Gastrointestinal signs and symptoms, in order of frequency, include chronic diarrhea, Giardia lamblia infestation, malabsorption, chronic vomiting, lactose intolerance, other disaccharide intolerances, vitamin B_{12} malabsorption, protein-losing enteropathy, atypical colitis, and malignancies.

B LYMPHOCYTE DEFECTS

Infantile X-Linked Agammaglobulinemia

Very low values of all immunoglobulins in a male child are associated, in this condition, with complete absence of plasma cells throughout the body, including the gastrointestinal tract. Bowel complaints are rare. Giardiasis is uncommon (24) compared to that found in common variable hypogammaglobulinemia. Although bacterial overgrowth has been noted in duodenal aspirates, no related clinical manifestations have been reported. Pseudomembranous colitis associated with Clostridium difficile has been noted following antibiotic therapy.

IgA Defects

Selective IgA deficiency is a relatively common finding, occurring in as many as 1:700 persons (25). The majority of these individuals do not suffer any adverse effects, despite the widespread reduction of IgA-containing plasma cells throughout the gut. This depletion involves mainly subclass IgA_1.

In those patients who are symptomatic, diarrhea, steatorrhea, food intolerances, nodular lymphoid hyperplasia, and giardiasis may be found in one combination or another. Subtotal villous atrophy and a dramatic response to a gluten-free diet has been reported in some of these patients. A secretory component defect has been found in an adolescent with absence of secretory IgA in the presence of normal serum IgA (26). The association of isolated IgA deficiency with circulating food antibodies, lactose intolerance, and inflammatory bowel disease is greater than would be expected by chance alone.

A compensatory proliferation of IgM-producing plasma cells and a complement of subclass IgA_2 have been noted in intestinal biopsies (27).

Intestinal nodular lymphoid hyperplasia (NLH). In the absence of IgA, with or without other immunoglobulin deficiencies, lymphoid nodules throughout the small

TABLE 3   Immunodeficiencies Affecting the Gastrointestinal Tract

Abnormality	GI Disorders	Presumed Cell Defect		
		B Cell	T Cell	Stem Cell
1. Primary Immunodeficiency				
a) Infantile X-linked agammaglobulinemia	– Malabsorption; diarrhea; giardiasis	+		
b) Selective IgA deficiency	– Celiac-sprue, giardiasis, malabsorption, diarrhea, Crohn disease, nodular lymphoid hyperplasia (NLH), pernicious anemia	+		
c) Secretory IgA deficiency	– Intestinal moniliasis, aphthous ulcers	?		
d) Thymic hypoplasia (DiGeorge syndrome)	– Stomatitis and esophagitis due to herpes simplex, cytomegalovirus, and monilia		+	
e) X-linked immunodeficiency with hyper IgM	– GI malignancy, NLH, diarrhea	+	?	
f) Severe combined immunodeficiency	– Diarrhea (occasionally intractable and bloody), salmonellosis, shigellosis; malabsorption, disaccharidase deficiency, mucocutaneous candidiasis	+	+	+
g) Common variable hypogammaglobulinemia	– Diarrhea, giardiasis, NLH, atrophic gastritis, disaccharidase deficiency, malabsorption	+	+−	
h) Immunodeficiency with thrombocytopenia and eczema (Wiskott-Aldrich syndrome)	– Melena, diarrhea, reticulosis	+	+	
i) Immunodeficiency with ataxia telangiectasia	– Diarrhea, reticulosis	+	+	
j) Nezelof syndrome	– Chronic diarrhea	+	+	
2. Secondary Immunodeficiency				
a) Protein-losing enteropathy	– Intestinal lymphangiectasia, Whipple disease, celiac-sprue, giant gastric rugal hypertrophy, (Menetrier), inflammatory bowel disease, Hirschsprung disease, and allergic gastroenteropathy		+−	
b) Malnutrition	– Diarrhea, intestinal infections			
c) Immunosuppressive agents	– Diarrhea, intestinal infections			
3. Miscellaneous Immunodeficiency				
a) Alpha-chain disease	– Diarrhea, malabsorption, abdominal pain, Ca and Mg malabsorption, lymphoma			
b) Kappa-chain deficiency	– ? cystic fibrosis			
c) Chronic granulomatous disease	– Diarrhea, malabsorption, rectal inflammation, perianal fissures, esophageal or gastric outlet strictures			
d) Hyper IgE syndromes	– Ascariasis, visceral larva migrans, capillariasis			

and large intestine may become markedly enlarged (1-3 mm), primarily because of the increased size of the germinal centers (28). The large follicles distort the villi and can be visualized on x-ray and by fiberoptic endoscopy. About 75% or more of the patients harbor Giardia lamblia, and a significant number ultimately develop a gastrointestinal malignancy. Much less commonly, nonspecific colitis, Crohn disease, and protein-losing enteropathy have been noted.

T-LYMPHOCYTE DEFECTS

DiGeorge Syndrome or Thymic Hypoplasia

Although defective cell-mediated immunity is the main problem, other congenital abnormalities related to developmental disturbances of the third and fourth pharyngeal pouches often are prominent and may be the presenting problem. These include neonatal hypoparathyroidism and cardiovascular anomalies, particularly involving the great vessels. Gastrointestinal manifestations include tracheoesophageal malformations, chronic diarrhea, malabsorption and intestinal moniliasis.

B- AND T-LYMPHOCYTE DEFECTS

Severe Combined Immunodeficiency

Hereditary severe deficiencies of B and T lymphocytes may be of both autosomal recessive or X-linked varieties. Adenosine deaminase is frequently deficient in circulating red and white blood cells in the recessive type and this may be a useful marker.

The consequences of severe deficiencies of B- and T-cell function, mainly found in young infants, are resistant, recurrent infections of all types, particularly, mucocutaneous candidiasis, as well as diarrhea and malabsorption. Resistant infections with Salmonella, cytomegalovirus, and Pneumocystis carinii are common (29). The mortality has been high; however, the recent use of bone marrow, thymus, or fetal liver transplants has restored some degree of immunocompetence in selected patients. Unfortunately, the occurrence of graft-vs-host reactions has been unusually frequent in these transplanted cases.

Common Variable (Acquired) Hypogammaglobulinemia

Most cases of immunodeficiency fit into this category, which involves many combinations of immunoglobulin deficiencies. Most patients have normal amounts of B and T lymphocytes in the peripheral blood. Tissue plasma cells are decreased in number. The basic defect(s) is possible due to immature function or excessive T-cell suppression.

Cases may be sporadic or follow an autosomal recessive mode of inheritance. Familial cases of autoimmune disorders are common. Some patients additionally have T-cell function deficits of variable severity, and about half of them eventually develop pernicious anemia, beginning in the second decade or later. Biopsy of the gastric mucosa reveals a loss of parietal and chief cells, as well as an infiltration of mononuclear cells without plasma cells. Giardiasis is common and may account for some vitamin B_{12} malabsorption. About two-thirds of the patients have diarrhea and malabsorption. Bacterial overgrowth in the proximal intestine occurs in the majority of cases; however, the signs and symptoms usually do not subside with antimicrobial therapy. Although intestinal malignancies involving any part of the bowel occur with increased frequency in young adults, they have never been reported in the pediatric age group.

Wiskott-Aldrich Syndrome

This X-linked disorder, with occasional sporadic cases, is characterized by eczema, thrombocytopenia, a bleeding tendency, and recurrent infections. Bloody diarrhea is relatively frequent with occasional reports of cases of malabsorption and mild pernicious anemia (30).

Various B cell disturbances have been noted, the most common being elevated IgE and decreased IgM. Impaired cell-mediated immunity appears to develop with time.

Ataxia-Telangiectasia

In this autosomal-recessive condition, the patients have deficient cell-mediated immunity and about half the patients develop IgA and IgE deficiency. Progressive cerebellar ataxia occurs from infancy, and the telangiectatic lesions are noted a few years later. Gastrointestinal symptoms are infrequent, except for occasional mild generalized malabsorption and a selective malabsorption of vitamin B_{12}. Most of the plasma cells in the lamina propria are IgM producing (31).

Nezelof Syndrome

This syndrome is characterized by a severe defect in cell-mediated immunity and B cell deficiency of varying degrees. Thymic hypoplasia, and hepatosplenomegaly and generalized lymphadenopathy usually are found. Gastrointestinal manifestations usually are found, and are like the cases with severe combined immunodeficiency, particularly involving nutriment malabsorption, enterocolitis, and intestinal candidiasis. Exceedingly high serum IgE values have been noted in some patients.

PROTEIN-LOSING ENTEROPATHY (Also see Chap. 18)

The presence of persistently ectatic intestinal lymphatics may be a primary condition, or may be secondary to a proximal obstruction of lymph flow. This usually is associated with a protein-losing enteropathy, and often a loss of lymphocytes which may result in an impaired cell-mediated immunity (see Table 3).

IMMUNOLOGIC ASPECTS OF GLUTEN-SENSITIVE ENTEROPATHY (CELIAC-SPRUE) (Also see Chap. 15)

Gluten-sensitive enteropathy (GSE) is a small-intestinal mucosal disease induced by the gliadin alcohol-soluble fraction of wheat gluten, in an unknown manner. This occurs in about 1:3000 persons in the United States, and with greater frequency in Great Britain. Initial interest in immunological factors centered around the finding of gluten antibodies in both serum and intestinal secretions. In untreated patients, serum IgA often is elevated and IgM frequently is decreased. These values revert to normal with successful dietary avoidance of gluten-containing foods. With gluten challenge immunoglobulin and complement are deposited in the basement membrane under the epithelial cells (32). Tissue organ culture techniques suggest that a humeral factor from damaged mucosa can cause the typical changes in susceptible mucosa (33). The mucosa from genetically predisposed individuals, particularly with the histocompatibility type HLA-B8, are most likely to develop an adverse reaction to gluten challenge (34).

IgA deficient persons (35) and patients with dermatitis herpetiformis (36), have an increased incidence of GSE. Additionally, some patients have developed severe ulcerative patchy lesions of the jejunum as well as the typical villous abnormalities;

others have an increased incidence of primary lymphomas (37). The latter may be the presenting manifestation of intestinal disease, and the patients are only subsequently shown to have GSE by the presence of atypical histology of the adjacent mucosa.

CHRONIC INFLAMMATORY BOWEL DISEASE (Also see Chap. 16)

A great deal of effort and paper has been spent in trying to define an immunological basis for the pathogenesis of both ulcerative colitis and Crohn disease. Unfortunately, the results have been either conflicting or inconclusive, and the various immunological phenomena demonstrated in these patients fail to resolve the etiological quandry (38).

PERNICIOUS ANEMIA

Although the predominant clinical features are hematological, pernicious anemia is truly a gastric autoimmune disorder, i.e., serum antibodies to parietal cells and intrinsic factor, and extensive lymphocytic infiltration of the stomach wall. The typical adult type of pernicious anemia rarely occurs in the pediatric age group. Most cases are of the juvenile type, i.e., congenital intrinsic factor defect. Others have coexistent primary immune deficiency (39) or familial juvenile polyendocrinopathy.

REFERENCES

1. Fubara, E.S. and R. Freter: Source and protective function of coproantibodies in intestinal disease. Am J Clin Nutr 25:137, 1972.

2. Williams, R. C. and R. J. Gibbons: Inhibition of bacterial adherence by secretory immunoglobulin A: A mechanism of antigen disposal. Science 177:197, 1972.

3. Gibbons, R.J. and J. van Houte: Bacterial adherence in oral microbial ecology. Ann Rev Microbiol 29:19, 1975.

4. Kraft, S.C., R.M. Rothberg, C.M. Kramer, A.C. Svoboda, L.S. Monroe, and R.S. Farr: Gastric output and circulating antibovine serum albumin in adults. Clin Exp Immunol 2:321, 1967.

5. Walker, W.A. and K.J. Isselbacher: Uptake and transport of macromolecules by the intestine: Possible role in clinical disorders. Gastroenterology 67:531, 1975.

6. Fallstrom, S.P., S. Ahlstedt, and L.A. Hanson: Specific antibodies in infants with gastrointestinal intolerance to cow's milk protein. Int Arch Allergy Appl Immunol 56:97, 1978.

7. Gryboski, J.D.: Gastrointestinal milk allergy in infants. Pediatrics 40:354, 1967.

8. Lebenthal, E.: Cow's milk protein allergy. Pediatr Clin N Am 22:827, 1975.

9. Clein, N.W.: Cow's milk allergy in infants. Pediatr Clin N Am 4:949, 1954.

10. Gerrard, J.W., J.W.A. MacKenzie, N. Goluboff, et al.: Cow's milk allergy: Prevalence and manifestations in an unselected series of newborns. Acta Pediatr Scand 234 (suppl):1, 1973.

11. Wilson, J. F., D. C. Heiner, and M. E. Lahey: Studies on iron metabolism. IV. Milk induced gastrointestinal bleeding in infants with hypochromic microcytic anemia. JAMA 189:568, 1964.

12. Wilson, J. F., M. E. Lahey, and D. C. Heiner: Studies on iron metabolism. V. Further observations on cow's milk induced gastrointestinal bleeding in infants with iron deficiency anemia. J Pediatr 84:335, 1974.

13. Waldmann, T. A., R. D. Wochner, L. Laster, et al.: Allergic gastroenteropathy: A cause of excessive gastrointestinal protein loss. N Engl J Med 276:761, 1967.

14. Gryboski, J. D., J. Katz, D. Reynolds, and T. Herskovic: Gluten intolerance following cow's milk sensitivity to milk and wheat proteins. Ann Allergy 26:33, 1968.

15. Davidson, M., R. C. Burnstine, M. M. Kugler, et al.: Malabsorption defect induced by ingestion of beta-lactoglobulin. J Pediatr 66:545, 1965.

16. Matthew, T. S. and J. F. Soothill: Complement activation after milk feeding in children with cow's milk allergy. Lancet 2:893, 1970.

17. Davis, S. D., C. W. Bierman, W. E. Peirson, et al.: Clinical non-specificity of milk coproantibodies in diarrheal stools. N Engl J Med 282:612, 1970

18. Goldmon, A. S., D. W. Anderson, Jr., W. A. Sellers, et al.: Milk allergy. 1. Oral challenge with milk and isolated milk proteins in allergic children. Pediatrics 32:425, 1963.

19. Powell, G. K.: Milk and soy induced enterocolitis of infancy. Clinical features and standardization of challenge. J Pediatr 93:553, 1978.

20. Shiner, M., J. Ballad, C. G. D. Brook, et al.: Intestinal biopsy in the diagnosis of cow's milk protein intolerance without acute symptoms. Lancet 2:1060, 1975.

21. Halpin, T. C., W. J. Byrne, and M. E. Ament: Colitis, persistent diarrhea, and soy protein intolerance. J Pediatr 91:404, 1977.

22. Klein, N. C., L. Hargrove, M. H. Sleisenger, and G. H. Jeffries: Eosinophilic gastroenteritis. Medicine 49:299, 1970.

23. Caldwell, J. H., S. H. Mekhjian, P. E. Hurtubise, and F. M. Beman: Eosinophilic gastroenteritis with obstruction: Immunological studies of seven patients. Gastroenterology 74:825, 1978.

24. Ochs, H. D., M. E. Ament, and S. D. Davis: Giardiasis with malabsorption in X-linked agammaglobulinemia. N Engl J Med 287:341, 1972.

25. Ammann, A. J. and R. Hong: Selective IgA deficiency: Presentation of 30 cases and a review of the literature. Medicine 50:223, 1971.

26. Strober, W., R. Krakauer, H. L. Klaereman, H. Y. Reynolds, and D. L. Nelson: Secretory component deficiency. A disorder of the IgA system. N Engl J Med 294:351, 1976.

27. Andre, G. , F. Andre, and M. C. Fargier: Distribution of IgA$_1$ and IgA2 plasma cells in various normal human tissues and in the jejunum of plasma IgA-deficient patients. Clin Exp Immunol 33:327, 1978.

28. Heremans, P. E. , K. A. Huizinga, H. N. Hoffman, and A. L. Brown: Dysgammaglobulinemia associated with nodular lymphoid hyperplasia of the small intestine. Am J Med 40:78, 1966.

29. Ochs, H. D. and M. E. Ament: Gastrointestinal tract and immunodeficiency. in Immunologic Aspects of the Liver and Gastrointestinal Tract. A. Ferguson and R. N. M. McSween (eds.). MTP, Lancaster, 1976.

30. Ament, M. E. , H. D. Ochs, and D. D. Starkey: Structure and function of the gastrointestinal tract in primary immunodeficiency syndromes. A study of 39 patients. Medicine 52:227, 1973.

31. Eidelman, S. , and S. D. Davis: Immunoglobulin content of the intestinal mucosal plasma cells in ataxia-telangiectasia. Lancet 1:884, 1968.

32. Loeb, P. M. , W. Strober, Z. M. Falchuk, and L. Laster: Incorporation of leucine-14 C into immunoglobulins by jejunal biopsies of patients with celiac sprue and other gastrointestinal diseases. J Clin Invest 50:559, 1971.

33. Katz, A. J. , and A. M. Falchuk: Definitive diagnosis of gluten-sensitive enteropathy. Use of an in-vitro organ culture model. Gastroenterology 75:695, 1978.

34. Falchuk, Z. M. , G. N. Rogentine, and W. Strober: Predominance of histocompatibility antigen HLA B-8, in patients with gluten sensitive enteropathy. J. Clin Invest 51:1602, 1972.

35. Asquith, P., R. A. Thompson, and W. T. Cooke: Serum immunoglobulins in adult celiac disease. Lancet 2:129, 1969.

36. Scott, B. B. , S. Young, S. M. Rajah, J. Marks, and M. Losowsky: Celiac disease and dermatitis herpetiformis: Further studies of their relationship. Gut 17:759, 1976.

37. Freeman, H. J. , W. M. Weinstein, and T. K. Shnitka, et al. : Primary abdominal lymphoma. Presenting manifestations of celiac sprue or complicating dermatitis herpetiformis. Am J Med 63:585, 1977.

38. Sachar, D. B. , M. O. Auslander, and J. S. Walfish: Aetiological theories of inflammatory bowel disease. in Clinics in Gastroenterology. R. G. Farmer (ed.). W. B. Saunders, Ltd. 9:231, 1980.

39. Twomey, J. J. , P. H. Jordan, T. Jarrold, S. Trubowitz, N. D. Ritz, and H. O. Conn: The syndrome of immunoglobulin deficiency and pernicious anemia. A study of ten cases. Am J Med 47:340, 1969.

40. Walker, W. A., and K. J. Isselbacher: Intestinal antibodies. N Engl J Med 297:767, 1977.

8

NORMAL AND ABNORMAL GASTROINTESTINAL MOTILITY

Eugene Aronow, M.D. and Mervin Silverberg, M.D.

NORMAL GASTROINTESTINAL MOTILITY

INTRODUCTION

Physiological studies of gastrointestinal motility are found in the literature, but with the exception of esophageal and colonic conditions, precious little of this experimental data has been applied to the human condition.

In references to the pediatric sector, the clinical information is even less impressive. The main problem is the difficulty in placing tubes, balloons, and electrodes in infants and children, and leaving these instruments in place for extended periods of time without the use of heavy sedation. This has greatly restricted the ability to obtain both meaningful subjective and objective information from patients.

The gut has been described in terms of a biohydraulic system with the velocity of flow and the dimensions of the lumen dependent on the muscular wall movement (1). Movement is determined by the contractions of the three muscle coats of the gut, either rhythmic (consistent) or tonic (variable). Innervation of the striated muscle portions of the esophagus originates from the brain stem nuclei and are found in the ninth and tenth cranial nerves supplying the oropharynx and proximal one-third of the esophagus (2). Smooth muscle portions of the stomach, intestines, and the distal esophagus have primarily cholinergic innervation arising from intramural and submucosal plexuses (Fig. 1). Adrenergic innervation arises from sympathetic ganglia and possibly nonadrenergic inhibitory nerves. Sensory fibers responding to mechanical and chemical receptors are also present but are morphologically undetectable. Muscle membrane potential of the smooth muscle varies in each area of the gut; however, the resting potential is usually low and unstable, resulting in a regular slow-wave activity not associated with muscle contraction. Contraction is related to a rapid depolarization and a change in membrane potential.

This infinitely complex hydraulic propulsive system with its activity modified by an uninterrelated series of built-in locks, or sphincters, is continually and normally influenced by changes in nervous input and output, blood flow, and temperature, osmo-, chemo-, and baroreceptors, and hormonal sensitivity. The presence of systemic or localized disease adds yet another complicating factor in the study of motility of the gastrointestinal tract.

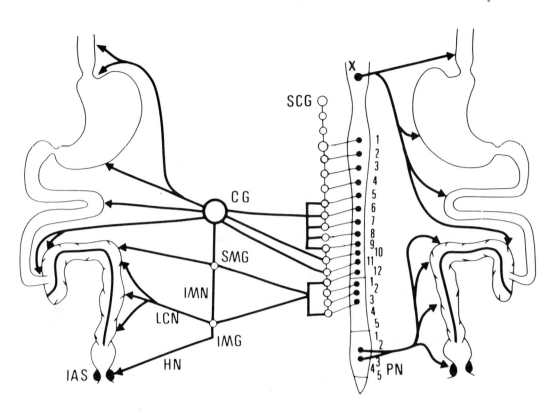

FIGURE 1   Schematic of the extrinsic efferent innervation of the gut.   The sympathetic innervation is represented on the left of the figure, the parasympathetic on
the right.   This representation is a synthesis of various data and may present variations according to different species.   (SCG) superior cervical ganglion; (CG) celiac
ganglion; (SMG) superior mesenteric ganglion; (IMG) inferior mesenteric ganglion;
(IMN) intermesenteric nerve; (LCN) lumbar colonic nerves; (HN) hypogastric nerves; (X) vagus dorsal motor nucleus and vagus nerve; (PN) pelvic nerves; (IAS) internal anal sphincter.   (From ref. 46.   Reprinted with permission.)

PHYSIOLOGY OF THE SWALLOWING MECHANISM
OF THE OROPHARYNX AND ESOPHAGUS

Although the fetus can swallow by the eleventh week, sucking and swallowing are
relatively inefficient during the first few days of life in the full-term infant, and for
about 2-3 weeks in the small premature infant.   At 35 weeks of gestation, the newborn makes weak sucking efforts and swallows in an incoordinate fashion.   With
"maturity," the sucking process consists of 10-30 consecutive sucks, with swallowing occurring during this period (3).   The liquid is kept in the mouth by the raised
posterior part of the tongue pressing on the soft palate.   With reflex closure of the
glottis, the tongue is lowered and the bolus of liquid or solid passes into the pharynx.   After 8 months of age, this reflex closure disappears and the infant must stop
sucking to breathe.   Air, present in the pharynx, is usually pushed ahead by the
bolus and both enter the esophagus to be swallowed.   The volume of air swallowed
may be equal to that of the liquid or solids.

Swallowing is an act initiated in the central nervous system reticular formation and coordinating nucleii of the trigeminal, facial, hypoglossal, and nucleus ambiguous nerve centers (Fig. 2). This activity is necessary for the pharyngeal component of swallowing. The upper esophageal sphincter (UES) and upper (striated muscle) portion of the esophagus receive innervation from both vagi and can function independently of the central nervous systems (2). Intrinsic muscular activity is of no importance in the contraction of the striated muscle portion of the esophagus. Areas of esophageal smooth muscle contract independently of the central nervous system's integrity, and lower esophageal sphincter (LES) tone apparently is not dependent on the vagal, hormonal, or central nervous systems. The UES is defined as mainly the striated cricopharyngeus muscle located posteriorly and attached to the cricopharyngeal cartilage, anteriorly; the resting pressure of 30-40 mmHg is sufficient to prevent free passage of air into the esophagus. Relaxation of the sphincter of 1- to 2-seconds duration occurs with presentation of a pharyngeal bolus to the sphincter area (Fig. 3). During the first 2-3 days of life, peristalsis to a great extent is nonpropagative, with many simultaneous contractions, and an extremely rapid peristaltic rate without any adverse effects on swallowing. With maturation, the body of the esophagus contracts with the swallowing or sudden distention, and the contraction then proceeds distally along the esophagus over 6-8 seconds, independent of gravity. The upper one-third, or skeletal muscle segment of the esophagus, is excited by vagal fibers. In the lower two-thirds of the smooth muscle esophageal segment, excitatory innervation is unknown. The LES encompasses the distal 3-4 cm of the esophagus in older children and is morphologically and histologically indistinguishable from the rest of the lower esophagus. There is a resting zone of high pressure, 20-30 mmHg, which relaxes upon initiation of a swallow. During the first 3-6 weeks of life, the infant has a relatively incompetent LES and the relaxation following deglutition is prolonged; regurgitation is common. Adult LES pressures are recorded at 3 months of life. Relaxation persists until the esophageal peristaltic wave traverses the length of the esophagus. Relaxation is mediated by an unknown intramural neuron-inhibitory neurotransmitter (4).

EVALUATION OF ESOPHAGEAL MOTILITY

The study of esophageal motor function has been accomplished by radiographic and intraluminal esophageal manometry. The former, with the added use of cineradiography, provides an accurate account of the sequential activity of swallowing, especially in the upper esophageal sphincter where muscular activity is more rapid and manometry is somewhat limited by technical factors. Manometry is presently performed with an assembly of polyvinyl tubes of varying number (see Fig. 3), continuously perfused with water by means of a hydraulic pump system at a rate to minimize system compliance and obtain accurate pressures (5). Pressures are recorded through strain gauge transducers and a suitable multichannel direct-writing recorder. The tube assembly is passed through the mouth or nose so that all side openings are within the stomach and the patient is in the supine or decubitus position. Respiration and swallowing activity may be recorded with a pneumograph and cervical myograph. Lower esophageal sphincter pressure is evaluated by either withdrawing the catheter openings through the LES by 1-cm increments, station pull-through techniques, or a rapid pull-through technique, withdrawing the tube at a rate of 0.5-1 cm/sec while the subject ceases breathing for 15-20 seconds (Fig. 4). The latter technique, without stopping respiration, is generally used in infants and younger children. Basal conditions are difficult to come by in the infant, and sedation will alter physiological responses. A recent tube-within-a-tube assembly may provide a better opportunity to study these infants (6). Since the LES pressure profile (as well as the UES) is radially asymmetrical, sequential station

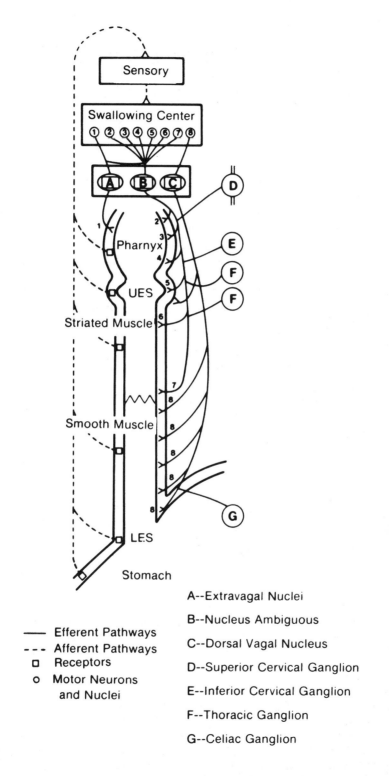

FIGURE 2   Neurological innervations of the esophagus. (From ref. 2. Reprinted with permission.)

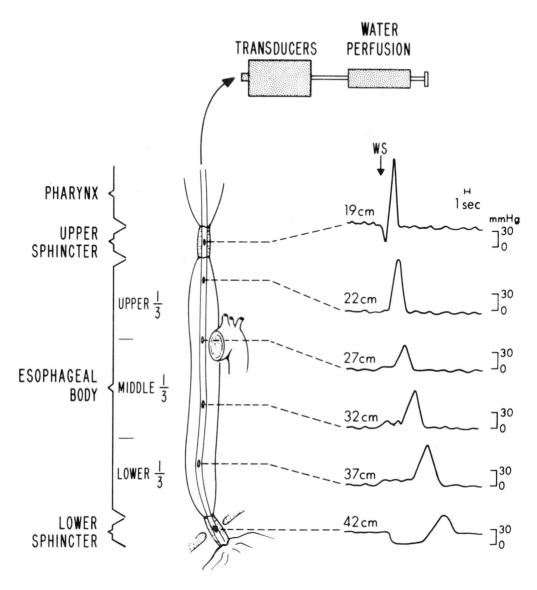

FIGURE 3   A schematic of the esophagus containing recording tube with side
openings at various distances from the incisors (in cm) and connected to individual transducers and perfusion pump. To the right of the figure a composite of the
pressure waves and resting pressure at various levels of the esophagus are noted.
Note the high resting pressures at the upper sphincter (UES) 30 mmHg, and at the
lower esophageal sphincter (LES) 20 mmHg.   At the initiation of a wet swallow (WS)
there is relaxation of the UES and LES pressures to intraesophageal and gastric
pressures, respectively. A peristaltic stripping wave of 40-60 mmHg proceeds distally along the body of the esophagus reaching the LES in 6-8 sec, as the LES
pressure returns to the resting level.   Note the contraction wave at the LES follow
ing relaxation.   There is a slightly lower amplitude in the contraction wave at the
level of the aortic arch, and the duration of the peristaltic wave increases at the
lower third of the body of the esophagus.

NORMAL RAPID PULL THROUGH

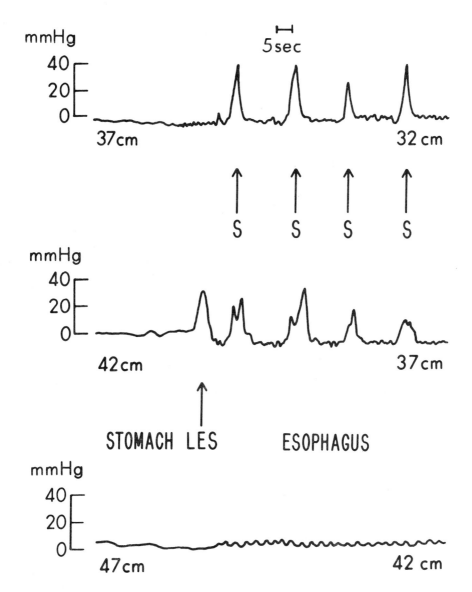

FIGURE 4   A record from a three tube assembly with side openings at 5 cm apart which is positioned with the most proximal opening intraesophageally (37 cm from the incisors) and the distal two openings intragastrically (42 and 47 cm). With respirations suspended, the middle opening is withdrawn from the stomach and through the LES into the esophagus to a (37 cm level).   At the level of the LES a 35 mmHg rise in pressure is noted.   Swallow(s) produce a peristaltic contraction wave in the intraesophageal recording sites.

pull-through and rapid pull-through pressure values of the LES vary in each tube opening, and either an average of the pressures or the lowest value may be used as the LES pressure. Resting LES pressure relaxes to gastric fundic pressure 1-2 seconds after initiation of the swallow in the oropharynx. Relaxation is maintained for 6-10 seconds or until the esophageal peristaltic wave reaches the LES. The other significant factor in resting LES pressure is the outer diameter of the catheter assembly. The larger the diameter of the tube assembly, the higher the LES pressure recorded. Normal resting LES pressure is 20-30 mmHg. This appears to be the normal value in children as well as adults (7-9).

Contractions in the body of the esophagus are measured with the tube assembly stationary following a single dry or wet swallow, since repetitive swallows may interrupt peristalsis. This makes evaluation of the body of the esophagus most difficult in children under 6-8 years of age. The peristaltic wave moves down the esophagus (more rapidly in the proximal esophagus) at a rate of 1-5 mm/sec. The amplitude of contraction is highest, and the duration of contraction shortest, in the proximal esophagus as opposed to the broader and lower pressure waves in the lower esophagus. The amplitude of the peristaltic wave varies from a high of 100 mmHg proximally, to 40 mmHg distally. Radial asymmetry of the UES is more pronounced than the LES, making an accurate measurement exceedingly difficult. Rapid longitudinal movements change the pressure during swallowing and breathing, and the high rate and volume of perfused fluids needed during manometry of the UES, add to the difficulty in obtaining meaningful and reproducible pressure readings. Resting UES pressure, averaging 80 mmHg in the anteroposterior plane, appears to be the present normal standard (10, 11). Relaxation to intraesophageal pressure occurs within 1 second of the arrival of the pharyngeal bolus.

All manometry values seem to be influenced by the rate of perfusion and the compliances of the tube and pump system. Compliance is affected mainly by the type of infusion pump. Until the equipment available to investigators achieves some uniformity, comparison of pressure values of different authors must be made with caution (5). Assessment of intraesophageal pH also is used in conjunction with manometry in both adults and children (12). A recording pH probe is placed in tandem with the esophageal manometry tube, or alone in the body of the esophagus. A pH recording below 4 indicates gastric acid reflux (13).

GASTRIC MOTILITY

There is little evidence of true peristalsis during the first few days of life. Gastric emptying appears to be achieved by the weight of the bolus and generalized tonic contractions of the stomach. In most newborns, emptying occurs within 2 hours and is most rapid when the infant is in the prone or right lateral position. Hypertonic feedings and high-fat contents within the lumen will delay gastric emptying.

In the mature infant, gastric motility can be divided into proximal and distal stomach (Fig. 5). The proximal portion of the stomach exhibits tonic contractions which subside only with swallowing, allowing filling of the proximal stomach during eating. There is no proximal mixing. Contractions and relaxation appear to be under neural control. The distal stomach has a 20-second cycle of peristaltic contractions mainly of the circular muscle, increasing in amplitude at the distal antrum. Movement is turbulent with a to-and-fro movement of solid contents and only liquid material passing the pylorus. Control of stomach contractions is both myogenic and neurogenic. However, control of the emptying of the stomach is mediated by chemoreceptors found in the duodenum. Control of pyloric opening and closing is controversial and uncertain. Closure coincides with arrival of the contraction wave, much like the LES, and relaxation follows. Decreased pyloric pressure has been postulated to result in gastric reflux of bile salts causing gastric mucosal injury with back diffusion of hydrogen ions. This may play a role in the

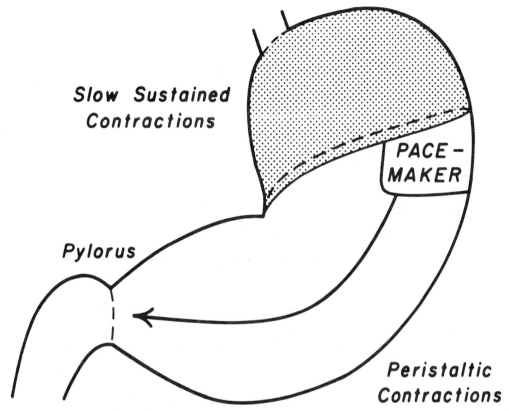

FIGURE 5   Proximal (shaded area) and distal gastric motor regions. The dividing line between the two gastric regions has been established by myoelectric and motor criteria. The line of division between the two regions does not correspond to the usual anatomical divisions of the stomach. The proximal motor regions including all of the gastric fundus and about the proximal third of the gastric body. (From ref. 47. Reprinted with permission.)

etiology of gastric ulcers. Healing of gastric ulcers has been shown to correlate with the return of pyloric sphincter pressure to normal.

SMALL-INTESTINE MOTILITY

Small-intestine motility in man is not well studied.   Apparently, segmental myogenic contractions occur rhythmically at 5-second intervals proximally, increasing to 8-second intervals at the ileum.   These ringlike or slow-wave contractions, originating in the circular muscle, propel chyme both caudad and aborad.   The net effect is caudad because segmentation is asymmetrical and frequency decreases downstream in the intestine.   These are the so-called type I waves.   Peristaltic contractions of type III waves move contents a few centimeters downstream.   These waves originate in the longitudinal muscle layers.   Cholinergic and possibly chemo- or mechanoreceptors initiate peristaltic movement or type III waves.   There have been few studies of small-bowel motility in clinical disease states, since long-term intubation with tube assemblies requiring perfusion is both difficult to tolerate and introduces artifacts in itself.   Infants and children tend to have more type I and fewer type III waves. Transit time through the small intestine averages 3-6 hours, as measured by radiographic techniques (1, 14).

COLONIC MOTILITY

The colon, like the stomach, may be separated into proximal and distal segments insofar as motility characteristics. The proximal colon exhibits primarily slow, rhythmic, to-and-fro or turbulent activity with the colonic contents moving both distally and backward toward the cecum, with occasional emptying into the transverse colon. Contents of the proximal colon may remain stationary for long periods facilitating absorptive and secretory functions. Control of movement is not well understood. The distal colon exhibits standing and peristaltic contractions, with material remaining stationary between haustral or contractile segments for long periods, and then being moved short distances by peristaltic contractions, facilitating absorption of fluid from this portion of the colon. There is occasional peristaltic movement originating from the hepatic flexure area producing significant movement of contents to the rectum (15). Continence is maintained by involuntary and voluntary means. The sharp anatomical angle of the junction of the rectum and anus produced by the puborectalis portion of the levator ani muscle is a major involuntary tonic component of continence. Voluntary accentuation of the angle by contraction of this muscle enhances continence. The high pressure maintained by the involuntary contraction of the internal anal sphincter augmented by both involuntary and voluntary external sphincter contraction, is the second main component of continence. The mucosa of the rectum is exquisitely sensitive to perception of increased pressure or fullness. Such an increase in pressure results in reflex relaxation of internal sphincter pressure and a voluntary reinforcement of the puborectalis and external sphincter. The increase in pressure lasts several minutes. If defecation is not voluntarily supressed, a cascade of events will lead to defecation, i. e. , intraabdominal pressure is increased, a squatting position assumed, which straightens the anorectal angle, the levator ani muscle relaxes, and external sphincter contraction is inhibited (16).

DISORDERS OF MOTILITY

GASTROESOPHAGEAL REFLUX (GER)

Introduction

Gastroesophageal reflux (GER) or chalasia in infants and young children is being recognized with increasing frequency using new modalities of diagnosis (17). An ever-increasing number of clinical disorders is attributed to GER with varying degrees of certainty (Table 1). Many of the diagnostic techniques are being currently reexamined in view of conflicting results and the consequences of overzealous intervention (18).

The state of the art suggests that GER occurs most frequently in asymptomatic individuals and requires no therapy. About 80% of symptomatic cases are mild and may be treated successfully by the primary care physician with thickened feedings and postprandial positioning in the semireclining position at 60° for 30-60 minutes. These patients do not require any definitive studies and are normal, or nearly so, by 18 months of age.

In about one-fifth of the symptomatic cases the presenting clinical features are severe enough to be investigated for GER at a referral center (Fig. 6). A hiatus hernia often is found in these patients, as well (19). Ninety percent of these patients respond to medical management, while the remaining 10% require an opera-

TABLE 1   Gastroesophageal Reflux (GER)

Clinical features	% incidence
1. Regurgitation vomiting	95-97
2. Failure to thrive	20-80
3. Pulmonary disease—recurrent and/or resistant	10-25
4. Esophagitis Irritability/pain/pyrosis Anemia/GI bleeding Exudative enteropathy + finger clubbing Dysphagia Sleep disturbances—disacchariduria Stricture formation	5-10
5. SIDS "Near miss"/choking spell/apnea	< 5
6. Associated neuropsychiatric features Developmental retardation Dystonia/Sandifer's syndrome Irritability "Seizures" Personality changes	< 2
7. Rumination/merycism	< 5
8. Pyloric dysfunction	< 5

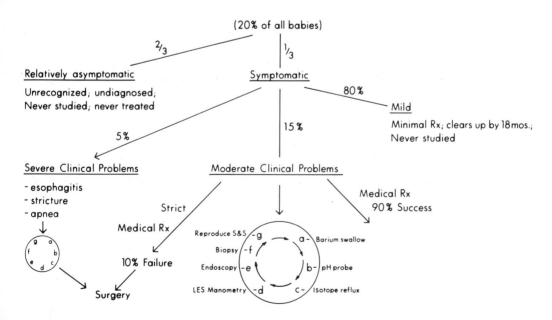

FIGURE 6   Management of patients with gastroesophageal reflux (GER).

tion. Whatever the etiology of GER, and in most cases there is no predisposing cause, it is now recognized that frequent and sustained reflux of gastric juice into the lower esophagus may produce a variety of problems.

Clinical Features

In infancy, postprandial vomiting and rumination account for 90% of the clinical presentations. Developmental failure, weight loss, failure to increase body length and weight, recurrent pulmonary infections, intractable or recurrent asthma, anemia, and esophageal stricture make up the remaining 10% of cases. In addition, GER may present with signs and symptoms suggesting neurological disease. Abnormal posturing of the head and neck (i. e. , torticollis), as well as spasms of the back and pelvis, can result from GER as observed fluroscopically (Sandifer syndrome).

Reflux may result in apparent seizures, which are in reality laryngospasm, and periods of apnea with a stiffening of the body ("dying spells"). These episodes may or may not be associated with pulmonary infiltrates. Whether GER is related to the sudden infant death syndrome is unclear. However, "near-miss" episodes have been recorded in infants with reflux and the apneic periods have been duplicated under experimental conditions. Infants with dysphagia, retardation, and behavorial abnormalities often are mislabeled as primary psychiatric disorders, when in fact GER is responsible for the clinical picture (20).

Only the older child will be able to communicate the subjective symptoms of heartburn to the clinician. The main symptoms of esophageal reflux in the older child are eructation and heartburn (pyrosis), a warm to frankly painful burning sensation located substernally. Reflux may present as a pressure or squeezing substernal sensation. It is occasionally confused with cardiac pain in the adolescent. Painful swallowing (odynophagia), intermittent dysphagia, stricture, and bleeding are less frequent problems (13, 21).

In large series of cases, 25% are noted to have some form of psychomotor retardation, and about 5% have an unrelated intestinal obstruction, e. g. , pyloric stenosis, duodenal obstruction, or malrotation.

Pathogenesis

The pathogenesis of reflux is thought to be primary loss of the entire reflux barrier, or lower esophageal sphincter (LES) incompetence. Development of the LES in infants is well documented by the age of 2-4 weeks. Lower esophageal sphincter pressure exceeding adult values has been noted in the first year of life, which may reflect methodology differences rather than real elevation of the LES pressure (8). As mentioned previously, the larger the diameter of the tube in relation to the size of the LES, the greater the pressure recording. The alteration of mechanical forces at the gastroesophageal junction (i. e. , a phrenoesophageal membrane), angle of entry of the esophagus into the fundus, and diaphragmatic pinch-cock effect, all play a lesser role. Lastly, defects in peristalsis of the body of the esophagus or impaired clearance of refluxed gastric contents also may play a role in symptomatology or signs. The presence of a sliding hiatus hernia has apparently little correlation with the presence of clinically significant esophageal reflux. It is also rare to find a congenitally short esophagus. The presence of esophagitis itself will further lower LES pressure. Causative agents include not only hydrochloric acid and pepsin, but alkaline substances such as bile salts and pancreatic enzymes. The etiology of the loss of the LES pressure is unknown, but there are multiple factors which are known to effect LES pressure. Certain food substances, drugs, hormones, etc. , all alter LES pressure (Table 2), but their clinical significance in maintaining the antireflux barrier is unknown.

TABLE 2   Agents Producing Changes in Lower Esophageal Pressure (LES)

Increased LES Pressure	Decreased LES Pressure
Gastrin/pentagastrin	Secretin
	Cholecystokinin
Motilin	Glucagon
	Gastric inhibitory
Substance P	polypeptide (GIP)
	Vasoactive intestinal polypeptide (VIP)
Prostaglandin F_2a	Prostaglandins E_1, E_2, A_2
	Beta-adrenergic antagonist
Alpha-adrenergic agonist	(isoproterenol)
(norepinephrine; phenylephrine)	Alpha-adrenergic antagonist
	(phentolamine)
Cholinergic agent	Dopamine
(bethanechol; methacholine)	Anticholinergic agent
	(atropine)
Anticholinesterase	Theophylline
(edrophonium)	Caffeine
	Gastric acidification
Histamine/betazole	Fat meal
	Chocolate
Gastric alkalinization	Smoking
	Ethanol
Metoclopramide	Peppermint
	Valium/Demerol/Morphine
Protein meal	Inflammation
Indomethacin	
Coffee	

Diagnosis

The diagnosis of esophageal reflux is made by demonstrating the presence of reflux directly or indirectly (Table 3, and see Fig. 6).

TABLE 3   Diagnostic Requirements for Gastroesophageal Reflux

1.   Demonstrate the presence of reflux: barium esophagram, pH probe monitoring, radioisotope reflux, and LES manometry

2.   Demonstrate the effects of reflux: esophagoscopy and mucosal histology

3.   Reproduce the symptomatology

Several tests may be required to be certain about the diagnosis. These, in order of accuracy, are:

1. Positioning of a <u>pH flexible electrode</u> (Microelectrodes, Inc. M. J. 506) in the lower esophagus above the lower esophageal sphincter for hours, with demonstration of a fall from pH 6 to less than 4, confirms the presence of reflux. (Tuttle test (22). Prolonged measurement of intraesophageal pH (12-24 hours), both in the upright and recumbent position, will also provide additional information as to esophageal clearance of acid or alkali (23). Failure to return to a pH over 4 within four swallows, or a pH of less than 4 for over 25% of the recorded time suggests, but does not prove, the presence of clinically significant acid reflux. The recommended use of pH monitoring combined with the instillation of 0. 1 N hydrochloric acid, intragastrically, is probably not physiological, since acidification of the stomach may itself decrease LES pressure.

2. The recent technique of adding <u>99mtechnetium sulfur colloid</u> to food, or directly into the stomach, may be used to detect reflux of gastric contents. A gamma camera isotope imaging should be followed for about 90-120 minutes. Both false-positive and false-negative tests have been reported (24). In some cases, pulmonary aspiration may be demonstrated.

3. A good radiologist will detect up to 90% of cases of GER by means of a barium swallow. However, others claim that the high density of the barium prevents more than a 50% accurate diagnosis. Many patients appear to have a coincidental sliding-type hiatus hernia.

4. <u>Manometric studies</u> in adults have shown a good correlation of low LES pressure with symptomatology and the presence of reflux. In infants, although the studies to date are limited and controversial, a decrease in LES pressure as demonstrated by the rapid pull-through technique, has shown reasonable correlation with symptoms of reflux (Fig. 7). Unfortunately, a normal pressure does not exclude reflux, and a low pressure is not synonymous with reflux (9).

5. <u>Flexible esophagoscopy</u> may reveal evidence of hyperemia, ulcers, erosions, stricture, or friability of the esophageal mucosa. However, a large number of patients with reflux esophagitis may have grossly normal appearing mucosa.

6. Examination of a properly oriented <u>suction biopsy</u>, taken at least 3 cm above the LES, will reveal distinctive histological changes which have over 90% correlation with detection of reflux of acid or alkalii (Fig. 8). The presence of (1) elongated dermal pegs extending over one-half the distance to the surface, (2) thickened basal layer of cells over 15% the width of the mucosal thickness, (3) an inflammatory cell infiltration of the lamina propria, are all histological criteria for the presence of esophagitis (25). The application of fiberoptic endoscopy and biopsy of the esophagitis has yet to be fully evaluated in the pediatric age group.

7. The determination of whether or not a symptom complex can be caused by an acid-alkali sensitive esophageal mucosa, may be determined by <u>intraesophageal perfusion of acid</u> (Bernstein test). Without knowledge of the patient or examiner, either 0. 1 N hydrochloric acid or normal saline is perfused into the midesophagus at 10-12 ml/min for 30 minutes. The test is considered positive if the patient's original symptoms are reproduced during the acid perfusion and relieved by saline instillation. This test may be combined with manometry. Because of the subjective nature of the responses, the test is often difficult to interpret. The ability of a child to describe symptoms limits the acid perfusion test in younger children, but has been used to reproduce apneic and coughing spells.

Treatment

The treatment of reflux in the infant frequently requires only propping in a reclining infant seat. This may be used for 30-60 minutes, postprandially, or up to 24 hours continuously for several weeks or months. Hypotensive sphincter pressures have

HYPOTENSIVE LES
RAPID PULL THROUGH

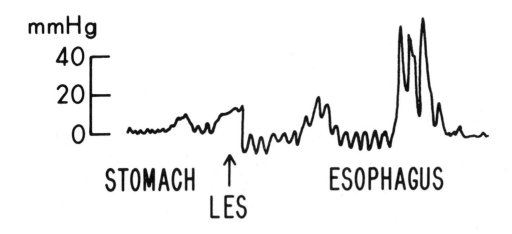

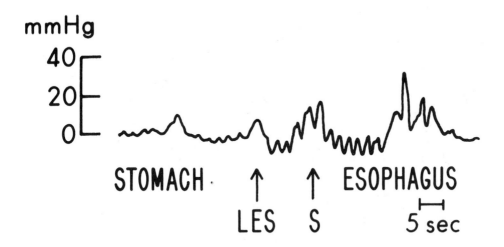

FIGURE 7   A 9-month-old infant with failure to thrive and radiographic evidence of barium reflux without hiatus hernia.   Rapid pull-through of the LES demonstrates a 12 mmHg rise in the proximal opening and a 8 mmHg rise in the distal opening.   Swallow(s) demonstrates low amplitude contractions.   Spontaneous high pressure repetitive contractions are seen to the right.   This indicates both spasm and ineffective acid clearance.

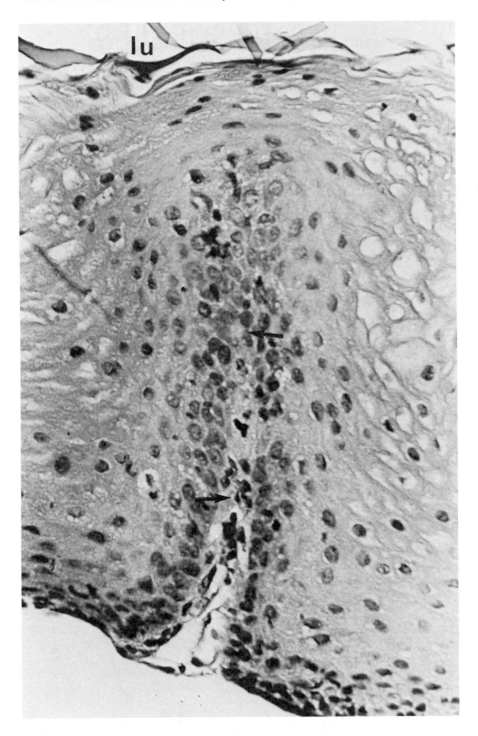

FIGURE 8   Chronic esophagitis in esophageal biopsy with upward extension of the papilla (arrow) reaching the upper third of the epithelial layer (lu = lumen). Hematoxylin-eosin stain. Original magnification x 306. (Courtesy of Dr. Ellen Kahn.)

been noted in these patients on manometry, as well as free GER on barium x-ray studies. The "spontaneous" cures in such infants might reflect "maturation" of LES pressure, which resolve by 9-12 months of age in the majority of infants. When symptoms persist, such as failure to thrive or recurrent pulmonary symptoms, antireflux surgery has apparently been beneficial (26). Creation of an intra-abdominal esophagus and a zone of high pressure with an anterior surrounding cuff of gastric fundus (the anterior fundoplication of Nissen) restores LES pressure to normal, as demonstrated by manometry. Repair of the hiatus hernia, creating a gastrostomy for debilitated patients, and a pylorplasty have all been recommended along with the fundoplication. Pyloroplasty is indicated in patients who have demonstrated preoperative delayed gastric emptying. Long-term effects on infants and children are unknown, but adults seem to have less than a 15% failure rate after 10 years (27). Good clinical improvements have been demonstrated. Relief of symptoms postoperatively in retarded children has been disappointing. The "gas bloat" syndrome, although rare, seems to be the major side effect of surgery and is the result of the relative inability to vomit or burp. Distal stricture formation of the esophagus is a late complication which usually responds to a single dilation.

Medical treatment in older children is preferred, unless major complications such as bleeding or stricture ensue (28). Treatment consists of elevation of the head of the bed to 6 in. , acid neutralization with adequate nonabsorbable antacids 1 hour after meals and at bedtime, and avoidance of food and drugs which lower LES pressure (see Table 2). Weight reduction, if appropriate, and avoidance of gastric secretagogues also are helpful. Bethanechol chloride (Urecholine) and metoclopramide have been shown to raise LES pressure. They increase gastric emptying, as well, and appear to be clinically effective in reducing symptoms. The group of H_2 receptor antagonists, such as cimetidine, reduce acid output without affecting LES pressure, and are useful in cases with superimposed esophagitis.

ACHALASIA

Achalasia of the esophagus is associated with (1) elevation of the LES pressure; (2) failure of complete relaxation of the LES on initiating a swallow; and (3) absence of peristalsis in the lower two-thirds or smooth muscle portion of the esophagus (29). Although achalasia is seen mainly in the adult population, up to 5% of the cases have been reported before age 15 (30). There have been cases reported under the age of 5, with the youngest reported at 2 weeks of age.

Etiology

The etiology of achalasia remains unknown, except when associated with the parasitic infection by Trypanosoma cruzi (Chagas disease), which results in aganglionosis of the myenteric plexuses of both the esophagus and colon. In idiopathic achalasia there probably is a decrease in the number of ganglion cells in the smooth muscle portion of the esophagus. Electron microscopic studies show changes in the myofilaments, degeneration of myelin sheaths, interruption of axons, and abnormalities of the dorsal motor nucleus of the vagus nerve. The muscle and neural structure of the LES generally have been reported to be normal in appearance and number (31).

Clinical Features

Symptoms are usually painless dysphagia, intermittent initially, but progressive over a variable period, ranging from months to years. Difficulty in swallowing solids followed by liquids is common, with exacerbation by emotional stress.

Progression to retention and regurgitation or vomiting of undigested food occurs often, with resultant weight loss or fear of eating. Pulmonary complications, such as bouts of coughing, nocturnal asthma, and aspiration pneumonitis, may be the main presenting clinical symptoms. Pulmonary problems initially are common in the pediatric age group. Retrosternal pain and pyrosis are rare symptoms in achalasia, except early in the course of the illness. Delayed growth and development are not uncommon.

Diagnosis

The diagnosis of achalasia is most commonly made by barium swallow, except in early cases when the esophagus is not dilated, or the clinical picture is predominantly one of odynophagia which may result in confusion with diffuse esophageal spasm (see later). The x-ray examination (Fig. 9a) should be performed with the patient recumbent, seeking ineffective peristalsis or aperistalsis in the lower two-thirds of the esophagus. When esophageal dilatation is prominent, the lower portion of the esophagus has a long, gradual, smooth, and tapering appearance, the so-called "birds beak" appearance. Esophageal manometry will demonstrate an elevated resting pressure in the body of the esophagus, and a high resting pressure in the LES, usually above 30 mmHg, with failure to relax fully to fundic pressure with the majority of swallows (Fig. 9b). The upper one-third, striated muscle portion of the esophagus, usually will exhibit normal peristalsis and upper esophageal sphincter function. Since the smooth muscle portion of the esophagus may be regarded as a denervated organ, stimulation with a cholinergic drug such as methacholine, 2-4 mg subcutaneously, or bethanechol (Urecholine) 5-10 mg subcutaneously, will produce a marked rise in the LES pressure as well as spasm of the lower two-thirds of the esophagus. This is often accompanied by subjective symptoms of pain and regurgitation of esophageal contents. Except in unusual cases, the test is probably not warranted, inasmuch as false-positive results have been reported (31). Endoscopy of the esophagus may show some esophagitis caused by stasis. Characteristically, there is no difficulty in passing the instrument through the gastroesophageal junction with exertion of minimal pressure in this area.

Treatment

The treatment of achalasia in patients under the age of 12 years remains surgical, i.e., esophageal myotomy (Heller procedure). This is the procedure of choice and the results are excellent if reflux complications do not occur. It is now popular to combine the Heller procedure with a fundoplication of the lower esophagus, often with a gastric outlet drainage procedure. In children aged 12 years or older, forceful pneumatic dilatation or rupture of the muscle of the LES by means of an inflatable balloon (Moser or Brown-McHardy bag) placed fluoroscopically in the lower esophageal sphincter region, effectively reduces LES pressure, and results in long-term elimination of symptoms in approximately 80% of the cases after one, or a maximum of two dilatations. Reflux, following pneumatic dilatation, also requires prophylactic treatment as outlined for GER. Patients with achalasia have a higher incidence of squamous cell carcinoma of the esophagus later in life. This incidence is not altered by successful treatment, hence these patients require careful long-term evaluations (31).

ESOPHAGEAL SPASM

Diffuse spasm of the esophagus is characterized by esophageal pain and dysphagia with an abnormal x-ray appearance of the esophagus and abnormal manometry. Most patients will not have all of these criteria, but present with one or several of

the above symptoms or findings. Some cases of diffuse spasm with positive methacholine tests have progressed to the clinical and manometric picture of achalasia,
and there have been cases of complete regression of symptoms and findings. Adolescent patients may present with severe chest pain, mimicking the pain of coronary artery disease, with or without dysphagia. The symptoms are characteristically intermittent.

Diagnosis

A barium swallow may reveal abnormalities classified as "cork screwing," curling, or tertiary contractions of the lower two-thirds of the esophagus (Fig. 10).
Thickening of the muscular wall of the esophagus also may be apparent.
Manometry studies usually reveal a high peristaltic pressure, over 100 mmHg,
in the body of the esophagus. There are prolonged nonperistaltic or simultaneous
contraction waves of the lower two-thirds of the esophagus, high LES pressure,
with adequate but shortened duration of relaxation on swallowing (32).

Treatment

All therapeutic approaches have been relatively unsatisfactory and difficult to assess in view of the intermittent nature of the complaints. Nitrates, narcotics,
pneumatic dilatations of the LES, and long myotomy all have been tried with variable success.

CONGENITAL AGANGLIONIC MEGACOLON
(HIRSCHSPRUNG DISEASE)

INTRODUCTION

Megacolon, or large colon, may be classified either as congenital or acquired.
Aganglionic megacolon is due to a congenital absence of ganglion cells in both the
submucosal (Meissner) and myenteric (Auerbach) plexuses. In the newborn period
it accounts for 20-25% of intestinal obstruction. Its incidence is 1:5000 (0.2 per
1000) live births, or approximately 700 new cases each year in the United States.
A recent report summarized the national United States experience (33). Familial
occurrence has been reported in about 7% of the cases, particularly in the group
involving long aganglionic segments, i.e., extending proximal to the splenic flexure. A significant association is established with Down syndrome, as well as with
other congenital birth defects, e.g., deafness. A male preponderance in the most
common varieties is well established, occurring in approximately a 4:1 ratio. In
long-segment disease, i.e., proximal to the splenic flexure, the ratio is reduced
to 2.5:1. In the United States there is no racial predilection.

PATHOGENESIS

The exact cause of aganglionic megacolon remains unknown. Normal embryological
development of the autonomic parasympathetic myenteric and submucosal plexuses
is cephalad to caudad, beginning about the fifth week of gestation and completed by
the twelfth week. Interruption of this process leaves an aganglionic area extending
proximally from the external sphincter for a variable length. Normally, there is
a paucity of ganglion cells extending at least 1-1.5 cm above the anorectal margin,
and biopsy for diagnosis should be taken above this area to avoid confusion. In the
majority of patients (75%), the aganglionic segment involves both the rectum and
sigmoid colon; but any length of colon or small intestine may be involved ranging

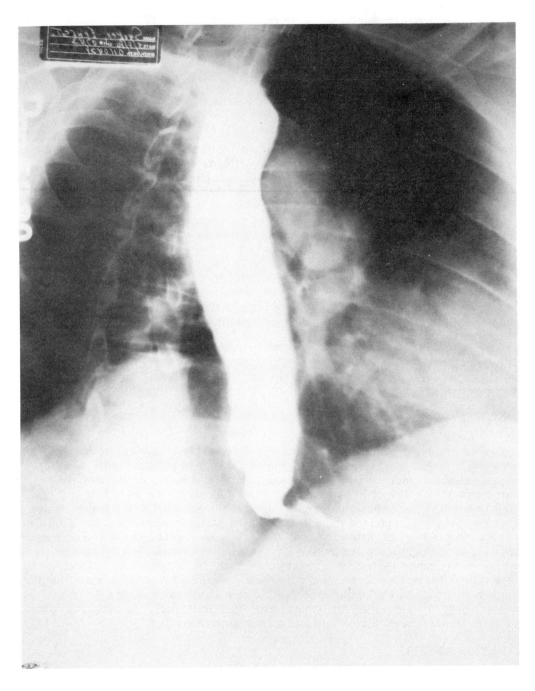

FIGURE 9a   X-ray of a patient with long-standing achalasia. (1) Note the dilated atonic esophagus with evidence of asymmetrical contours. (2) The tapered area at the gastroesophageal junction (so-called birds beak), with minimal trickle of barium through the nonrelaxing lower esophageal sphincter (LES).

ACHALASIA

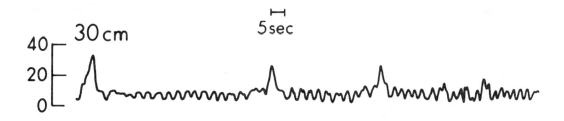

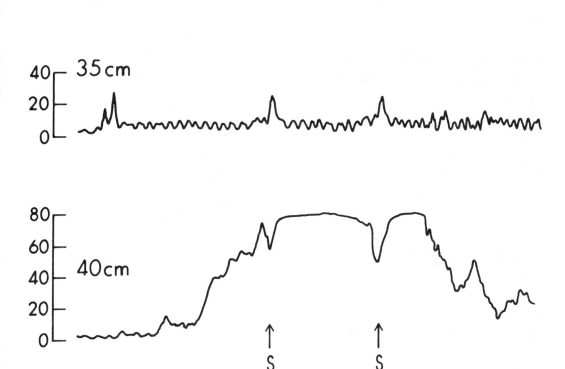

FIGURE 9b   A 14-year-old patient with the lower tube opening (40 cms) being moved (station pull-through technique) into the lower esophageal sphincter. Pressure in the sphincter is 80 mmHg and relaxation on swallowing(s) is minimal (20 mmHg). Peristaltic contractions in the body of the esophagus at 30 and 35 cm are simultaneous and of low amplitude.

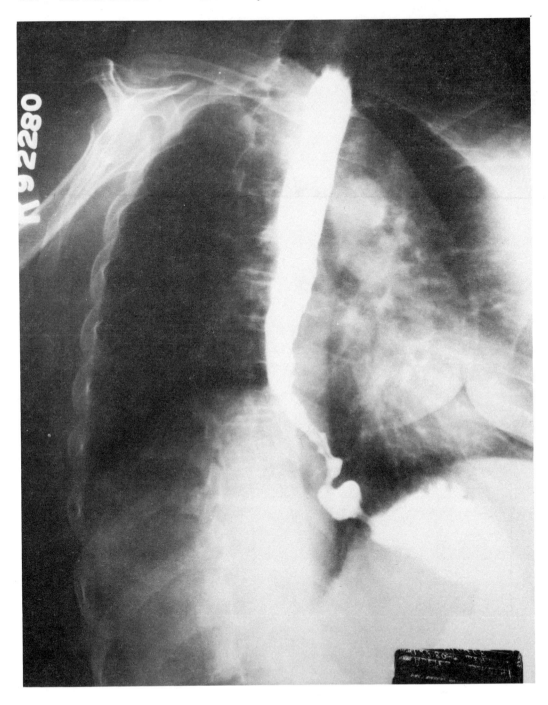

FIGURE 10   X-ray of esophageal spasm. Note the narrowing of the lower half of the esophagus with evidence of asymmetric contours of the esophagus corresponding to the nonperistaltic motility pattern. A hiatus hernis also is present.

from the ultrashort (less than 1%) to involvement of the entire colon with or without the small bowel (8%). Functionally, there is sympathetic hyperactivity in the affected segment leading to tonic contraction that is unaffected by parasympathomimetic agents such as methacholine chlorides.

CLINICAL FEATURES (Table 4)

The Newborn

With increased awareness and adequate facilities for diagnosis, the congenital form of megacolon usually is apparent in the first month of life in about 50-75% of the cases. Although unexplained, it occurs rarely in the preterm infant. The absence of, or delay in passage of meconium beyond 48 hours, followed by increasing abdominal distention and bilious vomiting within a few days of birth, is a classical clinical picture (34, 35). The newborn's appearance varies from looking relatively well to septic shock. Dilatation of the empty rectum by the first examiner, with an instrument or finger, will result in explosive expulsion of retained fecal material and decompression of the proximal normal bowel, in most patients. However, without repeated emptying or irrigation of the colon, obstructive symptoms promptly return. The development of diarrhea with enterocolitis occurs in approximately 20-25% of untreated cases, particularly in the first 3 months of life and in long-segment disease. No specific organism has been isolated in these cases. There

TABLE 4   Major Clinical Features of Congenital Aganglionosis
(According to Age at Diagnosis)

A. Newborn (50-65% of all cases)

   Meconium passage > 48 hours
   Meconium plug
   Intestinal obstruction
   Listless
   Cecal/appendiceal perforation

B. Infants 1-6 mo (33-48% of all cases)

   1. Severe constipation
       Impaction
       Intermittent intestinal obstruction
       Failure to thrive
       Enterocolitis

   2. Moderate constipation
       Abrupt intestinal obstruction
       Enterocolitis

   3. Mild to moderate constipation
       Failure to thrive
       Diarrhea
       Enterocolitis

C. Infants over 6 mo (< 2% of all cases)

   Mild chronic constipation
   Stool in rectal ampulla
   Soiling
   (Encopresis)

---

is a mortality of up to 30% with enterocolitis, and this is the major cause of death in Hirschsprung disease. The incidence and mortality have varied little during the last decade (33). Recurrent fecal impaction and stercoral ulcers of the colon, which occasionally result in colonic perforation, are additional superimposed problems. Appendiceal perforation is a rare complication.

Older Infants and Children (35)

If the aganglionic segment of colon is short, and manipulative measures are regularly undertaken, constipation and distention may become a way of life. The diagnosis in the older child is very often confused with acquired megacolon; however, with careful questioning the complaints always date from birth. The infant under 6 months of age continues to have variable but stubborn constipation punctuated by recurrent obstructive crises or impaction. The child fails to thrive, the abdomen is protuberant and frequently anemia and hypoproteinemia are noted. Fecal masses and peristaltic waves are easily noted. Enterocolitis may supervene and a significant mortality occurs in these unrecognized cases. In the rare patient who remains undiagnosed beyond the age of six months, constipation is still resistant to most routine measures, although soiling is unusual. The child usually is in a borderline nutritional status with gaseous distention and delayed puberty.

DIAGNOSIS

Motility Studies

Phasic motility of the dilated and often hypertrophied bowel proximal to the aganglionic segment remains normal. The absence of ganglion cells is associated with failure of the aganglionic segment to relax and permit passage of feces into the narrowed segment of colon. Manometric studies revealing a dissociation of the internal sphincter to rectal distention have proved to be an effective and simple means of eliciting a diagnostic tracing for aganglionic megacolon (36, 37). The patient is prepared by emptying the distal colon with cleansing saline enemas. Caution is required since occasional cases of water intoxication and hypertonic dehydration have been reported.
    The study involves placing in tandem three balloons in an empty rectum and sigmoid, with the patient in a decubitus position (Fig. 11) (38). The larger rectal balloon is inserted, with digital guidance, several centimeters into the rectum. Once all the balloons are within the rectum the middle smaller balloon is inflated and withdrawn until resistance indicates it is anchored within the internal sphincter. The external balloon should be visualized at the anus and is then also inflated. The nerve-rich mucosa of the rectum sets up a chain of reflex arcs which result in retention or selected passage of rectal contents through the sphincter areas, preserving continence. The normal physiological response to distention of the rectum is relaxation of the resting smooth muscle internal sphincter pressure, following a short low-pressure contraction (Fig. 12a); relaxation lasts 10-20 seconds. There is a simultaneous rise in external striated muscle sphincter pressure lasting 5-15 seconds. External sphincter pressure may be voluntarily prolonged until the rectum adapts to distention and the reflex relaxation of the internal sphincter ends. If no internal sphincter response to rectal distention with 30 cc of air is obtained, increasing volumes of air are used to inflate the rectal balloon. Rarely, as much as 150 cc of air has been used in markedly distended colons. In aganglionic megacolon, rectal distention not only fails to induce internal sphincter relaxation, but a paradoxical rise in sphincter pressure is often seen (Fig. 12b). The sphincter dissociation can only be considered diagnostic after the twelfth day of life (39). Identical results have been demonstrated by anorectal electromanometry.

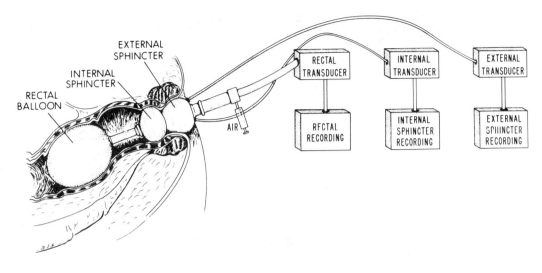

FIGURE 11   Schematic representation (38) of the triple balloon assembly and cannula positioned with the large balloon in the rectum and the smaller cannula-mounted balloons located at the internal and external sphincters.   A syringe containing air for inflating the rectal balloon is shown.   The balloons monitoring internal and external sphincter pressure are continuously inflated.   (From Ref. 38. Reprinted with permission.)

Radiographic Studies

A radiocontrast examination of the unprepared bowel of an enlarged colon will show the distal narrowed hypertonic segment of bowel, usually best seen in the lateral view (Fig. 13 a, b).   This transition zone will not be seen in the very long segments, and often is absent within the first 6 weeks of life.   However, failure to evacuate the barium completely within 24 hours is very suggestive in these infants. The radiograph may reveal a saw-toothed appearance of the contracted segment. In the ultrashort aganglionic megacolon, the narrowed area may be inapparent and the picture indistinguishable from the dilated bowel extending to the rectum, seen on x-ray in acquired megacolon.

Histologic Studies

A suction biopsy of the rectal mucosa is the most reliable and most available method of diagnosis.   The biopsy capsule should be placed at least 2 cm from the mucocutaneous junction in infants, and 3 cm above the junction in older children to avoid the physiological hypoganglionic zone.   The diagnosis of the absence of ganglion cells in the submucosal Meissner plexus requires meticulous review (up to 200 slide sections) by an experienced pathologist.   Hyperplastic sympathetic nerve fibers and proliferating Schwann cells are associated findings (Fig. 14).   An increase in acetylcholinesterase activity as determined by histochemical staining is noted to parallel the increased nonganglionic submucosal and neural elements and accumulation of acetylcholine.   The presence of this increased activity by staining can be sought to confirm the diagnosis of Hirschsprung disease (36).   In rare instances, all the studies are not clearly diagnostic, and a full thickness biopsy of the rectal wall is indicated to assess the normally more ubiquitous myenteric ganglion cells.

NORMAL RECTAL MANOMETRY

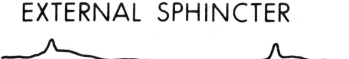

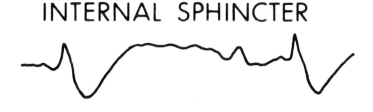

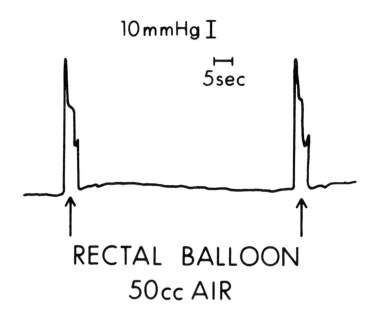

FIGURE 12a   Balloon manometry revealing a normal pressure response of both external and internal sphincter to inflation of rectal balloon with 50 cc of air. External sphincter shows a rise in pressure. Internal sphincter shows an initial rise in pressure then a drop in pressure to 20 mmHg lasting 15 sec.

HIRSCHSPRUNG'S DISEASE

EXTERNAL SPHINCTER

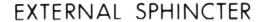

INTERNAL SPHINCTER

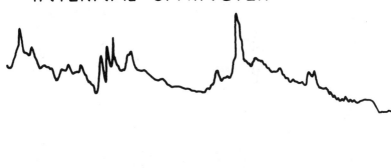

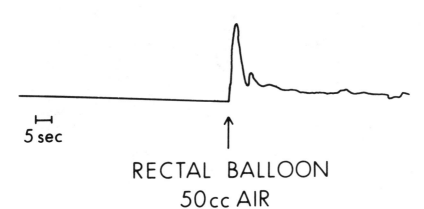

5 sec

RECTAL BALLOON
50 cc AIR

FIGURE 12b   The patient demonstrates a 25 mmHg rise in internal sphincter pressure following rectal distension without any relaxation of the internal sphincter. Note normal rise in external sphincter pressure. This is a characteristic response in Hirschsprung disease.

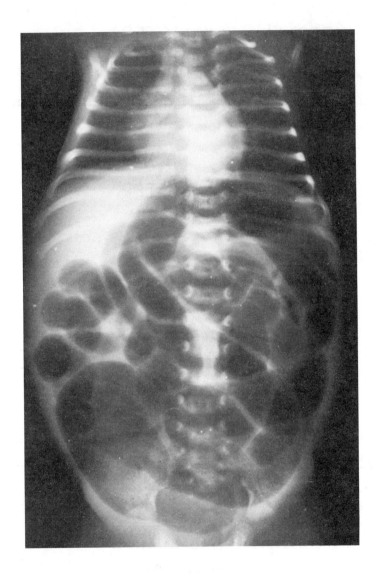

FIGURE 13a   Two-week-old male with severe abdominal distention and nonbilious vomiting. History of infrequent bowel movements since birth. X-ray reveals dilatation of colon and several small-bowel loops.

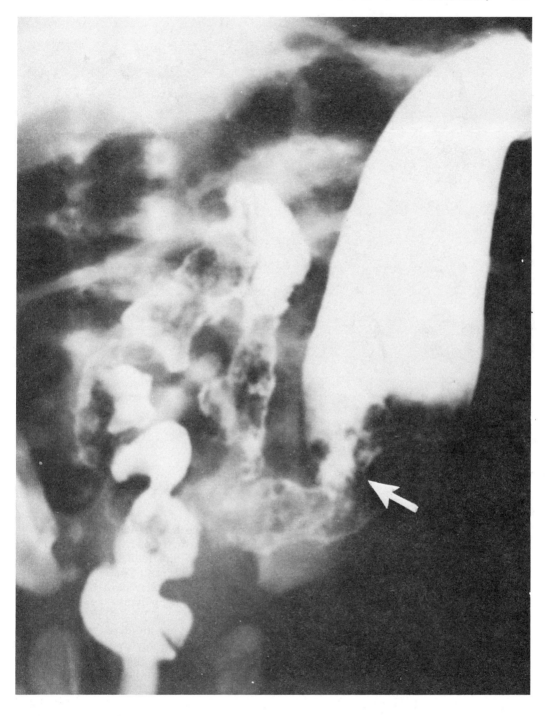

FIGURE 13b   Barium enema (AP view) demonstrates narrowed rectosigmoid and dilated left colon with a clearly defined transition zone (arrow).

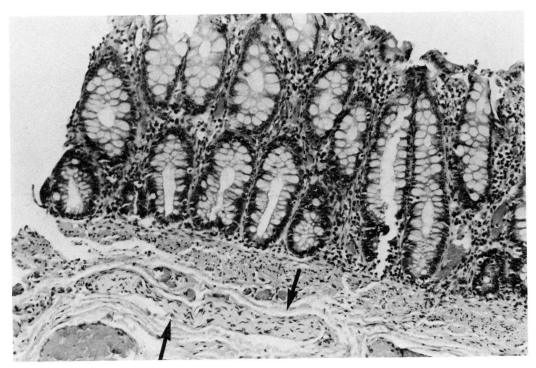

FIGURE 14   Rectal suction biopsy. Thickened nerve trunk (arrows) in the submucosa. No ganglia are seen. Hematoxylin-eosin stain. Original magnification
x 122. (Courtesy of Dr. Ellen Kahn.)

DIFFERENTIAL DIAGNOSIS

A wide variety of conditions are associated with severe megacolon and occur at
different ages (Table 5). In the newborn, when the majority of Hirschsprung cases
present, the major disorders to be excluded are meconium ileus, ileal atresia,
meconium plug syndrome, and the microcolon seen in infants of diabetic mothers.

In acquired megacolon, stool in a distended rectum is easily palpable and the
patient is usually older than 2 years of age. The internal sphincter responses to
rectal balloon distention are normal. Balloon manometry of the internal and external sphincter also may be helpful in differentiating systemic diseases such as
scleroderma, dermatomyositis, and myotonia dystrophica, involving either skeletal or smooth muscle, by observing altered responses of the sphincters. Quantitative measurement of external sphincter strength following injury is possible, as
is reflex conditioning to improve external sphincter strength following damage to
the external sphincter. The history of obstipation dating from the day of birth and
the presence of an empty rectum on digital examination, are more characteristic
of Hirschsprung disease.

During the past 15 years a number of disease entities have been reported which
clinically simulate Hirschsprung disease, but do not fit the histological and/or the
manometric criteria. In general, they are uncommon, often inadequately described,
and certainly poorly understood.

TABLE 5   Clinical Disorders Associated with Megacolon

---

1. Congenital

    Aganglionic (Hirschsprung disease)
    Achalasia of the distal colon*
    Pseudo-Hirschsprung (abnormal ganglions)*
       Neuronal colonic dysplasia (plexiform neurofibromatosis)
       Zonal aganglionosis
       Hypoganglionosis
       Immaturity
    Meconium ileus*
    Meconium plug*
    Microcolon*

2. Acquired

    Metabolic disease
       Myxedema (hypothyroidism, cretinism)*
       Porphyria
       Lead poisoning
       Hypokalemia
    Neurologic disease
       Chagas disease*
       Cerebral atrophy
       Parkinsonism
       Diabetic neuropathy
       Paraplegia
       Drug toxicity
       East African megacolon
    Obstructive lesions
       Rectal strictures secondary to repaired imperforate anus, trauma, etc. *
       Tumors
       Extracolonic compression
    Ischemic disease
       Postumbilical catheterization*
       Experimental
    Pseudo-obstructions
    Ulcerative colitis/toxic megacolon
    Functional/psychogenic

---

*Those disorders simulating Hirschsprung disease.

In those patients with abnormal or absent ganglion cells, hypoganglionosis refers to cases when only isolated ganglion cells are found, and requires a full-thickness biopsy for confirmation. In zonal aganglionosis (37), the aganglionic segment does not extend to the anal margin, or skip areas occur. Multiple biopsies are required to establish the diagnosis, and it is still a questionable entity, from an embryological point of view (37).
Neuronal colonic dysplasia may produce signs and symptoms similar to Hirschsprung disease, however its morphological features are very different, involving

hyperplasia of the parasympathetic innervation of the bowel wall. Giant ganglia in the submucosa are diagnostic. The presence of excessive histochemical acetylcholinesterase activity may be confused with Hirschsprung disease. This condition may be identical with plexiform neurofibromatosis of the colon which may simulate aganglionic megacolon in older children (40).

Degeneration and reduction in number of ganglion cells are found in Chagas disease. This condition is endemic to certain areas of South America and is associated with trypanosomiasis. Esophageal involvement is common.

Immature ganglion cells are noted in some premature infants and the relationship to disturbed motility is unclear.

Pseudo-Hirschsprung disease refers to a small group of conditions in which normal or abnormal ganglion cells are noted, associated with motility disturbances. An ultra-short aganglionic segment must be excluded. Achalasia of a distal rectal segment and East African megacolon are in this category. The etiologies are obscure.

TREATMENT

Medical Management

In most cases of Hirschsprung disease, the infant requires minimal preoperative intervention. Correction of dehydration, electrolyte abnormalities, and anemia are part of the early stabilization period. Enterocolitis is a critical complication which can develop within hours. As soon as the diagnosis of Hirschsprung disease is made, or suspected, a prophylactic program of colonic irrigation is instituted (41). A number 16 F Foley catheter is inserted into the rectum and gradually advanced into the right colon while 60 cc of warm saline is instilled. Progress may be confirmed by inspection and palpation of the infant's abdomen. The irrigation is continued until the effluent is clear. Distention and toxicity appear to abate almost immediately in most cases. Surgical intervention may be safely delayed until an ideal time for both patient and surgeon. Oral feedings can be instituted after 24-48 hours and a standard neomycin-erythromycin bowel preparation is begun just before surgery. When the child presents with diarrhea (often bloody), distention, fever, and vomiting, more aggressive measures are necessary, since septic shock and peritonitis are often imminent. Antishock measures and appropriate antibiotics are instituted and colonic irrigations are discontinued to avoid a perforation. A life-saving emergency colostomy should be considered as soon as possible.

Surgical Management

The treatment of aganglionic megacolon is primarily surgical. There are three basic types of correction currently used (Fig. 15), with many modifications being proposed. The Swenson rectosigmoidectomy procedure involves resection of the aganglionic bowel with anastomosis of ganglionic bowel to the area just above the internal sphincter. This is now usually combined with an internal sphincterotomy. The Duhamel retrorectal transanal pull-through is a side-to-side anastomosis of the innervated bowel to the posterior wall of the distal rectal segment. Portions of the innervated segment of bowel also is resected. The Soave endorectal pull-through procedure calls for mucosal stripping of the aganglionic segment with the pull-through of normally innervated proximal bowel. This may be performed with or without a primary anastomosis, preserving the aganglionic muscular coat which contains sensory receptors. The internal sphincter remains intact and pelvic nerves are exposed to no damage. Table 6 summarizes the results of a survey of the surgical section of the American Academy of Pediatrics between 1975 and 1976 (33). One or more postoperative complications occurred in about half of the cases

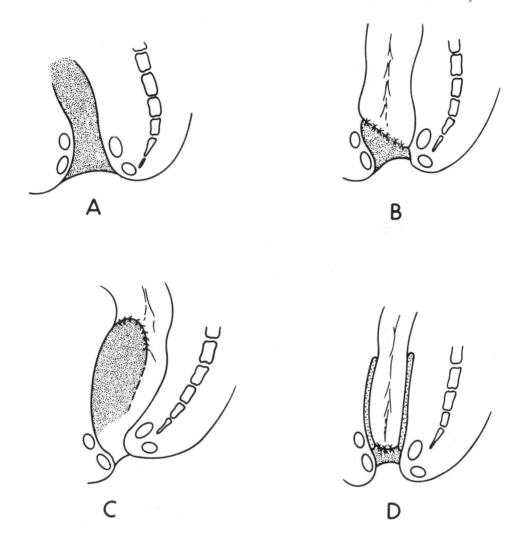

FIGURE 15   Abdominoperineal surgical procedures most commonly used in the management of Hirschsprung disease. (A) Before surgery–stippled area represents the aganglionic bowel. (B) Rectosigmoidectomy (Swenson). The resection leaves 1.5–2.0 cm of rectal wall anteriorly, with 1.0 cm or less posteriorly. May include a partial posterior internal sphincterotomy. (C) Retrorectal transcolonic pull-through (Duhamel, modified by Grob). The normal colon is pulled through the retrorectal space and anastomosed obliquely to the posterior wall of the aganglionic rectum. The anastomosis is above the internal sphincter to avoid incontinence. (D) Endorectal pull-through with primary anastomosis (Soave, modified by Boley). The mucosa and muscularis mucosae of the aganglionic segment are stripped off by submucosal dissection to the dentate line, and the normally innervated proximal colon is pulled through the remaining rectosigmoid cuff, and a primary anastomosis is performed.

TABLE 6   Results (%) of the Major Operative Procedures*

	Swenson rectosigmoidectomy (390 patients)	Duhamel rectorectal transanal pull-through (339 patients)	Soave endorectal pull-through without anastomosis (93 patients)	Boley endorectal pull-through with primary anastomosis (187 patients)
No complications	52.0	54.9	45.6	60.4
Mortality	2.5	1.8	3.2	1.1
postoperative	1.5	0.3	1.1	0.0
late	1.0	1.5	2.1	1.1
Postoperative enterocolitis	15.6	5.9	15.0	2.1
Incontinence	3.2	1.1	2.1	1.1
Disrupted anastomosis	11.2	2.4	1.1	5.8
Fecal fistula	6.2	2.9	1.1	1.1
Intestinal obstruction	9.0	7.1	3.2	1.6
Anal stenosis	9.5	5.5	15.1	9.4
mild	5.2	2.9	14.0	5.2
severe (requiring secondary procedure)	4.3	2.6	1.1	4.2

*Excluding patients with total colonic aganglionosis.   (Courtesy of Dr. Scott J. Boley)

in each procedure category. It is significant that the incidence of postoperative enterocolitis was about 15% in rectosigmoidectomy and endorectal pull-through without a primary anastomosis. This complication occurred much less frequently with the two other operations. In otherwise stable infants, a single stage Soave procedure can be done with little or no adverse effects. In preparation for a single operation, meticulous colonic saline irrigations are required. Most of these infants may be fed orally with a nutritious diet (41).

Over 40% of surgeons still prefer to perform an initial colostomy, the site varying with the length of the aganglionic bowel. The majority of the colostomies are removed at the time of the definitive procedure.

Ultrashort segments can be adequately treated by rectal myectomy and internal sphincterotomy (42). In infants with aganglionic segments extended proximal to the splenic flexure, a modified Duhamel procedure appears to provide the best results (43).

CHRONIC IDIOPATHIC INTESTINAL PSEUDOOBSTRUCTION (CIIP)

Another aberration of intestinal motility being recognized more often in the pediatric age group is idiopathic intestinal pseudoobstruction. The entity is characterized by the clinical picture of recurrent bowel obstruction, without any organic cause or associated medical condition, such as myxedema, porphyria, scleroderma, amyloidosis, Chagas disease, or hypoparathyroidism (44, 45). Symptoms of abdominal distention, vomiting, poor nutrition, abdominal pain, diarrhea, or constipation may begin anywhere from the first week of life through adolescence. The patients are of two basic varieties: (1) myopathies, which are both familial (hereditary hollow visceral myopathy) or sporadic, and (2) neuropathies, with abnormalities of the myenteric plexus including both familial and sporadic cases. The course is episodic with intervals of weeks or years marking the attacks. The physical findings are abdominal distention with variable bowel sounds. Megacystis and ureteral reflux are common in the myopathic forms.

DIAGNOSIS AND TREATMENT

X-ray studies show dilated loops of small and/or large bowel, with significant delays in barium movement, often characteristic of mechanical obstruction. Cineradiography of the esophagus may reveal poor contractions of the lower third and manometric tracings confirm motility disorders of the lower esophagus and low LES pressure. However, these esophageal findings as yet appear to have no clinical significance. Biopsy material of the small bowel, colon, rectum, and bladder usually show normal neuromuscular components in the myopathic disorders. The clinical course is unaffected by diet, steroids, or cholinergic drugs. Antibiotics may have some beneficial effect if bacterial overgrowth is causing diarrhea or malabsorption. Most of the patients undergo some surgical exploration or resection because of suspect mechanical obstruction, and this seems only to worsen the clinical course. Therefore, surgery is to be avoided. Total parenteral feeding maintains nutrition, but may entail an indefinite period of therapy, and it has not yet been fully evaluated.

REFERENCES

1.   Christensen, J.: The physiology of gastrointestinal transit. Med Clin N Am 58:1165, 1974.

2.   Weisbrodt, N.W.: Neuromuscular organization of esophageal and pharyngeal motility. Arch Intern Med 136:524, 1976.

3.   Gryboski, J. D. : Suck and swallow in the premature infant.   Pediatrics 43:96, 1969.

4.   Goyal, R. K. : The lower esophageal sphincter.   Viewponts Digest Dis 8: No. 3, December 1976.

5.   Dodds, W. J. : Instrumentation and methods for intraluminal esophageal manometry.   Arch Intern Med 136:515, 1976.

6.   Kenigsberg, K. , H. Aiges, G. Alperstein, and F. Daum: A unique device to measure lower esophageal sphincter pressure in unsedated infants.   J Pediatr Surg 16:370, 1981.

7.   Gryboski, J. D. : The swallowing mechanism of the neonate: Esophageal and gastric motility.   Pediatrics 35:445, 1965.

8.   Moroz, S. P. , J. Espinoza, W. A. Cummins, and N. E. Diamant: Lower esophageal sphincter function in children with and without gastroesophageal reflux.   Gastroenterology 71:236, 1976.

9.   Castell, D. O. : The lower esophageal sphincter: Physiologic and clinical aspects.   Ann Intern Med 83:390, 1975.

10.   Kilman, W. J. and R. K. Goyal: Disorders of pharyngeal and upper esophageal sphincter motor function.   Arch Intern Med 136:592, 1976.

11.   Christensen, J. : The controls of esophageal movement.   Clin Gastroenterol 5:15, 1976.

12.   Behar, J. : Reflux esophagitis.   Arch Intern Med 136:560, 1976.

13.   Hendrix, T. R. and J. H. Yardley: Consequences of gastroesophageal reflux. Clin Gastroenterol 5:155, 1976.

14.   Kalser, M. H. : Small bowel motility.   in Gastroenterology, Vol. II.   W. B. Saunders Co. , Philadelphia, 1976, pp. 188-193.

15.   Smith, F. W. and M. H. Sleisinger: Physiology of the colon.   in Gastrointestinal Disease.   W. B. Saunders Co. , Philadelphia, 1978, p. 1529.

16.   Fitzgerald, J. F. : Difficulties with defecation and elimination in children. Clin Gastroenterol 6:283, 1977.

17.   Darling, D. B. , J. H. Fisher, and S. S. Gellis: Hiatal hernia and gastroesophageal reflux in infants and children: Analysis of the incidence in North American children.   Pediatrics 54:450, 1974.

18.   Report of the Seventy-sixth Ross Conference on Pediatric Research: Gastroesophageal Reflux.   Ross Laboratories, Columbus, 1979.

19.   Willich, E. : Insufficiency of the cardia in infancy: Manometric and cineradiographic studies.   Ann Radiol 16:137, 1973.

20.   Bray, P. F. , J. J. Herbst, D. G. Johnson, et al. : Childhood gastroesophageal reflux: Neurologic and psychiatric syndromes mimicked.   JAMA 237:1342, 1977.

21. Herbst, J. J. , L. S. Book, D. G. Johnson, and S. Jolley: The lower esophageal sphincter in gastroesophageal reflux in children. J Clin Gastroenterol 1:119, 1979.

22. Christie, D. L. : The acid reflux test for gastroesophageal reflux. J Pediatr 94:78, 1979.

23. Strobel, C. T. , W. J. Bryne, M. E. Ament, and A. R. Euler: Correlation of esophageal lengths in children with height: Application to the Tuttle test without prior esophageal manometry. J Pediatr 94:81, 1979.

24. Heyman, S. , J. A. Kirkpatrick, H. S. Winter, and S. Treves: An improved radionuclide method for the diagnosis of gastroesophageal reflux and aspiration in children (milk scan). Radiology 131:479, 1979.

25. Pope, C. E. : Mucosal response to esophageal motor disorders. Arch Intern Med 136:549, 1976.

26. Johnson, D. G. , J. J. Herbst, M. A. Oliveros, and D. R. Stewart: Evaluation of gastroesophageal reflux surgery in children. Pediatrics 59:62, 1977.

27. Euler, A. R. , E. W. Fonkalsrud, and M. E. Ament: Effect of Nissen fundoplication on the lower esophageal sphincter pressure of children with gastroesophageal reflux. Gastroenterology 72:260, 1977.

28. Behar, J. , D. G. Sheahan, P. Biancani, et al. : Medical and surgical management of reflux esophagitis. N Engl J Med 293:263, 1975.

29. Elder, J. B. : Achalasia of the cardia in childhood. Digestion 3:90, 1970.

30. Magilner, A. D. and H. J. Isard: Achalasia of the esophagus in infancy. Radiology 98:81, 1971.

31. Castell, D. G. : Achalasia and diffuse esophageal spasm. Arch Intern Med 136:571, 1976.

32. Bennet, J. R. and T. R. Hendrix: Diffuse esophageal spasm: A disorder with more than one cause. Gastroenterology 59:273, 1970.

33. Kleinhaus, S. , S. J. Boley, M. Sheran, and W. K. Sieber: Hirschsprung disease. A survey of the American Academy of Pediatrics. J Pediatr Surg 14:588, 1979.

34. Ehrenpreis, T. : Hirschsprung's Disease. Year Book Medical Publishers, Chicago, 1970.

35. Raffensperger, J. G. : Hirschsprung's disease. in Gastroenterology. W. B. Saunders Co., Philadelphia, 1976, p. 816.

36. Boston, V. E. , G. Dale, and K. W. A. Riley: Diagnosis of Hirschsprung's disease by quantitative biochemical assay of acetylcholinesterase in rectal tissue. Lancet 2:951, 1975.

37.   MacIver, A. G. and R. Whitehead: Zonal colonic aganglionosis, a variant of Hirschsprung's disease. Arch Dis Child 47:233, 1972.

38.   Schuster, M. M.: Diagnostic value of anal sphincter pressure measurements. Hosp Prac 7:115, April 1973.

39.   Tobon, F., and M.M. Schuster: Megacolon: Special diagnostic and therapeutic features. Johns Hopkins Med J 135:91, 1974.

40.   Temberg, J. I. and K. Winters: Plexiform neurofibromatosis of the colon as a cause of congenital megacolon. Am J Surg 109:663, 1965.

41.   So, H. B., D. L. Schwartz, J. M. Becker, et al.: Endorectal "pull-through" without preliminary colostomy in neonates with Hirschsrpung's disease. J Pediatr Surg 15:470, 1980.

42.   Orr, J. D. and W. G. Scobie: Anterior resection combined with anorectal myectomy in the treatment of Hirschsprung's disease. J Pediatr Surg 14:58, 1979.

43.   Martin, L. W.: Surgical management of total colonic aganglionosis. Ann Surg 176:343, 1972.

44.   Schuffler, M. D., M. D. Lowe, and A.H. Bill: Studies of idiopathic intestinal pseudo-obstruction. I. Hereditary hollow visceral myopathy: Clinical and pathological studies. Gastroenterology 73:327, 1977.

45.   Schuffler, M. D., and C. E. Pope: Studies of idiopathic intestinal pseudo-obstruction. II. Hereditary hollow visceral myopathy; Familial studies. Gastroenterology 73:339, 1977.

46.   Schuffler, M.D., C.A. Rohrmann, R.G. Chaffee, et al.: Chronic intestinal pseudo-obstruction: A report of 27 cases and review of the literature. Medicine 60:173, 1981.

47.   Johnson, L.R.: Physiology of the Gastrointestinal Tract, Vol. 1. Raven Press, New York, 1981.

9

VOMITING

Mervin Silverberg, M. D.

Vomiting is a most ubiquitous complaint in the pediatric age group. It should always be viewed in relation to meals and other ingestants, nature of the vomitus, and associated physical examination. The serious implications of this symptom usually vary directly with age, with the exception of the newborn infant in whom vomiting is always a source of concern.

PATHOGENESIS (1)

The act of vomiting involves a series of responses to afferent stimuli which are mediated by a vomiting center, presumably in the lateral reticular formation in the medulla (Fig. 1). These stimuli are known to come from the pharynx, intestines, pleura, heart, urogenital and biliary tracts. Additionally, higher cortical centers, the vestibular apparatus, numerous metabolic factors such as azotemia, electrolyte imbalances, drugs (e. g. , chemotherapy, morphine derivatives, and cardiac glycosides), are all potent stimulants of this emetic center. The complex response to noxious stimuli involves nausea, accompanied by salivation, sweating, decreased gastric tone, and contraction of the gastric outlet and duodenum. Subsequently, the abdominal muscles and diaphragm contract and emesis occurs when the cardia and esophagus relax and gastric contents are forced upward by reverse antral peristalsis. The younger the child, the more likely that nausea and retching will be absent or of short duration.

NEWBORN

Vomiting in the newborn period, particularly within the first 24-48 hours requires careful examination and review. Mucoid nonbilious vomiting often is associated with the presence of excessive swallowed maternal amniotic fluid. Blood in the vomitus can be proved to be maternal by the Apt test (see Chap. 11) which may be performed in the nursery. If it proves to be the baby's blood, it is usually associated with overzealous resuscitation; however, gastric and esophageal erosions or perforations and coagulation disorders should be sought. Regurgitation of the initial

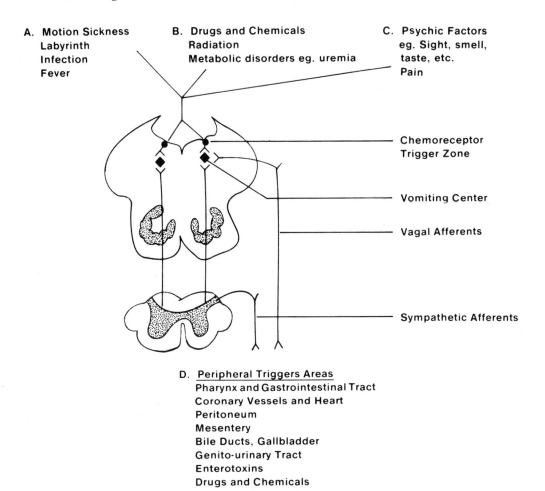

A. Motion Sickness
   Labyrinth
   Infection
   Fever

B. Drugs and Chemicals
   Radiation
   Metabolic disorders eg. uremia

C. Psychic Factors
   eg. Sight, smell,
   taste, etc.
   Pain

Chemoreceptor
Trigger Zone

Vomiting Center

Vagal Afferents

Sympathetic Afferents

D. Peripheral Triggers Areas
   Pharynx and Gastrointestinal Tract
   Coronary Vessels and Heart
   Peritoneum
   Mesentery
   Bile Ducts, Gallbladder
   Genito-urinary Tract
   Enterotoxins
   Drugs and Chemicals

FIGURE 1   The vomiting center and trigger areas.   The vomiting center is located in the dorsal portion of the lateral reticular formation of the medulla.   It presumably coordinates an integrated pattern of the vomiting process with adjacent medullary centers, e. g. , respiration.   The floor of the fourth ventricle (area postrema) contains the chemoreceptor trigger zone which responds to peripheral trigger areas.   All vomiting reactions are mediated via reflex arcs passing through the vomiting center from both central (trigger areas A, B, and C) and peripheral origins.   Trigger areas A and B act via the chemoreceptor trigger zone. Trigger areas C and D act via the forebrain/diencephalon and visceral afferent levels.   (Modified from Ref. 2.)

feeding, plus excessive drooling, should alert the examiner to the possibility of an esophageal atresia.

After 48 hours of age, in numerous malformations of the gastrointestinal tract, the vomiting may be bilious and unrelated to feeding (see Chap. 5).   These infants often have delayed passage of meconium, i. e. , beyond 36 hours, and rapidly develop distention, varying with the site of obstruction, i. e. , minimal distention with high intestinal obstruction; significant distention with distal obstructions.   Neonatal sepsis, intracranial disorders, e. g. , bleeding or subdural effusions, narcotic withdrawal, and the adrenogenital syndrome, may all present with vomiting at this early age. Numerous inborn errors of metabolism with retention of toxic metabolites such as ammonia, organic acids, and nitrogenous waste products may develop during this time, but usually are seen by the physician at a later date.

INFANCY

Infants are more likely to indulge in "spitting," regurgitation, and even projectile vomiting, with little more than a feeding disorder as the underlying factor. However, relatively "minor" causes of vomiting in infancy, e. g. , overfeeding, inadequate burping, upper respiratory infections, and disorganized domestic conditions, all may eventually result in failure to thrive and occasionally dehydration. In acute forms, gastroenteritis caused by infectious or toxic agents may present with vomiting initially and diarrhea supervening. The same is true for parenteral infections in the young. Intussusception occurs mainly in this age group, and is associated with abdominal pain and bloody "current jelly" stools. Projectile vomiting is common in gastric outlet obstructions, particularly hypertrophic pyloric stenosis, and in infants with a variety of conditions associated with intracranial hypertension, e. g. , meningitis, tumors, and bleeding.

Chronic effortless regurgitation of relatively unmodified ingested foods or formula is characteristic of gastroesophageal reflux (GER). Position or posture is important in this common condition. In the supine position, with the cardia and gastroesophageal junction dependent, reflux occurs with ease. Less than 5% of these patients require intensive investigation or intervention (see Chap. 8).

OLDER CHILDREN

Vomiting is usually of relatively greater concern in this age group, and is often associated with some form of organic disease. Mechanical obstruction and inflammation of an abdominal viscus, classically demonstrated by acute appendicitis, causes both vomiting and abdominal pain. Nausea usually is present, and occasionally diarrhea supervenes. Other common causes are gastroenteritis, hepatitis, and severe lower respiratory tract disease, e. g. , pneumonia and asthma.

UNUSUAL CATEGORIES OF VOMITING SYNDROMES

Reye syndrome is associated with a sudden onset of vomiting, usually accompanied by an upper respiratory infection (3). The patient subsequently develops encephalopathy and hepatic dysfunction. The latter is characterized by hepatomegaly and elevated blood ammonia and aminotransferase levels. The exact etiology is unknown. The encephalopathic features are associated with cerebral edema, which is the major cause of death if inadequately treated. There is a significant incidence of neurological sequelae (20-25%), and the mortality has ranged from 10-50%. The patients are usually between 2-15 years of age with a median age of 6.

Vomiting is more common than recognized in psychiatric disorders. This is particularly important in anorexia nervosa, where the patient appears unconcerned and will often hide the vomitus and withhold the information. Life-threatening deficiencies may ensue.

Rumination is a form of regurgitation occurring preponderantly in infants. The vomitus is held in the mouth, rechewed, and reswallowed. It is often effortless and associated with self-induced movements of the hands and tongue. With fre -

quent spillage and loss of oral contents, malnutrition may result. The etiology is supposedly related to psychogenic factors (4), e. g. , disturbed maternal-child interaction; however, many of these patients today are considered to have underlying gastroesophageal reflux.

Cyclic vomiting refers to recurrent bouts of vomiting, with no obvious cause, interspersed with periods of perfectly normal health. The majority of cases occur between 2-12 years of age, with sudden onset and recovery, often requiring intravenous therapy. Headache is common and emotional factors are often cited. Abdominal migraine, epilepsy equivalents, and a defect in gluconeogenesis should be excluded (5).

TREATMENT

A wide variety of drugs are useful as antiemetics; however they are generally more effective when used as prophylactics and early in the evaluation of the vomiting disorder (6). These agents include members of the phenothiazines, antihistamines, and components of marijuana.

REFERENCES

1.   Borison, H. L. , and S. C. Wang: Physiology and pharmacology of vomiting. Pharmacol Rev 5:193, 1953.

2.   Wang, S. C. , and H. L. Borison: A new concept of organization of the central emetic mechanism: Recent studies on the sites of action of apomorphine, copper sulfate and cardiac glycosides. Gastroenterology 22:1, 1952.

3.   Pollack, D. J. (ed.): Reye's Syndrome. Proceedings of a Symposium: Diagnosis, Pathology, Etiology and Management. Grune and Stratton, New York, 1975.

4.   Meuking, M. , J.G. Wagnitz, J.J. Burton, R.D. Coddington, and J. F. Sotos: Rumination—a near fatal psychiatric disease of infancy. N Engl J Med 280:802, 1969.

5.   Hayt, C. S. , and G. B. Stickler: A study of 44 children with the syndrome of recurrent (cyclic) vomiting. Pediatrics 25:775, 1960.

6.   Drugs for relief of nausea and vomiting. Med Let 16:46, 1974.

10

CONSTIPATION

Mervin Silverberg, M. D.

INTRODUCTION

Constipation refers to the passage of hard stools, usually associated with difficulty and infrequency. The layman's emphasis on the number of bowel movements may be deceptive, since the normal pattern of defecation varies widely (Table 1). The percentage of stool water content tends to be relatively constant. Generally, the infant under 6 months of age tends to pass a stool after each feeding, and during the next 3-4 years, the child has at least one stool per day. Less frequent patterns are only of concern when the fecal masses are hard, dry, and difficult to expel.

Anorectal continence is maintained by the physiological interaction of (1) mechanical muscular and (2) sensory motor nervous factors (2).

1. The rectum is usually empty and kept closed by the normal tonic contractions of the smooth muscle of the internal sphincter and the postural tone of the striated muscle of the muscular pelvic diaphragm. The latter includes the levator ani and the external sphincter (Fig. 1). Additionally, unpremeditated egress of rectal contents is prevented by the 70-80° angulation of the anorectal angle which is maintained by the crucial puborectalis sling of the levator ani (Fig. 2).

2. Visceral and somatic sensory components combine to complete the apparatus for fecal continence. The rectal mucosa is insensitive to intraluminal contents, but when stretched by stool or gas gives rise to a feeling of pelvic fullness, which at times may be variably painful. Afferent autonomic impulses are excited, mediated via the intrinsic myenteric plexus, resulting in reflex relaxation of the internal sphincter. The contents then move into the anal canal, where somatic sensory afferent fibers in the pudendal nerves are very sensitive to touch, temperature, and pressure, and are able to differentiate between stool and gas.

Although the host is now aware of imminent passage of stool, this may be obviated by the contraction of the levator ani which further angulates the anorectal junction and narrows the anal canal. Simultaneously, the external anal sphincter contracts clamping the anal canal further, preventing defecation, and the rectal wall temporariliy accommodates. These mechanisms are reflexly activated during acute episodes of increased intraabdominal pressure e. g. , sneezing and lifting, or by the presence of irritants in the anal canal, e. g. , proctoscope or suppositories. Continence may be further supported by the voluntary contraction of gluteal

TABLE 1   Stool Frequency, Weight, and Water Content in Normal Infants at Different Ages

	First Week	8-28 days	1-12 mo	13-24 mo
No. of infants	16	11	11	17
No. of stools	278	139	88	136
Stool frequency				
Mean interval between stools (hr) ± 1 SD	5. 2 + 1. 9	9. 9 ± 6.5	13. 2 + 9. 2	14. 9 + 8. 3
Range (hr)	0. 5 - 22	0. 7 - 38. 5	0. 5 - 53	2 - 120
No. of stools per 24 hr ± 1 SD	4 ± 1. 8	2. 2 ± 1. 6	1. 8 ± 1, 2	1. 7 ± 0. 6
Range	1 - 12	0. 6	0. 5	0 - 3
Wt. of individual stools (g)				
Mean	4. 3	11. 0	17	35
Range	0. 5 - 48	0. 3 - 40	2 - 98	4 - 180
Stool water content (%)				
Mean ± 1 SD	72. 8 ± 5. 0	73. 3 ± 2. 7	75. 0 ± 3. 0	73. 8 ± 3. 2
Range	65 - 84	72 - 77	72 - 80	66 - 81

(From Ref. 1. Reprinted with permission.)

muscles which secondarily cause contraction of the pelvic muscular diaphragm. In an advanced state, the child's gyrations and posturing to avoid soiling may be grotesque and this has been called the "duty dance. " When the stool or gas mass becomes critical, and the individual is able to find a toilet or a suitable squatting position, the levators are relaxed completely, a Valsalva maneuver moves the contents into the anal canal and subsequent contraction of the pelvic floor propels the material to the exterior.

Most of these mechanisms are operational by the beginning of the second year of life. "Toilet training" has nothing to do with organizing neuromuscular physiology. It represents the attempt of the infant's parents or surrogate, to make the child aware of the association of the signs of fecal presence in the rectum, and the voluntary defecation process, preferably in an appropriate receptacle.

CLASSIFICATION AND CLINICAL FEATURES (Table 2)

ACUTE CONSTIPATION

Acute constipation refers to episodes of stool retention of a relatively short duration. This often occurs following substantial changes in diet and environment, a prolonged or febrile illness, and postoperatively. Although most children recover spontaneously or respond to simple medication or dietary measures, some of these episodes are the forerunners of chronic conditions.

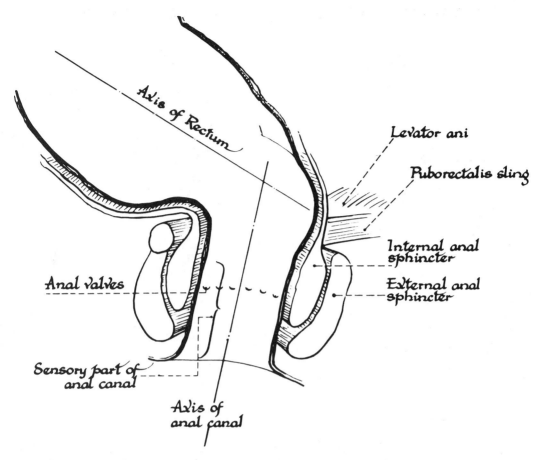

FIGURE 1   A longitudinal section of the pelvic floor around the anorectum.   The levator ani muscles consists essentially of two parts, the ileococcygeus and the more medial pubococcygeus.   The latter passes anteroposteriorly with its inner portion, the puborectalis acting as a sling around the rectum and anal canal.   It is intimately attached to the deep part of the external sphincter and to the fibers of the longitudinal muscle coat of the rectum.   If therefore forms an integral part of the anorectal ring, so essential for rectal continence. (From Ref. 3. Reprinted with permission.)

CHRONIC CONSTIPATION

Chronic constipation may be divided into four categories:

Mechanical

Mechanical is considered as any condition causing reduced or inspissated intestinal contents that result in constipation.   These conditions include inadequate intake of food or liquids, viscid stool as in cystic fibrosis, and the curdled milk syndrome due to hyperconcentration errors in mixing formulas.   Anatomic abnormalities are included in this category and involve congenital defects such as anorectal malformations (see Chap. 5), and extrinsic acquired masses such as tumors and

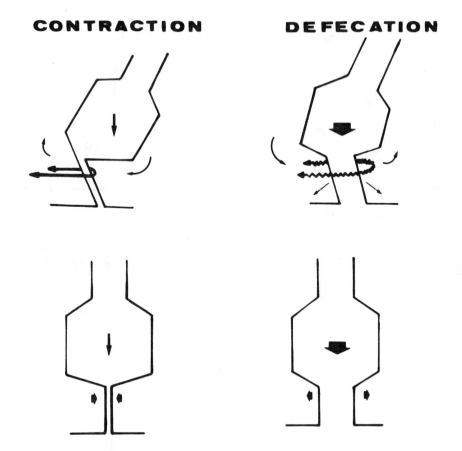

CONTRACTION   **DEFECATION**

FIGURE 2   Puborectalis muscle function in continence and defecation. The muscle encircles the upper most part of the anal canal and during contraction increases the angle and results in continence. During defecation, the muscle relaxes, straightening the canal. Above, is lateral view; below, anteroposterior view. (From ref. 10. Reprinted with permission.)

TABLE 2   Classification of Constipation

---

1.   Acute constipation: short duration; follows known precipitating factors, e. g. , post-bed rest, drugs, painful defecation

2.   Chronic constipation:

    a.   Mechanical: associated with inspissation of stools and intrinsic or extrinsic pressures (e.g. , abnormal diet, drugs, tumors, strictures, volvulus)

    b.   Intrinsic motility disorders: abnormalities of intramural ganglia (e.g., Hirschsprung and pseudo-Hirschsprung) and metabolism (e.g. , diabetic acidosis, diabetic neuropathy, porphyria, uremia, hypokalemia, hypopituitarism, hypothyroidism, hypercalcemia)

TABLE 2   (cont'd)

---

2.   Chronic constipation (cont'd)

    c.   Extrinsic neurological and muscular disorders: abnormalities of the brain, spinal cord, or sacral nerves; primary muscle diseases

    d.   Idiopathic/functional disorders: abnormalities of elimination without any specific cause; never starts at birth and eventually associated with overflow soiling, and megacolon. Rectal ampulla is distended with stool

---

abscesses. The diagnosis of anal stenosis and "tight sphincter" are overdone, since in fact they are extremely rare. In most of these infants therefore therapeutic digital dilatations are unnecessary or may cause actual harm. Mechanical factors occasionally underlie acute constipation, and may evolve into an intestinal obstruction.

Intrinsic Motility Disorders

Intrinsic motility disorders are often associated with a variety of conditions. Because of its potential morbidity and mortality, Hirschsprung disease must be excluded as early as possible (see Chap. 8). Although the majority of these cases will present during the first month of life with some disturbance of defecation, a high index of suspicion must be kept for mild or late onset cases usually due to aganglionic short segments and a variety of rare disorders called pseudo-Hirschsprung syndrome. A number of endocrine, metabolic, and pharmacologically induced conditions also should be included in the differential diagnosis. Congenital and acquired hypothyroidism may present with significant constipation and only subtle stigmata of thyroid insufficiency.

Extrinsic Neurological and Muscular Disorders

These disorders are frequently associated with constipation. Indeed, this may be an overriding problem in the rehabilitation of these patients. Abnormalities of the lower spinal cord or sacral nerves abrogate normal reflex and voluntary responses to stool passage in the anorectal region. Primary muscular disorders involving the abdominal wall, e. g. , prune belly syndrome, or paralysis of the diaphragm, prevent the child from effectively increasing intraabdominal pressure. Although sphincter tone may be decreased or absent, a weakened ability to initiate and maintain a Valsalva maneuver, and lack of awareness of intraluminal contents may prevent efficient defecation. Some of these patients are studied for spurious diarrhea caused by overflow incontinence.

Idiopathic/Functional Disorders

Constipation of unknown etiology incorporates the greatest number of clinical problems of fecal continence in children (Table 3).

    Functional constipation, the single largest subgroup, has an onset between 1-24 months of age in 75% of the cases, and is frequently complicated by fecal soiling or encopresis (4). The high frequency of concordance in identical twins (5) and the familial tendency of this complaint, suggests a genetic influence. The etiology is multifactoral, including neurodevelopment, personality, and parenting,

TABLE 3   Functional Constipation in 63 Patients*

	No (%)	Remarks
1. Age at onset: 0-1 yr	52	40% <25th percentile in weight
1-2 yr	14	13% <25th percentile in weight
2-3 yr	14	
4-10 yr	9	
> 10 yr	5	
2. Learning/psychosocial problems	45	12% in controls
3. At least one relapse with treatment: mineral oil	24	Followed up to 7 yr
laxatives	90	Only 2/3 were strictly compliant

*Followed in Gastroenterology Center at North Shore University Hospital

as contributing factors (6). Overzealous "training", unsympathetic attitudes, bribing, and a wide variety of punishments, play an important role in perpetuating the problem.   Early in the patient's history, there is preoccupation with the child's "rear-end" and frequent "assaults" occur with suppositories, laxatives, enemas, and digital stimulation.   The episodes of constipation are often intermittent, with periods of normal to loose stools in between.   This variability is more common when the child falls in the category of the irritable bowel syndrome, which some authors claim constitutes most of these cases.

Since most patients, excluding the newborn infants, are in the functional category, and there are few if any clear-cut features, the diagnosis is one of exclusion. A detailed history and meticulous physical examination are of paramount importance.   Deep abdominal palpation usually will reveal the extent and severity of stool retention.   A careful bimanual rectal digital evaluation must be performed with close inspection of the perineum.

Encopresis

Encopresis refers to the presence of soiling of the perineum and underclothing. It usually is associated with an overdistended rectum filled with stool of various consistencies.   This impaction with overflow incontinence occurs in more than 95% of encopretics.   A somewhat patulous anal orifice in these patients usually is not associated with any neurological deficits, but results from the large stool mass resting on the external sphincter.   Encopresis is frequently a psychogenic disorder, although rare cases of spinal cord anomalies may present in this manner.   Radiocontrast studies are generally of no value in the differential diagnosis.   In all doubtful cases, a short aganglionic segment can be excluded by manometric demonstration of a normal internal anal sphincter, or by the presence of ganglia in rectal suction biopsies taken serially at 3, 4, and 5 cm proximal to the anal verge (see Chap. 8).

TREATMENT

LAXATIVES

No discussion of constipation can avoid the debate on the value and effects of laxative drugs. Furthermore, we are now aware that the mechanism of action of many of these drugs requires reevaluation. Most irritant cathartics, e. g. , cascara, phenolpthalein, bisacodyl, castor oil, and oxyphenisatin, and bulk cathartics, e. g. , methycellulose, plantago seed, and semisynthetic cellulose act directly by increasing water and electrolyte secretion into the bowel contents. This is also true for the stool softener, dioctyl sodium sulfosuccinate (7). Those compounds containing stimulant cathartics often are not only ineffective, but cause significant discomfort and abdominal cramps.

Mineral oil remains alone as the standard lubricant (8), and is relatively harmless, except when the child is forced to take the oil. Aspiration pneumonia is the major complication of the aggressive use of mineral oil; however, forcible administration of any of the cathartics may prove to be counterproductive. Noncompliance is a problem with long-term use.

DIET

Dietary manipulation may be helpful; however, there is little objective evidence to prove that the roughage, or special diet alone, has been very effective in managing constipation. At best, the data at present support the conclusion that dietary fiber (not crude) will increase stool bulk. Many young infants will produce softer stools when excess dietary carbohydrate and prunes or prune juice are added. Adequate liquid intake is important in all age groups, particularly during acute or chronic illness. As a rule, changes in diet should be unobtrusive, and under no circumstances is it worth making the dining table into a battleground.

SPECIFIC THERAPY

Short-term use of dietary changes and laxatives are useful in acute or subacute constipation; however, chronic disorders require a more complex organized approach. This is particularly true for the patient with fecal impaction. The fecaloma should be evacuated before any oral medication is administered. A mineral oil enema followed within 1-2 hours by a hypertonic phosphate enema, 2-3 ml/kg, is effective. If unsuccessful, the paired enemas may be repeated once or twice at 12-hour intervals. Isotonic saline enemas should be used in resistant cases, to avoid hypertonic dehydration and hyperphosphatemia. Tap water enemas are absolutely contraindicated in the pediatric age group because of the real danger of water intoxication. Digital disimpaction is rarely necessary. Occasionally, bisacodyl (suppositories or by mouth) may be required to clear the colorectum.

Oral use of light-grade mineral oil is started as soon as the rectum is effectively cleaned out. In compliant children, the usual starting dose is 15 ml/kg of body weight, given in one or two divided doses. The tasteless mineral oil is best taken cold with citrus fruit juice to remove the aftereffect of oiliness in the mouth. The amount of oil is increased slowly until the dose is effective in producing two to three loose bowel movements, preferably in the immediate postprandial period, with minimal leakage of oil. This regimen is continued for 6-8 weeks to permit the distended rectum to return to normal size and sensitivity. The long-term success of the program occurs after weaning from the mineral oil and the gastrocolic reflex becomes the major stimulus for defecation, with little or no cathartic requirements. Although the reputed losses of fat-soluble vitamins in the mineral oil has never been substantiated, it is recommended that the child be given a daily water-soluble multivitamin preparation 1 hour before or more than 2 hours after the oil is administered.

The chronic use of laxatives in children is rarely, if ever, indicated. Unlike adults, reports of abuse and medical complications are very uncommon, i. e. , dependency, melanosis coli, cathartic colon, secretory diarrhea, or hypokalemia.

The use of a proper squatting position is stressed by most, but not all, workers in the field. Permitting the child to sit on a "potty" or toilet seat, with feet adequately supported, will facilitate the neuromuscular features of the defecation process. The physician must orchestrate the parent-child interaction, and in very complex cases, psychiatric consultation is usually necessary.

BIOFEEDBACK

Biofeedback is a new modality in the treatment of children with stool retention who have anorectal malformations. Some success also has been reported in patients with functional constipation (9).

REFERENCES

1. Lemoh, J. N. , and O. G. Brooke: Frequency and weight of normal stools in infancy. Arch Dis Child 54:719, 1979.

2. Fleisher, D. R. : Diagnosis and treatment of disorders of defecation in children. Pediatr Ann 5:70, 1976.

3. Duthie, H. L. : Dynamics of the rectum and anus. Clin Gastroenterol 4:470, 1975.

4. Fitzgerald, J. F. : Encopresis, soiling, constipation: What's to be done? Pediatrics 56:348, 1976.

5. Bakwin, H. , and M. Davidson: Constipation in twins. Amer J Dis Child 121:179, 1971.

6. Levine, M. D. : Children with encopresis: A descriptive analysis. Pediatrics 56:412, 1975.

7. Donowitz, M. , and H. J. Binder: Effect of dioctyl sodium sulfosuccinate on colonic fluid and electrolyte movement. Gastroenterology 69:941, 1975.

8. Davidson, M. , M. M. Kugler, and C. H. Bauer: Diagnosis and management in children with severe and protracted constipation and obstipation. J Pediatr 62:261, 1963.

9. Olness, K. , F. A. McFarland, and J. Piper: Biofeedback: A new modality in the management of children with fecal soiling. J Pediatr 96:505, 1980.

10. Ihre, T. : Studies on anal function in continent and incontinent patients. Scand J Gastroenterol 9(suppl 25), 1974.

11

GASTROINTESTINAL BLEEDING

Arnold Schussheim, M. D.

INTRODUCTION

Gastrointestinal bleeding is a relatively common problem in all pediatric age groups. It may be massive and a life-threatening emergency, or only apparent by chemical tests of the stool (occult bleeding). The bleeding may originate at any level from the mouth to the anus and is caused by a great variety of primary gastrointestinal and systemic disorders. The bleeding course may be unabated or intractable, but it is usually intermittent and stops spontaneously. Recurrent gastrointestinal bleeding in children is a difficult problem (1).

Hematemesis is the vomiting of blood which may be bright red, or if altered by the action of gastric acidity, "coffee ground" in appearance. In either case it originates proximal to the ligament of Treitz. When sufficient upper gastrointestinal bleeding progresses downward, it appears by rectum as black or "tarry" stool (melena). Hematochezia is the passage of red blood rectally and this usually originates in the lower gastrointestinal tract. Gastrointestinal bleeding is frightening to both the patient and the family and is often brought to the physician's attention on an emergency basis. Occult gastrointestinal bleeding also should be considered in the differential diagnosis of anemia with no other obvious origin.

Classification of gastrointestinal bleeding can be based on age, severity, location, etiological agents, etc. , as discussed in Chap. 4, Diagnostic Approach. One possible grouping is by etiological factors. (Table 1). These etiological agents can be thought of as acting directly on the intestinal mucosa, on the blood vessels, or via disturbances in the bleeding or clotting mechanism.

ETIOLOGY

CONGENITAL MALFORMATIONS (See Chap. 5)

Meckel Diverticulum (An Omphalomesenteric Duct Remnant)

This bleeding usually presents as dark red, massive, painless, recurrent, rectal bleeding in infancy, with greater frequency in males, and occasionally familial. It is the most frequent cause of serious gastrointestinal bleeding in children found

TABLE 1   Etiology of Gastrointestinal Bleeding

1. Congenital malformations
   a. Meckel diverticulum
   b. Duplication of the bowel
   c. Hiatal hernia and intrathoracic stomach
   d. Heterotopic gastric mucosa

2. Trauma
   a. External trauma
   b. Foreign bodies
   c. Mallory-Weiss syndrome
   d. Iatrogenic trauma (biopsy)

3. Infection/inflammation
   a. Enterocolitis
   b. Acute gastritis
   c. Esophagitis
   d. Proctitis

4. Tumors
   a. Polyps
   b. Vascular malformations
   c. Other: lymphosarcoma, Hodgkin disease, etc.

5. Metabolic-systemic
   a. Acid/peptic ulceration
   b. Inflammatory bowel disease
   c. "Allergies"
   d. Drugs
   e. Nonspecific intestinal ulcerations

6. Collagen-vascular
   a. Disturbances in bleeding and clotting mechanisms
   b. Henoch-Schonlein purpura
   c. Hemorrhagic disease of the newborn
   d. Volvulus and mesenteric vessel insufficiency
   e. Periarteritis nodosa

7. Anatomical
   a. Portal hypertension
   b. Intussusception
   c. Anal and perianal disorders

8. Spurious gastrointestinal bleeding
   a. Coloring agents
   b. Swallowed blood: maternal, mouth, nose, throat, hemoptysis
   c. Vaginal bleeding, pink urinary sediment

9. Undetermined causes

at laparotomy, after the usual diagnostic measures have not revealed a specific etiology.   Its demonstration by barium enema or upper gastrointestinal series is
most unusual.   The dictum that Meckel diverticulum is frequently sought, and infrequently found, has recently been modified by the use of preoperative angiography
and radioisotope imaging (2, 3).   The latter procedure has been found useful, with
due note of possible false-positive and false-negative studies.   Technetium-99m
pertechnetate is injected intravenously and subsequent radioimaging of the abdomen
will demonstrate the ectopic gastric mucosa in the Meckel diverticulum (Fig. 1).
Bleeding from this diverticulum is due to ulceration of the adjacent ileal mucosa
on the mesenteric border.   In the absence of gastric mucosa, the diverticula are
not associated with intestinal bleeding, except in the presence of an intussusception
(see Chap. 5).

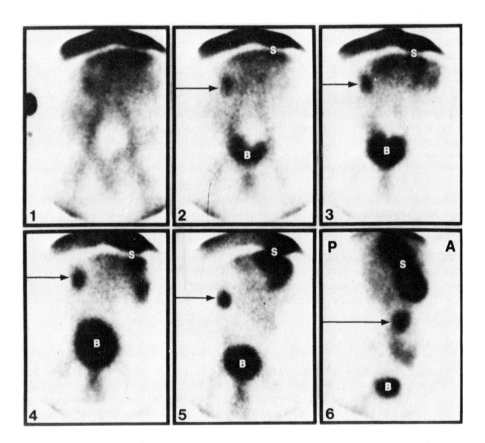

FIGURE 1   Interval abdominal imaging after intravenous injection of technetium
99m pertechnetate: (S) stomach; (B) bladder; (arrows) Meckel diverticulum with
ectopic gastric mucosa.   Section 5 is postvoiding and section 6 is lateral view.

Duplication of the Bowel (See Chap. 5)

Duplications may be found at all levels in the gastrointestinal tract, most commonly involving the small bowel; less than 50% communicate with the lumen. Bleeding
is due to heterotopic acid-secreting tissue or necrosis. A mass may be found on
abdominal examination or an extrinsic filling defect noted on radiographic bowel
studies. The heterotopic gastric mucosa found in both the Meckel diverticulum and
in duplications secretes hydrochloric acid and therefore may cause bleeding from
sites low in the gastrointestinal tract.

Hiatal Hernia (See Chap. 8)

Both hiatal hernia and esophageal reflux may be associated with hematemesis and/
or occult blood in the stools. The diagnosis of esophagitis may be difficult at
times even with endoscopy, and histological examination of bite-biopsies are necessary for confirmation.

TRAUMA

A blunt or penetrating wound of the abdomen may cause immediate or delayed gastrointestinal bleeding due to perforation or subsequent rupture of an intramural
hematoma. The latter occurs most commonly in the fixed retroperitoneal duodenum. Foreign bodies may be swallowed, or inserted into the rectum, and are frequently radiopaque. Indwelling nasogastric tubes or a rectal thermometer may be
the source of iatrogenic gastrointestinal bleeding, and an intramural hematoma
should be suspected in a battered child. Prolonged vomiting or retching may
cause an esophageal tear, i.e., retching erosions or Mallory-Weiss syndrome.

INFECTION/INFLAMMATION

This wide-ranging group is frequently associated with fever and diarrhea. Enteric
infection with invasive organisms such as Salmonella, Shigella, Yersinia, or Campylobacter, or pathogenic amebae are frequent causes of rectal bleeding in
children. Heavy infestations with trichuria or schistosomes may also cause rectal
bleeding. Other bacteria, viruses, and parasites are less common causes. The
clinical course is usually of short duration and the bleeding nonmassive. The enterocolitis of Hirschsprung disease, pseudomembranous colitis (postantibiotic),
and necrotizing enterocolitis of the neonate also should be considered in this group
(4).

Acute Gastritis (See Chap. 13)

Pathologically, this may be hemorrhagic or erosive and caused by infectious
agents, chemical substances, or uremia. It also may occur as a complication of
some more obvious systemic illness such as hepatitis or bronchopneumonia. Ra-
diologic studies of the gastrointestinal tract are frequently negative, owing to the
superficial nature of the lesions, and a more accurate diagnosis is accomplished
with flexible endoscopy. The bleeding often stops spontaneously and many previously undiagnosed cases of upper gastrointestinal bleeding may have been due to
this entity. The association with the ingestion of acetylsalicylic acid is probably
one of the most common causal factors.

TUMORS (See Chap. 17)

Polyps

Polyps are solitary or multiple and they are almost always benign in children. The majority may be seen by endoscopic examination, and about one-third felt by digital rectal examination. The bleeding is usually nonmassive and the most frequent age of occurrence of juvenile polyps (inflammatory or retention polyps), the most common type, is approximately 3-5 years of age (5). Polyps produce painless, usually red, recurrent rectal bleeding, often sufficient to cause anemia. The blood is frequently on the surface of a formed stool or seen on the toilet tissue. They also may be demonstrated radiographically with or without air contrast studies. Less common polyposis syndromes (6) are outlined in Table 2 (also see Chap. 17). Familial colonic polyposis usually presents clinically in adolescents. Peutz-Jeghers polyps involve predominantly the small bowel and the typical buccal pigmentation may be diagnostic (Fig. 2). Nodular lymphoid hyperplasia, pseudopolyps of ulcerative colitis, pneumatosis, etc., should be considered in the differential diagnosis of filling defects of the bowel. Nodular lymphoid hyperplasia may involve the small intestine (often associated with IgA deficiency and malabsorption); terminal ileum (possible association with abdominal pain); or colon and rectum (frequently a nonpathological finding). The lymphoid follicles may show apical umbilication on barium contrast studies (7).

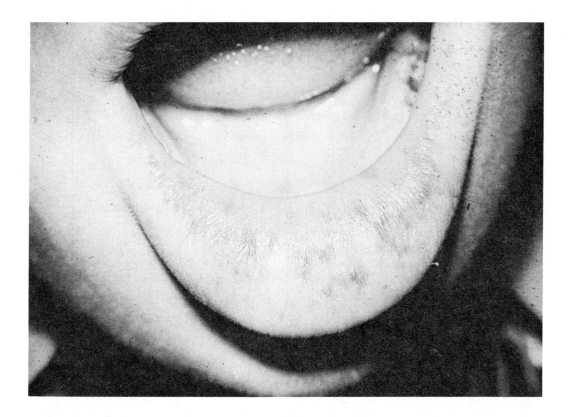

FIGURE 2   Peutz-Jeghers syndrome showing orobuccal pigmentations.

TABLE 2   Intestinal Polyposis Syndromes

Syndrome	Pathology	Major symptoms	Malignant potential	Inheritance	Location*	Associated lesions
Familial colonic polyposis	Adenoma	Bloody diarrhea	+ (± 100%)	Autosomal dominant	R, C	None
Generalized polyposis of the GI tract	Adenoma	Bloody diarrhea	+ (? incidence)	?	S, SB, C	Reported desmoid
Gardner syndrome	Adenoma	Bloody diarrhea	+ (± 100%)	Autosomal dominant	C, R	(1) Bony tumors (2) Soft tissue tumors
Turcot syndrome	Adenoma	Bloody diarrhea, CNS symptoms	probably +	? Recessive	C, R	CNS malignant tumors
Peutz-Jeghers (P-J) syndrome	P-J polyp (hamartoma)	Recurrent SB obstruction	very rare	Autosomal dominant	SB, S C	Mucocutaneous pigmentation Ovarian Ca
Juvenile colonic polyposis	Juvenile	Bloody diarrhea	0	?	C	None
Diffuse gastrointestinal juvenile polyposis (Cronkhite-Canada variant)	Juvenile	Diarrhea, edema, pain	0	?	S, SB, C	Alopecia, onchotropia, pigmentation

*S = stomach, SB = small bowel, C = colon, R = rectum

Vascular Malformations

These lesions are uncommon causes of gastrointestinal bleeding in children and are very difficult to diagnose. They vary from multiple phlebectasias of the bowel, as in Osler-Weber-Rendu disease or Turner syndrome, to cavernous hemangiomas. Vascular skin lesions frequently are associated. Phleboliths may be seen on flat plate examination of the abdomen and are diagnostic. Selective angiography may be useful in demonstrating these lesions.

METABOLIC/SYSTEMIC

Acid/Peptic Ulceration (See Chap. 13)

These lesions may occur in the lower esophagus, stomach, duodenum, or along surgical anastomotic lines. They may be primary or associated with stress, central nervous system disease, burns, hypercalcemia, gastrin-secreting tumors, or drug use. The exact incidence of these acute and chronic lesions as a cause of gastrointestinal bleeding in children varies among many reporting institutions. The bleeding is frequently occult, may be painless, and often the diagnosis is delayed until pallor and weakness are noted. With the increasing number of children being treated in intensive care units, the number of stress ulcerations of the gastrointestinal tract seems to be increasing.

Inflammatory Bowel Disease (See Chap. 16)

Rectal bleeding is more frequent in ulcerative colitis than Crohn disease. Hematochezia may be an initial manifestation of ulcerative colitis, even before the onset of diarrhea, particularly in the group with involvement restricted to the rectum, i. e. , proctitis. Sigmoidoscopy and radiographic findings in addition to biopsy establish the diagnosis. Many other disorders enter into the differential diagnosis of inflammatory bowel disease, also causing gastrointestinal bleeding, such as irritation colitis, hemolytic uremic syndrome, etc.

Cow's Milk Protein-Sensitive
Enteropathy (See Chap. 7)

Sensitivity to bovine proteins may cause gross gastrointestinal bleeding or occult blood loss in children from the newborn period onward. Good response to the removal of milk and occasionally other bovine protein products, as well, is diagnostic. Other food protein "allergies" are less commonly involved in gastrointestinal bleeding except for soy proteins.

Drugs

A large variety of drugs have been implicated in causing gastrointestinal bleeding. These include aminophylline, alcohol, anticoagulants, corticosteroids, reserpine, iron and some antibiotics. Some anticoagulant drugs may cross the placenta or appear in breast milk. The most common offender, however, is aspirin and it deserves special attention (8). It is surely one of the most frequent causes of upper gastrointestinal bleeding in children; frequently suspected and often not proved. It may occur with physiological dosage and can be massive or occult. The pathology observed endoscopically or at tissue examination is acute, hemorrhagic gastritis. The physiological mode of action is not certain at present and current theories include physical contact, platelet effect, mucosal barrier damage with alteration of mucous secretion, or back diffusion of hydrogen ions. Serum salicylate levels, prolonged bleeding time, or loss of secondary phase of platelet aggregation may corroborate salicylate ingestion.

Nonspecific Ulceration

Primary nonspecific small-bowel ulceration, ingestion of enteric coated potassium and other rare causes of small-bowel ulceration (ZE syndrome, typhoid fever, ischemia) are nongranulomatous, usually solitary and frequenty not diagnosed before laparotomy. The ileum is frequently involved (9).

COLLAGEN-VASCULAR

Disturbances in the Bleeding and Clotting Mechanism

In this group of disorders there may be evidence of bleeding from multiple sites, both within and outside the gastrointestinal tract. Disorders affecting the bleeding mechanism are a more frequent cause of gastrointestinal bleeding than those affecting the clotting mechanism, except in the newborn period, where we see the effects of vitamin K deficiency and hypoprothrombinemia (10). This group should be thought of as a major cause of simultaneous upper- and lower-tract bleeding.

Henoch-Schonlein Purpura

Henoch-Schonlein purpura is usually associated with rectal bleeding, abdominal pain, hematuria, rash and joint manifestations (11). The bleeding rarely requires transfusion. Unfortunately, the appearance of the urticarial or purpuric skin lesions, predominantly on the lower half of the body, which are characteristic for this disease, may be delayed causing great difficulty in diagnosis. Henoch-Schonlein purpura may be associated with intussusception due to an intestinal intramural hematoma, thus confusing the clinical picture and creating an additional cause for bleeding. This intramural hemorrhage in the small bowel may give a "thumbprinting" filling defect on radiographic studies.

Volvulus and Mesenteric Vessel Insufficiency (See Chap. 5)

These disorders are associated with acute pain and signs of intestinal obstruction and are emergency situations. Anoxia and indwelling vascular catheters also may contribute to vascular insufficiency of the bowel.

ANATOMICAL

Portal Hypertension

Intra- and extrahepatic portal venous obstruction leads to portal vein hypertension with subsequent esophageal or gastric varices and potential bleeding from these sites. Hematemesis is frequently followed shortly thereafter by melena. There may be a history of previous jaundice, umbilical manipulation, sepsis, dehydration, or the various causes of hepatic cirrhosis. Liver function tests are abnormal with intrahepatic causes. On physical examination, the liver and spleen are usually enlarged, although the latter may contract in response to blood volume loss. In the absence of a concurrent coagulation defect, most episodes are self-limited. The varices may be demonstrated on barium examination. Visualization of varices and bleeding sites by flexible endoscopy and selective angiography also is possible.

Intussusception (See Chap. 5)

This is a leading cause of intestinal obstruction during the first 2 years of life. It is two to three times more common in males. The most common variant is the ileocolic invagination with impairment of venous return. There is a sudden onset of rhythmic pain and subsequently, an abdominal mass may present. Currant jelly stools or frank hemorrhage may occur. A barium enema is diagnostic as well as often therapeutic.

Anal and Perianal Lesions

Perianal fissures are the most common cause of nonmassive, red, rectal bleeding in children, particularly noted in office practice. Bright red blood streaks the stools, the latter tending to be harder than normal. One or more slitlike mucosal tears can usually be seen by spreading the buttocks, or by the insertion of a small anoscope. Hemorrhoids are a distinctly uncommon lesion in childhood and are almost always of the external variety. Stercoral ulceration and rectal prolapse are additional examples of anal diseases that may cause rectal bleeding, and are usually associated with predisposing causes, i.e., constipation, malnutrition, cystic fibrosis, etc. It is important to inquire regarding painful defecation or "hyper-wiper" habits.

SPURIOUS GASTROINTESTINAL BLEEDING

Blood in the stool or vomitus may be simulated by a variety of coloring agents. Blood that is acid-altered may be simulated by iron, bismuth, charcoal, beets, licorice, etc. Red coloring matter may appear from various antibiotics, artificially colored drinks, ketchup or tomatoes in excess, antihelminthic drugs or Jell-O. Maternal blood may be swallowed during delivery or by sucking at a breast with fissured nipples. Maternal blood is differentiated by the Apt test—1 ml is dissolved in 10 ml of distilled water and filtered; add 2 ml of 1% sodium hydroxide; fetal blood remains pink, due to the alkaline resistance of fetal hemoglobin, while maternal blood will turn brown. A dark green diarrheal stool is frequently incorrectly described as melanotic, especially when viewed in subdued light. Dilution of the stool with water brings out the true green color. Blood entering the stomach from dental, nose, and throat sources may be difficult to differentiate, but one should obtain a detailed history to look for these very carefully. Rarely, one may ingest blood for psychiatric reasons. Hemopytsis may be distinguished by its presentation with coughing, frothy appearance, and alkaline reaction. Unsuspected "menses" in the newborn or initial menstruation of the adolescent may be confused with rectal bleeding. In infants, one frequently sees a pinkish urinary sediment (amorphous urates), or relatively harmless bleeding from a penile meatal ulcer appearing in the diaper.

UNDETERMINED CAUSES

Even after intensive investigations, many episodes of gastrointestinal bleeding defy definitive diagnosis; especially in the newborn period, over half of the presentations are not specifically diagnosed.

DIAGNOSIS

Some initial generalizations may be made on the basis of the patient's age, severity of the bleeding, the presence of pain, fever, or systemic disease, together with the determination of the anatomical level of the bleeding. Many classifications of gastrointestinal bleeding are made on the basis of age. For example, rectal fissures and intussusception are the number 1 and 2 causes of rectal bleeding in the first two years of life, while portal hypertension is more common in adolescents. This statistical correlation is helpful, but usually a precise etiological diagnosis must await stabilization of the patient and more refined techniques (12). The ease of diagnosis varies from the instantaneous visual diagnosis, as in Peutz-Jeghers syndrome (see Fig. 2), to the complex radioisotopic studies (see Fig. 1) and angiography (Fig. 3). A schematic approach is illustrated in Fig. 4.

In taking the history it is necessary to describe all stools and vomitus specifically as to color, intimacy of the blood to stool, and the estimation of blood loss. Upper-tract bleeding may be red or dark colored, depending on gastric emptying and acid contact time. Lower-tract bleeding is usually red and may often appear as streaks of blood on formed stools or blood alone. The exact relationship to defecation should be elicited. Pain and fever in the history serve to make one think of several groups of causes of gastrointestinal bleeding, as remarked on previously. As in the usual history, familial and systemic diseases, especially bleeding tendencies, polyps, and inflammatory bowel disease, should be elicited. Trauma, retching, travel, etc. , have already been noted as diagnostic factors. It is important that all administered medication be recorded, especially aspirin, which may be present in a great variety of proprietary products. Try to document a recent hematocrit for comparison. Gastrointestinal bleeding may be concealed and remain internal for a period. It also has been observed that children vomit blood less often than adults.

In the physical examination, the skin and mucous membrane should be carefully inspected for pigmentations, angiomas, and evidence of a bleeding tendency. Hepatosplenomegaly, abdominal masses, and abdominal tenderness are found in diseases such as portal hypertension, intussusception, and intestinal duplications. A careful perianal and digital rectal examination is always indicated. Pallor, pulse rate, blood pressure, and historical data as well as laboratory values are used to estimate blood loss. Determination of the severity of bleeding is important for the institution of treatment, as well as for the consideration of the statistical probability of certain diagnoses. A Meckel diverticulum is a much more likely source of rectal bleeding in massive rather than intermittent occult bleeding or with streaks of blood with no change in the hematocrit. One must be aware of the possible delay in changes of the hematocrit in acute bleeding. An elevated serum BUN (with normal creatinine) and ammonia may be due to resorption of large amounts of blood from the gastrointestinal tract. This blood also may cause marked hyperperistalsis, slight temperature elevation, and leukocytosis. Tachycardia greater than 100, hematocrit less than 30, a blood pressure drop, or estimated blood loss in excess of 25% of the circulating blood volume is considered to be a massive hemorrhage. On the other hand, estimation of blood loss by visual inspection or testing of the stool is a very inaccurate process. Small amounts of blood-stained water or tissue may give the appearance of large blood losses, and a maximum stool chemical test of 4+ for blood can be obtained with only moderate blood loss in the gastrointestinal tract.

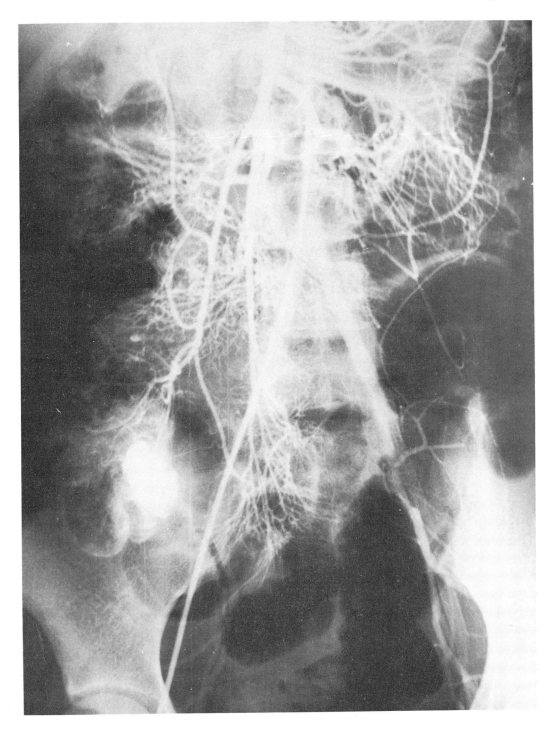

FIGURE 3   Superior mesenteric angiogram demonstrating extravasation of dye into the cecum; later identified as an arteriovenous malformation.

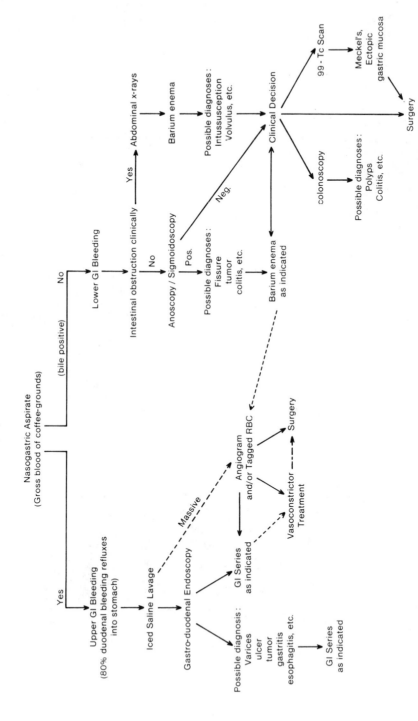

FIGURE 4   General management and diagnostic procedures in significant gastrointestinal bleeding based on available nasogastric (NG) aspirate. Dotted lines refer to options when bleeding is brisk, massive, or does not cease.

INVESTIGATIONS

First Phase

Blood is taken simultaneously for a complete blood count, the bleeding and coagulation studies that are indicated, as well as type and cross-match. In those cases without obvious hematemesis, a nasogastric tube should be carefully inserted into the stomach to determine if blood is present, and thereby establish upper gastrointestinal localization. About 80% of patients with a bleeding duodenal ulcer will demonstrate refluxed blood in a gastric aspirate. Division at this point into upper and lower gastrointestinal hemorrhage is important since this will direct much of the further investigation (13). The clinical establishment of upper or lower hemorrhage has some difficulties. It has been noted that rapid passage of upper gastrointestinal tract blood through the intestinal tract may appear via rectum as red or maroon bleeding. On the other hand, during delayed passage of blood through the gastrointestinal tract, even colonic bleeding may be sufficiently altered to appear rectally as dark stool. A chemical test should be done to document blood. Chemical tests for blood (14) include the o-tolidine (Hematest), benzidine, and guaiac (Hemoccult). These tests vary in sensitivity to normal amounts of blood in the diet (meat) as well as to other substances such as iron and nonheme peroxidases to give false results. The Hemoccult slide test is gaining wide office use, but one should be aware of false-negative results due to prolonged storage of these cards. They are very convenient to use in ambulatory patients, who must return stool specimens to the physician. Recently the ingestion of vitamin C by the patient has been reported to cause false-negative stool guaiac tests. Further on in the phase 1 investigation, proctosigmoidoscopy will reveal causes of lower-tract bleeding such as colitis and polyps. Rectal biopsy and stool cultures as well as stool smear may be done at this time. Radiographic studies of the esophagus, stomach, small bowel and colon are often needed. Important lesions of the gastrointestinal tract such as polyps, duodenal ulcers, colitis, and Meckel diverticulum may be present despite normal-appearing radiographic studies.

Second Phase

The more complex investigations follow as needed.

Liver function tests and measurement of portal venous pressure will be required if one considers portal hypertension probable. Gastric hyperacidity may be found in some children with duodenal ulcer, but is generally not a useful diagnostic test. Measurements of red blood cell loss with radioactive chromium-tagged erythrocytes may be indicated in some cases of long-standing undetermined occult blood loss into the gastrointestinal tract. Selective angiography is now being used with increasing frequency. It may localize the source of active bleeding that is greater than 1 cc/min, or identify an abnormal vascular pattern of a vascular malformation, abnormal mesentery, etc. The wider use of fiberoptic flexible endoscopy has made direct visualization of the esophagus, stomach, and duodenum more frequently available in children and has been responsible for identifying a substantial number of previously undiagnosed lesions. Colonoscopy is useful for lesions that cannot be visualized by normal proctosigmoidoscopic techniques.

TREATMENT

The initial treatment of a patient with gastrointestinal hemorrhage depends on the degree of blood loss. This would be quite different in the patient with shock as opposed to a patient with chronic occult blood loss. The briskly bleeding child is an emergency and should be hospitalized immediately. An adequate intravenous route then should be established and maintained, and replacement with whole blood (5-10 ml/kg) or plasma expanders started, as necessary. Serial documentation of the pulse, blood pressure, urine output, and hematocrit, as well as fluids administered and estimation of blood loss, are mandatory. Monitoring of central venous pressure may be helpful.

Established surgical and medical diseases should be specifically treated. Tamponade of bleeding esophageal varices with a triple lumen tube (Sengstaken-Blakemore) offers only temporary relief and is hazardous in inexperienced hands. Continuous aspiration with a nasogastric tube as well as lavage with iced saline irrigations is advisable in upper gastrointestinal hemorrhage.

A number of patients defy specific diagnosis after all tests are completed. Joint management by a surgeon and the medical team is advisable, and expectant care instituted. Transfusion of whole blood is indicated in shock, falling hematocrit, or in preparation of patients for surgery with hematocrits below 30%. Blood should be given over a period of time and in amounts depending on the rate of loss. One should be aware of the small circulating blood volume in young children and the critical situation with even small-volume blood losses. In acute episodes, when replacement is not adequate or in the presence of recurrent massive bleeding, exploratory surgery may be justified for diagnostic and therapeutic reasons. In chronic, nonmassive bleeding of undetermined etiology, there should be some reluctance to do a diagnostic laparotomy, since no cause is found in many cases. This is particularly true in the newborn infant. Newer techniques of preoperative diagnosis have significantly diminished the number of idiopathic bleeders. These newer methods include more elaborate isotopic techniques for Meckel diverticulum, selective angiography, and flexible upper and lower endoscopy. Selective angiography also has widened the therapeutic field with direct use of vasoconstrictive substances or embolization techniques to control bleeding (15). Prevention and treatment of nonspecific "gastritis" bleeding with cimetidine or antacids is under study.

REFERENCES

1.   Spencer, R.: Gastrointestinal hemorrhage in infancy and childhood. Surgery 55:718, 1964.

2.   Rutherford, R. B. and D. R. Akers: Meckel's diverticulum. Surgery 59:618, 1966.

3.   Schussheim, A., G. W. Moskowitz, and L. M. Levy: Radionuclide diagnosis of bleeding Meckel's diverticulum in children. Am J Gastroenterol 68:25, 1977.

4.   Schussheim, A., and E. J. C. Goldstein: Antibiotic-associated pseudomembranous colitis in siblings. Pediatrics 66:932, 1980.

5.   Holgersen, L. O., R. E. Miller, and H. A. Zintel: Juvenile polyps of the colon. Surgery 69:288, 1971.

6.   Schwabe, A. D., and K. J. Lewin: Gastrointestinal polyposis syndromes. Viewpoints Dig Dis 12:No. 1, 1980.

7.   Madewell, J. E. , and M. M. Reeder: Multiple filling defects in the colon. JAMA 232:172, 1975.

8.   Gartner, A. H. : Aspirin-induced gastritis and gastrointestinal bleeding. J Am Dental Assoc 93:111, 1976.

9.   Harrison, H. E. , G. S. Spear, and J. P. Dorst: Chronic idiopathic ulcerative ileitis in infancy. J Pediatr 78:538, 1971.

10. Thomas, J. , P. J. Collipp, A. Schussheim, et al.: Vitamin K deficiency in infants with chronic diarrhea. Clin Med 79:25, 1972.

11. Allen, D. M. , L. K. Diamond, and D. A. Howell: Anaphylactoid purpura in children. Am J Dis Child 99:147, 1960.

12. Shandling, B. : Laparotomy for rectal bleeding. Pediatrics 35:787, 1965.

13. Cox, K. , and M. E. Ament: Upper gastrointestinal bleeding in children and adolescents. Pediatrics 63:408, 1979.

14. Ford-Jones, A. E. A. , and J. J. Cogswell: Tests for occult blood in stools of children. Arch Dis Child 50:238, 1975.

15. Baum, S. , and M. Nussbaum: The control of gastrointestinal hemorrhage by selective mesenteric arterial infusion of vasopressin. Radiology 98:497, 1971.

12

FUNCTIONAL GASTROINTESTINAL DISORDERS

Mervin Silverberg, M. D.

IRRITABLE BOWEL SYNDROME

INTRODUCTION

The irritable bowel syndrome (IBS) is essentially a disorder of intestinal motility. The etiology is unknown, although it is likely multifactorial with a commonly observed familial incidence. About 75% of cases have a positive family history of a functional bowel disorder (1). It is still a syndrome which is not clearly defined in children, and there are no specific diagnostic tests. There are many similarities between the disease in adults and children, and up to one-third of adult patients claim to have had their complaints since childhood. The two main differences in children, compared to adult patients are (1) painless diarrhea is much more common, and (2) the female preponderance is either absent or even reversed. A preponderance of Jewish patients is evident in all age groups (2) (Table 1), which is similar to reports in adults.

TABLE 1   IBS Cases at North Shore University Hospital, NY (1972-1978)

Type and age	No.	Sex (M/F)	Mean age at onset (yr)	Jewish origin (%)
Diarrhea-predominant	215	127/88	$1\frac{1}{2}$	60. 2
0-4 yr	182			
5-18 yr	23			
Pain-predominant	156	86/70	7-3/4	64. 3
0-4 yr	16			
5-19 yr	140			

(From Ref. 2. Reprinted with permission.)

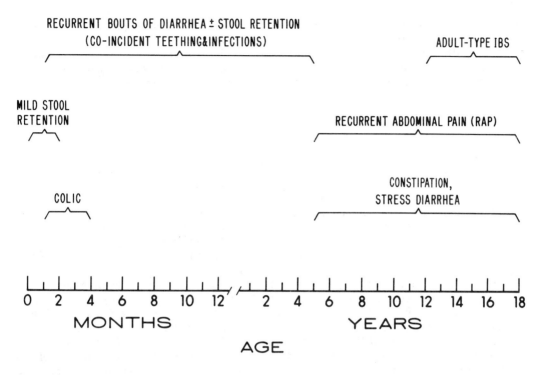

FIGURE 1   The clinical spectrum of IBS varies with age.   The child may demonstrate each of the clinical features in an orderly progression, or experience
only part of the spectrum, most commonly recurrent abdominal pain.   The older
adolescent usually presents with stress-related pain, altered bowel habits, dys-
pepsia, and symptoms of vasomotor instability, which are typical of adult IBS.
(From Ref 2. Reprinted with permission.)

There are two major clinical varieties which differ in their manifestations and
age incidence.   In each case, the definition requires complaints of a minimum 3-
week duration (Fig. 1).

Diarrhea-Predominant Group or Chronic Nonspecific Diarrhea

This group includes painless, usually intermittent diarrhea in an otherwise normal
patient.   It occurs mainly in the preschool child, particularly between 6-30 months
of age (1).   The stools vary from watery to mush, often contain mucus and undigested food particles, and usually number less than five times each day.   More
than 50% of the patients have a pattern of nearly normal stools in the morning,
progressing to looser stools later in the day, but never waking the child from
sleep.

Pain-Predominant Group or Recurrent Abdominal Pain (RAP)

This variety occurs mainly in the school aged child.   The median age group is 7-9
years (3).   The pain is localized most often to the periumbilical area in the young-

er child and to the left lower quadrant in the adolescent.   The pains are crampy, and worse postprandially, particularly after the evening meal.

Constipation or stool retention is common in the pain-predominant group, and occasionally alternates with diarrhea, particularly when associated with stress. Headache and limb pains frequently are reported in adolescents (4).

DIAGNOSIS

A detailed, careful history and a thorough physical examination are very helpful in the diagnosis of IBS.   The children nearly always appear to be in relatively good health.   The preschoolers are usually well nourished, while the older children tend to be lean, but have appropriate sexual development.   In the school aged group, the descending colon is frequently palpable, contains palpable stool, and is tender in over half of the cases (5).   Rectal examination should never be deferred. Commonly, patients who claim to have normal bowel habits, are found to have distended rectal ampullae with hard or soft stool, to everyone's surprise.   In post-pubertal girls, a gynecological assessment is mandatory, particularly if there is a history of sexual activity or delayed menarche.

Laboratory studies are kept to a minimum.   Diarrhea-predominant patients should have a complete blood count and stool examination for culture and occult blood.   A stool passed within 30 minutes may be examined for eosinophils and neutrophils by a Wright stain, and the fresh stool liquid (centrifuged, if mixed with particulate matter) tested for pH and reducing substances.   A pH less than 5. 0 and reducing substances in excess of 0. 25% are indications for definitive studies of carbohydrate malabsorption.   The random screening examinations of the stool for fat and starch can be misleading and frequently lead to the mistaken diagnosis of malabsorption of these nutriments.   If the child appears with unexplained malnu-trition, sweat electrolytes should be analyzed to exclude cystic fibrosis, the most common cause of malabsorption in children.

Pain-predominant patients should have a complete blood count, erythrocyte sed-imentation rate, immunoglobulin studies, and routine urinalysis.   The urinary tract is the most common site of inapparent organic disease in these children.   The patients with significant weight loss or extraintestinal manifestations suggestive of inflammatory bowel disease, e. g. , unexplained fevers, arthropathy, erythema nodosum, oral apthous ulcers, receive a sigmoidoscopic examination, and a rectal biopsy is always obtained.

The proctoscopic examination often reveals only excess intraluminal mucus. Occasionally, IBS and chronic inflammatory bowel disease coexist.   Histologically, there is an increase in mucous-secreting cells and a decrease in the cell popula-tion in the lamina propria.   Lactose intolerance is claimed to be an important con-tributing factor by some authors, i. e. , up to 50% of the cases in older adolescents (6), while most workers in the field have not been as impressed.   The breath hy-drogen analysis appears to be the most accurate procedure to demonstrate carbo-hydrate intolerance, but may lack specificity.

Radiocontrast studies of the bowel or urinary tract are indicated only when there are specific reasons, i. e. , fevers, weight loss, or when routine therapy is unsuccessful.   It should be noted that it is unusual to find radiographic evidence of disordered motility, particularly areas of colonic spasm, as described in adults. In teenage girls with perplexing lower abdominal pain, laparoscopy has been use-ful in establishing a diagnosis in carefully selected cases (7).

TREATMENT

Although the therapeutic measures differ for the diarrhea-predominant and the pain-predominant groups, both require a sympathetic interviewer and an awareness of the difficulties that parents and older children have in accepting the diagnosis of a psychosomatic disorder. The discussion must be free of diversions and interruptions. The teenager should have the opportunity to speak to the physician alone, and the language used should be comprehensible to the teenager. Since both parents and teenagers have the possibility of critical illness uppermost in their minds, it is rewarding to specifically exclude this early. Discussion of the heredofamilial nature of the disorder usually helps patients to accept the diagnosis, but it must be handled tactfully without instilling guilt or culpability. Periodic follow-up visits should be offered, since about 50% have complaints that last more than 1 year.

Discussion of all the diagnostic possibilities in the diarrhea-predominant group is essential, and using a diagram of the gastrointestinal tract will often help. The discussion might emphasize the problem as a "disturbance of packaging of waste products, which rarely affects the utilization of nutriment for adequate growth and development." Furthermore, water losses are usually modest and rarely result in dehydration or electrolyte deficiencies.

Dietary restrictions are rarely indicated, particularly since the parents will present a long list of frustrated dietary modifications that occasionally seem to help, but only in a transitory fashion. When lactose intolerance is suspected a lactose-free diet must be instituted sometimes for up to 4 weeks to confirm the diagnosis (5). The slow successful introduction of a normal diet for the patient's age is very reassuring to the family and at worst will have no more adverse effects than the restrictive diet. It is not uncommon that after starting a normal diet a complete remission ensues, thus obviating the need for extensive studies. This is particularly true in cases who are on a low-fat diet. The addition of a normal fat-containing diet results in fewer and firmer stools (8). During very active diarrhea, cold liquids should be avoided, since there is some evidence linking cold stimuli in the stomach with increased colonic propulsive activity. Caffeine-containing beverages such as colas have been known to exacerbate diarrhea. If increased flatus is a concern, gas-producing foods such as mushrooms, cabbage, and beans should be avoided.

Antidiarrheal compounds have very little therapeutic value in IBS. Diphenoxylate hydrochloride (in Lomotil) is considered a narcotic and should never be used in preadolescents. It should be reserved for the older child when all else has failed and the diarrhea interferes with special events in school or social occasions. Diiodohydroxyquin (Diodoquin) has been used successfully in more than half of the patients (9), although effects were suppressive and not curative. Its therapeutic value has never been established and a small controlled study showed no advantage over a placebo (10). Because of the temporary effects of this drug, coupled with its potential for ophthalmotoxity, its use is not recommended. Cholestyramine was reported to be used in cases with active diarrhea, presumably by sequestering an unknown noxious agent. Most of the successes are anecdotal and no controlled studies have been published. Additionally, the complications of the preparation, e. g. , steatorrhea, hemorrhagic diathesis, intestinal obstruction, do not justify its use in a relatively benign condition such as IBS.

In the pain-predominant group, the initial approach is to "open up the bowels." The short-term use of stool softeners such as light-grade mineral oil (15 ml/kg) or dioctyl sodium sulfosuccinate (1-3 mg/kg per dose, three times daily), to the point of producing one to three stools each day, is ideal. The two should not be used together since the surface-wetting agent may enchance the absorption of oil. The use of light mineral oil is limited to children over the age of 18 months who are resistant to the more palatable dioctyl sodium sulfosuccinate. The mineral oil is taken cold with juices, in single or divided amounts. The initial daily dosage is usually increased by 30 cc increments until the desired effect is achieved. When combined with a postprandial defecation pattern, this regimen will result in significant improvement in two-thirds of the patients. A high-roughage nutritious diet and regular eating habits are suggested. Dietary manipulation is of limited value and parents are cautioned against compounding the problems by making the dinner table a battleground.

The physician must be aware of the emotional background of this disorder, particularly in the older child. There is very little proven value for the use of psychotropic drugs. An attentive ear and honest responses are important for the suffering child. Abdominal cramps and erratic bowel habits are not benign to the child who finds it difficult to attend school or social functions without knowing the locations of the nearest bathroom. A psychiatric consultation may be valuable in selected cases. Long-term follow-up of this latter group showed that they were able to cope better with their symptoms, and were less restricted in their activities, compared to a control group of nonreferrals.

GASTROINTESTINAL GAS

Excessive gastrointestinal gas is a relatively common complaint heard from both children and their parents. Only recently, has the study of intestinal gas revealed the scientific background to the three main complaints of eructation, bloating, and flatus. Nitrogen, oxygen, carbon dioxide, hydrogen, and methane are reported to comprise more than 99% of gaseous intraluminal material anywhere in the bowel (11).

ERUCTATION, BELCHING, OR BURPING

Eructation, belching, or burping is almost always related to swallowed air. In the young infant, gastric gas is associated with air that is swallowed during sucking on the bottle. Release of the gastric bubble in the fundus permits the child to continue feeding and avoids regurgitation of other gastric contents. Excessive eructation in the older child is usually associated with a nervous habit of "air swallowing" and usually represents air which is in the esophagus and has never reached the stomach. Antigas medications are of little value.

BLOATING

Bloating is frequently associated with abdominal pain and has always spuriously been attributed to excessive gas. In fact, both by direct gas analysis and by abdominal x-ray studies, excessive gas has not been found, nor is there any correlation between the amount of gas and the degree of bloating or discomfort. These patients, however, are similar to irritable bowel patients in that they appear to be more sensitive to experimental distention of the bowel with air than are controls. Additionally, there is a disorder of motility, since the air tends to move in a retrograde fashion. Organic etiologies of abdominal distention must be excluded, including electrolyte imbalance, partial intestinal obstruction, and intestinal pseudo-obstructions. Dietary manipulation and medications such as charcoal, antacids, and antiflatulents are of little value. Reassurance and a clear understanding on the part of the patient that this is a benign condition is usually helpful.

FLATULENCE

Flatulence or excessive rectal gas frequently is associated with stool retention. Some older children may appear to be unduly flatulent with no evidence of constipation. There appears to be a wide range in gas constituents in the normal bowel. Most of the gas consists of hydrogen, carbon dioxide, and methane, i.e., gas produced by bacterial flora in the bowel (12). Truly excessive rectal gas is mainly due to unabsorbed carbohydrates. This would occur in patients who are lactose intolerant and in normal individuals with dietary excesses involving wheat, beans, etc. Simple dietary restriction is the treatment of choice.

REFERENCES

1. Davidson, M., and R. Wasserman: The irritable colon of childhood. (Chronic nonspecific diarrhea syndrome). J Pediatr 69:1027, 1966.

2. Silverberg, M. , and F. Daum: Irritable bowel syndrome in children and adolescents. Pract Gastroenterol 3:25, 1979.

3. Apley, J.: The Child with Abdominal Pains, 2nd ed. Blackwell Scientific Publications, Oxford, 1975.

4. Oster, J.: Recurrent abdominal pain, headache and limb pains in children and adolescents. Pediatrics 50:429, 1972.

5. Stone, R. T. , and G. J. Barbero: Recurrent abdominal pain in childhood. Pediatrics 45:732, 1970.

6. Barr, R. G. , M. D. Levine, and J. B. Watkins: Recurrent abdominal pain of childhood due to lactose intolerance: A prospective study. N Engl J Med 300:1449, 1979.

7. Kleinhaus, S. , K. Hein, M. Sheran, and S. J. Boley: Laparoscopy for diagnosis and treatment of abdominal pain in adolescent girls. Arch Surg 112: 1178, 1977.

8. Cohen, S. A. , K. M. Hendricks, R. K. Mathis, S. Laramee, and W. A. Walker: Chronic non-specific diarrhea: Dietary relationships. Pediatrics 64:402, 1979.

9. Cohlan, S. Q.: Chronic non-specific diarrhea in infants and children treated with diiodohydroxyquinoline. Pediatrics 18:424, 1956.

10. Silverberg, M. , and R. Goldbloom. Unpublished data.

11. Levitt, M. D. , and J. H. Bond: Volume, composition and source of intestinal gas determined by means of an intestinal washout technique. N Engl J Med 284:1394, 1971.

12. Levitt, M. D. , R. B. Lasser, J. S. Schwartz, and J. H. Bond: Studies of a flatulent patient. N Engl J Med 295:260, 1976.

13

DISORDERS OF THE STOMACH AND DUODENUM

Mervin Silverberg, M. D.

INTRODUCTION

The stomach is one of the most variable portions of the gastrointestinal tract. It may assume many forms depending on its contents, body habitus, and position of the body. Lean people tend to have a J-shaped stomach, whereas a stocky individual's stomach tends to have a transverse location. The latter is also true for younger infants. The stomach is the most dilated portion of the gastrointestinal tract, and various degrees of distention can occur, particularly with gastric outlet obstruction. The normal adolescent has a maximum stomach capacity of about 1 L. The approximate area of the normal stomach in a child may be represented by the size of his hand. The cardia of the stomach is fixed to the diaphragm about 1-2 cm to the left of the midline posteriorly at the level of the ninth vertebra. The pylorus is the most distal portion of the stomach and enters the duodenum about 2 cm to the right of the midline at the level of the first lumbar vertebra posteriorly, just anterior to the neck of the pancreas, and it lies just posterior to the quadrate lobe of the liver.

The stomach is the main reservoir of ingested material and it controls the egress of small portions following the mixing of foodstuff with the acid digestive enqymes, e. g. , pepsin, lipase, gelatinase, and a cathepsin. Only about 10-15% of available aminonitrogen is liberated by peptic digestion of proteins in the stomach. However, these peptones and other amino acid complexes play an important role in gastrin and cholecystokinin-pancreozymin (CCK-PZ) secretion. The lipase is mainly lingual in origin and is active at relatively acid pHs (1). A variable amount of carbohydrate digestion by salivary amylase takes place in the stomach after the food is swallowed. This action is effective only as long as the pH remains relatively high, which may occur within the center of the food mass. In addition to these major secretory functions, the stomach secretes the following:

1. Gastrin, from the G cells in the antrum (2), is a polypeptide hormone which stimulates the secretion of hydrochloric acid, pepsin, and intrinsic factor (IF). More distally, gastrin has similar functions with CCK-PZ on the pancreas, and stimulates intestinal motility and causes contraction of the gastroesophageal sphincter mechanism.

2. Histamine, is an effective stimulator of acid and pepsin secretion. It is found in most cells throughout the gastric mucosa, particularly along the course of small blood vessels.

3. Intrinsic Factor (IF), is a glycoprotein, secreted mainly by parietal or oxyntic cells, which is essential in the absorption process of dietary vitamin B_{12}. The factor combines with the vitamin to form complexes which are able to bind to receptors in the terminal ileum. Generally, the secretion of IF is closely bound to acid secretion. Patients with achlorhydria usually develop vitamin B_{12} deficiency, in time, although the degree is variable, since excess amounts of IF are excreted in the normal individual.

GASTRITIS

Many conditions and agents have been alleged to contribute to gastritis; objective endoscopic and histological evidence is sparse. Diagnosis based on radiographic studies are usually inaccurate. Flexible fiberoptic endoscopy may be helpful, but should have confirmatory biopsy evidence to be certain.

ACUTE GASTRITIS

Acute gastritis refers to a fairly extensive mucosal injury characterized by superficial ulcerations and hemorrhagic phenomena, such as petechiae and friability. More severe lesions may be associated with deeper ulcerations, which may be indistinguishable from a peptic ulcer. Most cases are caused by drugs and medications, such as acetylsalicylic acid, alchohol, nonsteroidal anti-inflammatory drugs, calcium chloride, bile salts, as well as irradiation, in order of frequency. Salicylates appear to act by altering the gastric mucosal barrier resulting in back diffusion of H^+ and other changes in mucosal permeability (3). Most infectious agents, e. g. , gastroenteritis, do not appear to cause any visible evidence of gastritis, and the vomiting is due to other mechanisms. Staphylococcal food poisoning is an exception, although the noxious agents is probably an enterotoxin.

Clinical Features

The major manifestation is acute upper gastrointestinal bleeding, usually preceded by epigastric discomfort and anorexia. Vomiting, which usually contains coffee-ground material is common, and proceeds to temporary relief from symptoms. The bleeding is rarely massive, tends to be self-limited, and all evidence of mucosal damage may be gone in 3-5 days.

Treatment

Treatment is usually conservative, and most cases stop bleeding spontaneously. A well-lubricated nasogastric tube will provide evidence of bleeding and its duration. Ice cold saline lavages, with 30-60 ml aliquots, keep the stomach empty, and the effluent indicates termination of the bleeding when it is clear or slightly pink. If bleeding persists for more than 4 hours, liquid antacid (Table 1) is instilled intermittently or by drip, in amounts adequate to keep the gastric pH greater than 5. The antacid should be given orally every 1-2 hours after the tube is withdrawn. Cimetidine has been used, anecdotally, in more severe cases with good success.

TABLE1   Relative Potency of Liquid Antacids

Antacid	Contents	mEq/ml[a]	mEq/15 ml[b]	ml/140 mEq Dose[c]
Delcid	Al and Mg hydroxides	8.5	128	16
Ducon	Al and Mg hydroxides, Ca carbonate	7.0	105	20
Mylanta II	Mg and Al hydroxides, simethicone	4.1	62	34
Titralac	Glycine, Ca carbonate	3.9	59	36
Camalox	Al and Mg hydroxides, Ca carbonate	3.6	54	39
Basaljel	Al carbonate	3.3	50	42
Aludrox	Al hydroxide gel, Mg hydroxide	2.8	42	50
Maalox	Mg and Al hydroxide gel	2.6	39	54
Creamalin	Hexitol stabilized Al hydroxide gel, magnesium hydroxide	2.6	39	54
Di-Gel	Al and Mg hydroxides, simethicone	2.5	38	56
Mylanta	Mg and Al hydroxides, simethicone	2.4	36	58
Silain-Gel	Mg and Al hydroxides, simethicone	2.3	35	61
Marbien	Mg and Ca carbonates, Al hydroxide, Mg phosphate, Mg trisilicate	2.3	35	61
WinGel	Al and Mg hydroxides, hexitol stabilized	2.3	35	61
Gelusil M	Mg trisilicate, Al hydroxide, Mg hydroxide	2.2	33	64
Riopan	Mg and Al hydroxides	2.2	33	64
Amphojel	Al hydroxide gel	1.9	29	74
A-M-T	Mg trisilicate, Al hydroxide gel	1.8	27	77
Kolantyl Gel	Benty1, Al hydroxide, Mg hydroxide, methylcellulose	1.7	26	82
Trisogel	Mg trisilicate, Al hydroxide gel	1.7	26	82
Malcogel	Mg trisilicate, Al hydroxide gel	1.6	24	88
Gelusil	Mg trisilicate, Al hydroxide gel	1.3	20	108
Robalate	Dihydroxyaluminum aminoacetate	1.1	17	127
Phosphaljel	Al phosphate gel	0.4	6	350

[a]These figures, multiplied by 10, are the volumes of 0.1 N HCl added to 1 ml of each antacid to maintain a pH of 3.0 for 120 minutes.
[b]These figures indicate the neutralizing capacity, in mEq. of 15 ml of each antacid.
[c]These figures indicate the volume, in ml, of each antacid necessary to provide 140 mEq of neutralizing capability.
(From ref. 13. Reprinted with permission.)

CORROSIVE GASTRITIS

Corrosive substances, when ingested accidentally or purposely, usually cause most of the tissue injury in the esophagus. These include acids, alkali, drugs, and detergents. However, when excessive amounts of these substances are ingested, gastric corrosive effects are noted, particularly involving the antrum where the agents usually pool. The spastic pylorus protects the duodenum and exaggerates local effects in the antrum.

Pain, vomiting, and hematemesis are common, as a result of local inflammation, erosions, and occasionally perforation. The bleeding may be intermittent, but the pain is usually persistent. Antral stenosis may be noted over a 2- to 6-week period, with progressive signs and symptoms of gastric outlet obstruction. Fatal gas emboli in the portal circulation have been reported.

Treatment is directed toward supportive measures, general and specific antidotes, as well as close observation with fiberoptic endoscopy. Areas of gangrene should be considered for surgical excision.

PEPTIC ULCER

INTRODUCTION

Peptic ulcers are uncommon problems in the pediatric age group, although the amount of time and effort spent in looking for these cases is disproportionately larger. In part, this is due to the ubiquitous nature of abdominal pain in children. Although the reported frequency of ulcer disease varies in different parts of the United States, most large centers do not see more than two or three proven new cases each year (4). About 2% of adults with peptic ulcer report that they have had symptoms since childhood.

PATHOGENESIS

All age groups are affected, although the disease is different in the very young and in those patients where it is secondary to another illness, a drug, or a metabolic disorder. A genetic factor plays a significant role in a manner that is unknown at the present time. Concordance in monozygotic twins is less than 100%, but consistently exceeds that in dizygotic twins (5). This concordance is also true for the ulcer site, i. e., duodenal vs gastric. Generally, a proven family history is reported in about 50-60% of the cases. The influence of psychosocial factors is controversial; however, there is considerable evidence to suggest that these children have higher levels of anxiety and sensitivity to stress than control subjects. Obvious emotional disturbances are not seen in more than 25% of the patients, most of which are school related (6). Abnormal levels of gastric acid and pepsin and defective acid disposal by the duodenum are believed to occur in some combination with local impairment of mucosal resistance. Hypergastrinemia accounts for a very small portion of increased acid-pepsin secretion (7). Unfortunately, few studies are available in children and often they have not been revealing.

CLINICAL FEATURES

There are three clinical subdivisions of peptic ulcer that can be recognized.

Acute Infantile and Secondary Ulcers

This type of ulcer presents mainly in the preschool child, particularly during the first 2 years of life. The newborn infant may be vulnerable during the first 48 hours of life, owing to a large parietal cell mass during this time. Hemorrhage and perforation are not uncommon early manifestations (8). The ulcers occur with equal frequency in the stomach and duodenum. Stress-related ulcers fall into this category, occurring with severe infections, burns (Curling ulcer), and central nervous system diseases (Rokitansky-Cushing ulcer). Many drugs are claimed to be ulcerogenic, e.g., acetylsalicylic acid, nonsteroidal anti-inflammatory drugs, caffeine, amino acid mixtures, and calcium compounds; however, corticosteroids, one of the most commonly accused drug groups have not been clearly shown to be related to an ulcer diathesis. A number of diseases have been associated with an apparent increased frequency of peptic ulcers. These include cirrhosis, chronic pulmonary disease, hypoglycemia, and congenital pyloric stenosis. However, no large series in any category in children have been reported. Generally, all these patients tend to present with acute signs and symptoms, and most do not recur once the precipitating circumstances are controlled or removed. Pain, if present, is usually periumbilical and not related to meals. Vomiting and failure to thrive are not uncommonly found.

Adult Type or Chronic Ulcers

Most cases of peptic ulcer of the school-aged child or adolescent are not related to underlying diseases. Pain is the most common complaint varying in location from periumbilical in the younger child, to the epigastrium in the teenager. Pain often is aggravated by food intake and frequently accompanied by vomiting in the younger child. In contrast, the older patient has the typical rhythmicity of pain-food-relief, often occurring during the night and characterized as "hunger pains." There is a higher incidence of peptic ulcers in heroin users, and the use of coffee or alcohol will exacerbate the discomfort (9). The physical examination reveals epigastric tenderness, often to the right of the midline. Signs of pallor and tachycardia may be evident in those cases with significant chronic blood loss. Asymptomatic, subclinical bleeding occurs in about 15-20% of the patients. Occult blood in serial stools is diagnostic.

The ulcer is located in the duodenal bulb in 90% of the cases, the posterior wall being the site of predilection. Although not as marked, the prevalence of adult males is evident, with a male/female ratio of about 1.5:1. Most children respond to a sustained antiulcer regimen. However, when followed for longer than 1 year, as many as 50% are reported to have persistent or recurrent complaints (10). The incidence of complications is high; however, most of these are due to delayed diagnosis or poor management.

Zollinger-Ellison and Related Disorders

The Zollinger-Ellison syndrome is associated with a secreting non-beta cell adenoma. The ulcers in this syndrome may be clinically and radiographically indistinguishable from the more common variety. However, ulcers which are usually large, persistent, progressive, and unresponsive to good management are most suspect. Although the majority are in the duodenal bulb, they represent a more significant proportion of multiple, distal, and stomal ulcerations. Gastrin has been identified as the putative secretagogue and is found in large concentration in the serum and tumor (gastrinoma) extracts, and can be demonstrated in the tumor cells by immunofluorescent techniques. Blood gastrin levels usually exceed 300 pg/ml, often above 1000 pg/ml, whereas in other varieties of peptic ulcer disease, values are below 200 pg/ml. In patients with equivocal serum gastrin elevation, a calcium carbonate intravenous challenge may result in diagnostic levels of serum gastrin and increased acid secretion (7). Most patients demonstrate a maximal gastric hypersecretion that is relatively unresponsive to histamine augmentation. In patients with other varieties of peptic ulcer disease, basal gastric acid secretion per hour is usually less than 60% of the amount secreted after a maximal dose of histamine or betazole (Histalog). Severe watery diarrhea and malabsorption of fat and Vitamin B_{12}, resulting from excessive gastric secretions entering the upper small bowel, may complicate the already difficult course for these patients.

A number of rare related ulcerogenic syndromes have been described (11). These include multiple endocrine adenomatosis (type 1), multiple endocrine islet cell tumors, islet cell hyperplasia and hyperparathyroidism. The adenomas are hormonally active in various combinations. The ulcer disease may be associated with a severe choleralike illness and profound hypercalcemia.

DIAGNOSIS

A careful radiocontrast study of the upper gastrointestinal tract is the main diagnostic aid, although as many as 25% of the cases may have negative findings. The diagnosis depends on the demonstration of an ulcer crater (Fig. 1) or a persistently deformed duodenal bulb as a result of scarring. Gastric ulcers are best seen with small amounts of barium and proper positioning so that all stomach regions are visible in profile and "en face." Better visualization of the duodenal bulb may be achieved with hypotonic radiography using intramuscular propantheline bromide (15-30 mg). Descriptions of an irritable bulb, duodenitis, pylorospasm, and retained gastric secretions are presumptive signs and of little value, since they can be seen in normal very frightened children. Flexible gastroduodenoscopy is a valuable procedure in patients with very suggestive complaints, and a negative radiographic examination. It is still unclear as to the degree of improvement in diagnostic accuracy that is thus achieved. This form of endoscopy also may be very useful in patients with acute episodes of bleeding ulcers.

Gastric acid studies in children, including the augmented histamine stimulation test, shows an unusually broad range of normal values. Although ulcer patients often are not distinguishable, these tests may help to identify these children (12) and those who are more likely to have recurrences. Basal secretory values may be useful in the diagnosis of gastrinoma.

Fasting serum gastrin levels show a great overlap with normal controls. However, gastrin studies are useful in differentiating ulcers associated with secretory adenomas, i. e. , Zollinger-Ellison syndrome.

TREATMENT

The major goals of therapy are to control gastric acidity, peptic activity, treat complications, and prevent relapses. A variety of measures are used, but few have been examined with controlled studies, particularly in the pediatric age group. Acute ulcers should be treated vigorously, preferably in a hospital if the complaints are very severe, or if complications such as bleeding or penetration develop that require very close observation.

Antacids (13)

Frequent neutralization of gastric acid is still the mainstay of treatment for all ulcers. A wide variety of antacids are available commercially, and the appropriate choice should depend on buffering capacity, quantity required, palatability, and side effects (see Table 1). Ideally, the volume of antacid equivalent to 80 mEq of

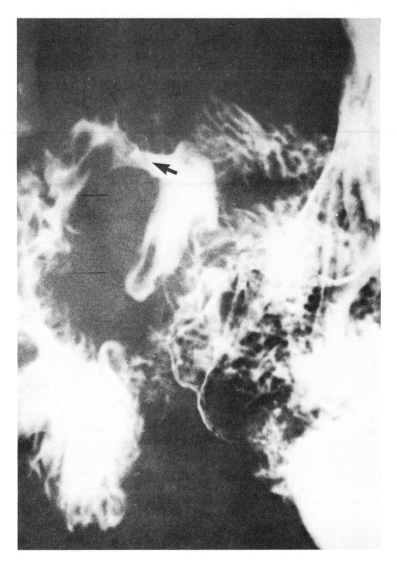

FIGURE 1   Duodenal ulcer. Ulcer crater in apex of the deformed duodenal bulb
in an 8-year-old child with painless iron-deficiency anemia. Crater retains barium and is surrounded by edematous folds (arrow).

acid neutralizing capacity per hour provides the optimal therapeutic regimen. In
general, liquid preparations are superior and the best effects are achieved when
the preparation is taken 1 hour after eating (14) since the food itself will neutralize acid for about 1 hour. In the acute symptomatic patient, hourly administration of 5-60 ml of the antacid is given according to age. Mixtures of aluminum
and magnesium hydroxides or magnesium trisilicate are most effective. The magnesium compounds tend to balance the constipating effects of aluminum hydroxide;
however, they must be used with caution in patients with renal insufficiency to
avoid hypermagnesemia. As the patient improves, and in less severe cases, the
antacid is given 1 hour and 3 hours postprandially and again just before bedtime
for 2-3 months, or longer, if the complaints are resistant. Although there are no

supporting studies, the patients are encouraged to continue the 1-hour postprandial and night dosage for another 3 months plus occasional dosage supplements when episodes of pain occur. The asymptomatic patient who after this time has no ulcer on radiographic and/or endoscopic examination is considered healed, but should be examined periodically. Although still controversial, cholinergic blocking agents have been shown to be effective in reducing ulcer pain. The optimal dosage of drugs such as propantheline bromide (1. 5 mg/kg/24 hr) appears to be close to the level at which side effects, such as dryness of the mouth, are produced. The medication is given postprandially and at bedtime throughout the symptomatic period and for an additional 3-4 months. In those patients who respond slowly, the nocturnal dose should be continued for a full year. Patients with delayed gastric emptying should not be given any anticholinergic agents since gastric retention may be exaggerated.

Diet

There is no evidence that bland diets contribute to ulcer healing. All foods, including milk, elicit an acid secretory response (15). "Fast-foods" such as hot dogs, pizza, and hamburgers are equally acceptable in the child's diet. Generally, children should be permitted to eat a diet appropriate for age and only those foods which cause symptoms need be avoided. Adolescents should be cautioned to refrain from the use of alcohol, caffeine-containing products, and smoking.

H_2- Receptor Antagonists

The use of the histamine H_2-receptor antagonist cimetidine has been reported in all age groups including the newborn, with few, if any, of the serious side effects noted in adults (16). However, since all the complications are not known in children, and since its overall superiority over antacids has not been demonstrated, antacids are still the drugs of first choice. Cimetidine has been shown to decrease pain due to various acid-peptic disorders including ulcers and esophagitis, and to promote ulcer healing. Recurrence of ulcer complaints, after discontinuing cimetidine, is not uncommon (20-25% of cases), but is no more likely than with antacids. The recommended dosage for children is 20-40 mg/kg/day, with meals and at bedtime, with a maximum of 1600 mg/day given for 2-3 months.

SPECIAL PROBLEMS

Blood Loss

Mild bleeding is usually chronic and will result in an iron deficiency anemia. These patients should be treated with an appropriate ferrous sulfate preparation given with food to avoid gastric upset. Hemorrhage will cause hematemosis and melena, and may result in hypovolemic shock. Packed erythrocytes or whole blood should be used as replacement to keep the hematocrit at about 30%.

A nasogastric tube should be inserted and the stomach lavaged frequently with 30-50 ml of cold saline until the bleeding is stopped. Intractable bleeding is rare in children and usually suggests a complicating hemorrhagic diathesis.

Intractable Pain

Persistent pain is usually due to inadequate therapy, noncompliance, or penetration of the ulcer through the wall of the viscus. Antacids given intragastrically by a continuous perfusion to keep the gastric pH over 5, have been successful. Cimetidine also has been effective.

Obstruction

Pylorospasm, edema, anticholinergic drugs, and scarring all may cause sufficient luminal narrowing to result in a high intestinal obstruction. In most cases, discontinuing oral feedings and placing the stomach at rest by continuous nasogastric suction for 2-4 days should resolve the acute problem. Before removing the indwelling tube, 200-500 ml of saline (according to age) may be instilled, and less than 10% should be retained after 1 hour.

Surgical Intervention

Perforation, obstruction, and intractable bleeding or pain are all indications for emergency surgery, which is an uncommon occurrence in children. More commonly, recurrent episodes of bleeding and pain, relatively resistant to medical management, will raise the possibility that surgical intervention may be more effective in limiting the disease process. This should be a joint decision involving both medical and surgical consultations (17, 18). Vagotomy and pyloroplasty are the procedures of choice for children. Vagotomy and antrectomy have been used in some patients as the initial operation, while others reserve these procedures for vagotomy failures. The use of selective vagotomies has been used in too few children to be properly evaluated.

REFERENCES

1.   Hamosh, M.: A review. Fat digestion in the newborn: Role of lingual lipase and preduodenal digestion. Pediatr Res 13:615, 1979.

2.   McGuigan, J. E., M. H. Greider, and L. Grave: Staining characteristics of the gastrin cell. Gastroenterology 62:959, 1972.

3.   Fromm, D.: Gastric mucosal "barrier." Gastroenterology 77:396, 1979.

4.   Singleton, E. B., and M. H. Faykus: Incidence of peptic ulcer as determined by radiological examinations in the pediatric age group. J Pediatr 65:858, 1964.

5.   Rotter, J. I.: The genetics of peptic ulcer: More than one gene, more than disease. Prog Med Genet 4:1, 1980.

6.   Tudor, R. B.: Peptic ulceration in childhood. Pediatr Clin N Am 14:109, 1967.

7.   Schwartz, D. L., J. J. White, F. Saulsbury, and G. A. Haller, Jr: Gastrin response to calcium infusion: An aid to the improved diagnosis of Zollinger-Ellison syndrome in children. Pediatrics 54:599, 1974.

8.   Rosenlund, M. L., and C. E. Koop: Duodenal ulcer in childhood. Pediatrics 45:283, 1970.

9.   Friedman, G. D., A. B. Siegelaub, and C. C. Seltzer: Cigarettes, alcohol, coffee and peptic ulcer, N Engl J Med 290:469, 1974.

10.   Milliken, J. C.: Duodenal ulceration in children. Gut 6:25, 1965.

11.   Ballard, H. S. , B. Frame, and R. J. Hartsock: Familial multiple endocrine
       adenoma-peptic ulcer complex.   Medicine 43:481, 1964.

12.   Christie, D. L. , and M. E. Ament: Gastric acid hypersecretion in children
       with duodenal ulcer.   Gastroenterology 71:242, 1976. '

13.   Sleisenger, M. H. , and J. S. Fordtran (eds.): Gastrointestinal Disease—
       Pathophysiology-Diagnosis-Management, 2nd ed. W. B. Saunders Co. ,
       Philadelphia, 1978, p. 896.

14.   Fordtran, J. , and C. T. Richardson: In-vivo and in-vitro evaluation of li-
       quid antacids.   N Engl J Med 288:923, 1973.

15.   Ippoliti, A. F. , V. A. Maxwell, and J. I. Isenberg: The effect of various
       forms of milk on gastric acid secretion.   Studies in patients with duodenal
       ulcer and normal subjects. Ann Intern Med 84:286, 1976.

16.   Henn, R. M. , J. I. Isenberg, V. Maxwell, and R. L. Sturdevant: Inhibition
       of gastric acid secretion by cimetidine in patients with duodenal ulcer.   N
       Engl J Med 293:371, 1975.

17.   Johnston, P. W. , and W. H. Snyder, Jr. : Vagotomy and pyloroplasty in in-
       fancy and childhood.   J Pediatr Surg 3:238, 1968.

18.   Curci, M. R. , K. Little, W. K. Sieber, and W. B. Kiesewetter: Peptic ulcer
       disease in childhood re-examined. J Pediatr Surg 11:329, 1976.

14

CHILDHOOD DIARRHEA

Fima Lifshitz, M.D.

Diarrheal disease is a leading cause of infant mortality and morbidity in all parts of the world. There are approximately 500 million episodes of diarrhea per year reported in children, and there are 5-18 million deaths caused by this illness (1). It also causes and/or contributes to malnutrition throughout the world (2, 3).

ETIOLOGY

Diarrhea may be infectious, metabolic, nutritional, allergic, chemical, neoplastic, and/or psychogenic in origin; it also may be idiopathic. The infectious causes are multiple, and include viral, bacterial, and protozoan diarrheas (4). Similarly, there are several inborn or acquired metabolic alterations which result in diarrhea such as celiac disease, familial chloride diarrhea, disaccharidase deficiencies, or monosaccharide intolerance. Allergic reactions to milk or other foodstuffs also are known to induce this disorder. Feeding hyperosmolar formulas or overfeeding normal formula may also result in loose stools. Generalized malnutrition and starvation as well as intake of inadequate diets, i.e., low fat, also may lead to diarrhea (5). There may be mechanical causes for the disease, as in gastrointestinal fistulas, obstruction, or short-gut syndrome. Several neoplasias may lead to chronic diarrhea as the primary manifestation, e.g., ganglioneuroma, lymphoma, and Whipple disease. Excessive intake of chemicals and heavy metals produce loose stools, too. Psychological stress also may result in diarrhea. In addition, there is diarrhea of an idiopathic nature in entities such as chronic inflammatory bowel disease.

PATHOPHYSIOLOGY

WATER TRANSPORT ALTERATIONS

Diarrhea may be considered to result whenever there is a decrease in the net movement of water from the intestinal lumen to plasma. Diarrhea occurs when the volume of liquid that is delivered to the colon surpasses the reabsorptive ability of the large intestine. The factors responsible for a decreased net movement of water in the intestine include a decreased time for adequate reabsorption, a decreased absorptive surface, and an altered transport capacity.

A decreased time for water reabsorption may occur in conditions where there is a short gut or a rapid transit time. A short gastrointestinal tract is rare and generally is a problem after major surgical resections. Much emphasis has been put on rapid transit as a cause of diarrhea. However, it has long been known that in many instances diarrhea is seen in patients with distended, fluid-filled loops, suggesting that adequate time does exist for reabsorption of water. It must be remembered that fluid remaining within the intestinal tract serves as a stimulus to peristaltic action, and hyperirritability may be the result, rather than the cause of decreased transport of water, and thus diarrhea. A diminished intestinal surface area may be of importance in chronic disease such as ulcerative colitis or celiac disease, with major scarring and loss of normal epithelium.

An altered intestinal transport capacity seems to be the most important factor leading to a net decreased transport of water. Under normal circumstances the conservation of water by the intestine is so efficient that usually less than 200 ml is excreted in the feces (6, 7) (Fig. 1). A slight change in water transport per unit of surface area can cause a very marked change in the net intestinal flow of water. Consequently, even relatively minor alterations that increase the secretion or inhibit the absorption of actively transported solutes by the intestine, principally sodium and glucose to which water transport is linked, may result in diarrhea (see Fig. 1).

TYPE OF DIARRHEA

The type of diarrhea may vary according to the primary alteration responsible for the decreased net movement of water by the intestine. Secretory diarrhea occurs when diarrhea persists after oral feedings are discontinued. The stools in this type of diarrhea contain large quantities of sodium (more than 80 mEq/kg body weight), since this electrolyte is secreted by the intestine together with water (8).

Absorptive diarrhea occurs when diarrhea improves after oral feedings are stopped. The stools of these patients usually contain smaller quantities of sodium but may contain unabsorbed carbohydrates. Absorptive alterations leading to diarrhea are frequently found in infants with this disorder. It has long been recognized that fasting reduces fluid loss in diarrhea.

Secretory and absorptive alterations may be ongoing simultaneously in a given patient and these alterations may be further complicated by motor and/or other abnormalities. Thus the type of diarrhea may vary in any one patient even when the primary alteration led to a specific intestinal transport abnormality. When diarrhea results from small-intestinal secretion of large quantities of water and electrolytes, the losses are somewhat compensated by the colonic reabsorptive capacity. Thus, the large intestine may modify the composition and reduce the total loss of ileal effluent in stools. The most important factor in determining the type of diarrhea is the luminal osmotic gradient (9). The presence of unabsorbed carbohydrates and other osmotically active molecules may determine the presence or absence of diarrhea and the type and severity of the illness, regardless of the initial event that triggered the disease. The details of the cycle of events that result whenever there is unabsorbed carbohydrate are discussed later.

PATHOGENIC MECHANISM

Diarrhea may result when there is a disruption of the intestinal epithelium with morphological damage and/or when there is a secretory enhancement with mucosal integrity being preserved. A brief review of the pathogenic mechanisms of common causes of diarrhea in children is noted below.

INTESTINAL WATER TRANSPORT

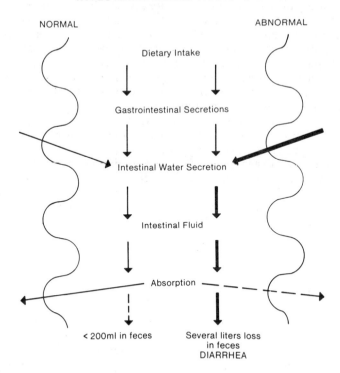

FIGURE 1   Intestinal water transport. In the course of a day the human intestine handles large quantities of water as indicated in the figure. The bulk of fluid input into the intestine comes from the dietary intake (2–3 L/day), and from various gastrointestinal secretions, included are saliva (1–2 L/day), gastric juice (2 L/day), bile (1 L/day), pancreatic juice (2 L/day), and succus entericus (1 L/day). In addition, there is fluid in the intestine derived from the enteric recirculation of water and solutes, namely, there is an ongoing movement by fluid through secretion and reabsorption which could account for several liters per day. Therefore, under abnormal circumstances, when there is a functional loss of alteration which results in an enhanced secretory or diminished absorption capacity of the intestine, the fluid losses may be enormous.

Diarrhea Caused by Disruption of Intestinal Epithelium (Table 1)

Bacillary dysentery is the classical model of pathogenicity resulting from invasion and penetration of the intestinal mucosa leading to mucosal inflammation and epithelial cell disruption. Common pathogens such as Shigella and the "pathogenic" strains of Escherichia coli have a similar mechanism (10). Although Salmonella also invades the epithelium, it does not induce extensive destruction of the mucosa. In such cases, the epithelial lining is left intact and organisms reach the lamina propria wherein an inflammatory response is elicited (11). The reverse can be seen in Entameba histolytica. The protozoa invade and destroy the intestinal mucosa but produce minimal inflammatory reaction. In invasive diarrhea the intestinal alterations in water transport may vary. Experimental infection with Salmonella typhimurium impaired the absorptive transport capacity of the jejunum, cecum, and colon and when diarrhea occurred it also induced a marked secretion of sodium and water by the ileum as seen in toxigenic diarrhea (12). On the other hand, in experimental Shigella flexneri infections in monkeys, there was an intestinal transport defect with net jejunal and colonic secretion of water and electrolytes. Ileal electrolyte transport was normal; therefore, unlike toxigenic diarrheas, dysentery results from a colonic transport defect, while diarrhea is secondary to jejunal secretion superimposed on the defective colonic absorption of water and electrolytes (13).

Proliferation of fecal and colonic flora in the small intestine also may produce a disruption of the intestinal epithelium leading to disease by altering foodstuffs and/or host secretions. Such bacterial metabolic activity generates a variety of substances, i.e., deconjugated bile salts (14), hydroxy fatty acids (15), short-chain organic acids (16), or alcohol (17, 18). These can be injurious to the intestine, with induction of alterations in the transport of solutes and water, resulting in diarrhea. Ultrastructural and functional abnormalities of the intestine all have been related to these bacterial metabolites. A wide spectrum of enteric microorganisms may alter intestinal function when present in excessive numbers in the small intestine (19). Bacterial overgrowth could be the primary cause of acute illness or it could be secondarily associated with diarrhea due to monosaccharide intolerance, gastrointestinal surgery, blind loop syndrome, achlorhydria, inflammatory bowel disease, and alterations of intestinal motility (20-25). However, it may play a most important role as a secondary pathogenic alteration of diarrhea, often causing prolongation and aggravation of the disease.

Campylobacter fetus subspecies intestinalis and Campylobacter fetus subspecies jejuni have been recently recognized with increasing frequency as a cause of diarrhea in all age groups, particularly after the first decade of life. In some areas as much as 15% of diarrhea patients have been attributed to this pathogen. It occurs more commonly during the warmer months and is transmitted primarily by the fecal-oral route. The most prominent features of Campylobacter infection are diarrhea, fever, transient vomiting, and cramps. The stools often contain mucus, blood and inflammatory cells. Atypical cases include arthralgias, arthritis, pseudoappendicitis, severe rectal bleeding, chronic weight loss, relapsing diarrhea, intussusception and toxic megacolon. Direct examination of a fresh stool by the dark field technique may reveal the organisms which have the characteristic "bumper-car" motility: they are not seen with the usual methylene blue preparation. Special simple isolation techniques and cultures are required.

Viral infections play a most important etiological role in gastroenteritis in children (26, 27). Over 70% of diarrheal infants were shown to have a virus detected by electron microscopy. Several viruses which differ morphologically and antigenically have been described (28, 29). They have been referred to as rheovirus, orbivirus, duovirus, coronavirus, and rotavirus.

Human rotavirus enteritis has a peak incidence between 6 months and 2 years, with few childhood cases occurring after 4 years of age. Stool volume may be minimal to massive, with various degrees of electrolyte and acid-base imbalance. It is usually a self-limited disease, and deaths in the United States are rare. Virus is shed for about 5-7 days and recovery is complete in 7-10 days. Work is in progress to develop a vaccine. They appear to have a worldwide distribution and principally affect infants. Other viruses and the Norwalk agent seem to be less common and are associated with periodic, brief community outbreaks with high attack rates affecting older children and adults.

Norwalk virus (agent) is a very small virus (27-32 nm) which rarely causes disease in preschool children. Outbreaks commonly occur in epidemics, often during winter months, and probably account for about one-third or more of outbreaks of nonbacterial gastroenteritis. Incubation period is less than 48 hours and there is an abrupt onset. Complete recovery appears to be the general rule. Immunocompromised patients appear to be more vulnerable and have more serious illnesses. Viral diarrheas also have been shown to induce morphological and functional changes in the jejunum. Following experimental virus infections, the intestinal

TABLE 1   Clinical Features of Infectious Diarrhea*

Organism	Seasonality	Mode of Transmission	Age	Other Findings	Duration	Stools	Diagnosis	Antibiotic Therapy
Enterotoxigenic E. coli	Warm season peaks; travelers' diarrhea	Food and water	Any	Abdominal pain	Brief	Large, watery; no cells	Elisa +, toxin production	Not indicated
Enteroinvasive E. coli	Unknown	Food (cheese)	Any	Bowel discomfort – cramping	Variable	Small, viscous; RBC-WBC	Guinea pig eye test	Colistin/Ampicillin
Enteropathogenic E. coli (11 serotypes)	Warm season peaks	Food, direct fecal-oral	<1 yr	Malaise	>7 days	Variable, slimy, variable RBC-WBC	Serotyping	Colistin
Salmonella	Warm season peaks	Food	Any	Generalized malaise	3–7 days	Slimy, RBC-WBC	Culture	Contraindicated except in young infants and septicemia
Shigella (small-bowel form)	Warm season peaks	Direct fecal-oral	<2 yrs	Generalized malaise	1–3 days	Large, watery; WBC	Culture	TMP/SMX or ampicillin
Shigella (large-bowel form)	Warm season peaks	Direct, fecal-oral; rarely food	Any	Bowel discomfort – cramping, tenesmus	>7 days	Small, viscous, RBC, WBC	Culture	TMP/SMX or ampicillin
Yersinia enterocolitica	Cold season peaks	Food; sporadic	Any	Severe abdominal pain, FTT, erythema nodosum, arthritis	>7 days; occasionally chronic	Small, viscous; RBC, WBC	Unusual media, cold enrichment culture technique	Possibly, aminoglycosides TMP/SMX

Campylobacter	All year, warm > cold	Food, water, animals, person to person	Any; usually >10	URI in 1/3	>7 days	Moderate, mucoid, WBC-RBC	Special antibiotic containing media; direct phase contrast-darting motility	Self-limited – 85%; possibly erythromycin
Human Rotavirus	Cold season peaks	Direct, fecal-oral, respiratory droplets	<2 yrs; >4 yrs rare	Unusual	2-8 days	Large, watery, no cells	Electron microscopy – 70 nm Elisa +, Rotazyme	Contraindicated
Norwalk Virus	Cold season peaks	Food, water	>5 years		2 days	Large, watery, no cells	Electron microscopy, 27-32 nm	Contraindicated

*Modified from table provided by Dr. Heinz Eichenwald

+Elisa = enzyme-linked immunosorbent assay; TMP/SMX = trimethoprin sulfamethoxazole

epithelial cells were penetrated by the viral pathogens which induced mucosal inflammation, villus shortening, crypt hypertrophy, increased epithelial cell mitosis, dilatation of endoplasmic reticulum, and an increase in intracellular multivesicular bodies (27-29). Brush border enzyme activities also were decreased. On
the other hand, the colonic mucosa was spared in this syndrome. Viruses also
were able to evoke intestinal water secretion by a mechanism which may be different from that induced by toxins (30).

Diarrhea Caused by Secretory
Enhancement of Intestinal Epithelium

This type of pathogenic mechanism, inducing diarrhea, has been extensively reviewed (8, 31). It may be implicated in many diarrheal disorders in children in
addition to the classic prototype, cholera. It should be pointed out that enterotoxin
formation and mucosal cell penetration are genetically transmissable factors which
may be inter-related, facilitating invasion of the host epithelium by the organisms.
E. coli may express enteropathogenic (11 serotypes), enteroinvasive (diarrhea epidemics associated with contaminated cheese), and enterotoxigenic properties in different strains and even in the same strain (10). The enterotoxigenic strains of E.
coli have been frequently implicated as a cause of traveller's diarrhea, when persons travel from low- to high-risk areas. The occurrence of severe abdominal
pain in this disorder differs from the finding in clinical cholera, where pain is generally absent. In a recent study, up to 72% of "turista" episodes in Mexico were
associated with heat-labile toxigenic strains of E. coli isolated from stools of
American students with diarrhea (32). However, the healthy students who had no
diarrhea also had these strains detected in 15% of their stool specimens. S. aureus,
P. aeruginosa, C. perfringens and even some Shigella and Salmonella strains have
also been found to produce enterotoxins (31). In toxigenic diarrhea, the organism
multiplies in the lumen or on the surface of the epithelium of the small intestine
and exerts its pathogenic effects by producing a toxin. In staphylococcal food poisoning, ingestion of preformed toxin produces the illness. Preformed toxin does
not seem too important in cholera or diseases caused by E. coli. Enterotoxins
cause the small intestinal epithelial cells to secrete electrolytes and water, while
the colon is usually impervious to its actions. Enteric toxins may produce these
reactions by a process of activation of intestinal secretory mechanisms which have
been associated with activation of the intracellular cyclic AMP system (31) (Fig. 2).
The entire process occurs after attachment of the toxin to a membrane receptor.
This effect can be blocked by agents which act at the receptor site or at the level of
activation of adenyl cyclase or protein synthesis, e.g., wheat germ and indometha-
cin, respectively.

Antimicrobial-associated diarrhea is caused by the toxin of C. difficile in the
vast majority of cases, with S. aureus accounting for no more than 1% of cases.
Pseudomembranes were the hallmark of this complication, hence the term pseudomembranous colitis; however, membranes are not found in mild or early cases. Antimicrobial-associated diarrhea may occur with almost all antimicrobial agents and
is reported at all ages. Generally, most cases are mild and resolve with cessation
of the antimicrobial therapy. The diarrhea is usually profuse and watery, and
bloody stools are actually uncommon. The diagnosis is made by obtaining a stool
culture for C. difficile using a special media and testing for C. difficile cytotoxin in
stools. As many as 10% of normal newborns and 50% of high-risk newborns will
have toxin in the stool, although most are asymptomatic.

Diarrhea Caused By a Variety of Factors

It seems reasonable that excessive rapid transit through the intestine may result
in diarrhea. Substances which increase gut motility such as bradykinin and pros-

ENTEROTOXIN PRODUCED DIARRHEA

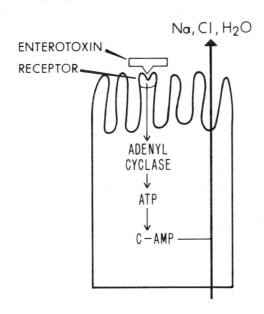

FIGURE 2   Enterotoxins are metabolic products of bacterial growth; therefore, gut colonization is a necessary prerequisite for its formation. Virulent strains of E. coli which produce enterotoxin possess a distinctive surface antigen K-88, whereas the avirulent strains are K-88 negative. This factor permits the adherence of E. coli to the intestine which is the initial stage in colonization of the intestine. The cell surface receptor is not well characterized but it is localized in a complex heterosaccharide layer called glycocalyx which coats the intestinal epithelial cell brush border. V. cholerae and E. coli toxins appear to bind to GM ganglioside in the membrane. Shigella enterotoxin binds to a different receptor which contains oligomeric B1-4 linked N-acetylglycosamine. The heat labile toxins of V. cholerae and E. coli have a capacity to stimulate adenylate cyclase, causing an increase in the intracellular content of cyclic AMP, the signal for intestinal cells to secrete. Other toxins (heat stable), activate other mechanisms, guanylate cyclase, resulting in increased cyclic GMP levels, which also seem to turn on a secretory response.

taglandin may be responsible for the diarrhea observed in some patients with carcinoid syndrome and with medullary carcinoma of the thyroid. However, prostaglandins also may act by inducing intestinal secretion of fluid. Disordered intestinal motility has been observed as the cause of diarrhea in diabetic patients with neuropathy. The mechanism of laxatives is not simple since they may have various absorptive and secretory effects. The principal effect of saline laxatives is to increase fecal water as a result of the slow and incomplete absorption of the polyvalent ions.

Protein absorptive defects may be associated with diarrhea since unabsorbed amino acids may act as osmotic cathartics. Fat malabsorption also has been linked with diarrhea. Excess fatty acids in the bowel can be associated with failure to reabsorb water; the best example is ricinoleic acid, a fatty acid which is the active principle of castor oil. This is chemically similar to oleic acid and shares the property of stimulating intestinal fluid excretion in the small and large bowel. Bile acids are also mucosal secretogogues and when present in excess in the colon, particularly following ileal resection, they may act as endogenous cathartics. Carbohydrate malabsorption possibly enhances the loss of water and electrolytes leading to diarrhea through a variety of mechanisms as described in detail next.

A specific alteration of chloride transport may result in familial chloride diarrhea. In this condition the ileum and colon cannot handle chloride normally and water is excreted with this anion. Acquired chloride diarrhea also has been recognized as a complication of marked potassium deficiency.

CARBOHYDRATE INTOLERANCE IN DIARRHEAL DISEASE

In diarrheal disease there is carbohydrate malabsorption frequently leading to carbohydrate intolerance (33). The mucosal damage of the small intestine, with depression of brush border oligosaccharidases and intestinal transport processes, results in carbohydrate malabsorption (34-36). The inflammation of the epithelial cell membranes also may contribute to this problem due to alterations in intestinal permeability. In diarrheal disease there may be other alterations leading to carbohydrate malabsorption even without a decrease in intestinal oligodisaccharidases. For example, there may be increased motility with reduced exposure of the carbohydrates to the action of these enzymes. Also, there may be interference with the binding of the substrate to the brush border enzymes due to epithelial cell inflammation, anatomical disturbances, or other alterations.

A small-intestinal injury in diarrhea may be the result of the pathogenesis of diarrhea per se and/or the complications of the disease. Mucosal damage may be achieved by the tissue invasion of the microorganisms with disruption of the enterocyte, or by the effects of injurious factors generated by the action of bacteria on foodstuffs and host secretions. It has been postulated that lactase is the receptor and uncoating enzyme for infantile enteritis viruses (37). These viruses seem to infect only gut epithelium rich in this enzyme. Local factors such as the hyperosmolality of intestinal fluid and decreased pH optimum also may account for possible enzymatic and mucosal alterations even in the absence of intestinal infection. In addition, dehydration, shock, and the nutritional state of the patient could lead to small-intestinal alterations.

Carbohydrate malabsorption in diarrhea is frequently specific for lactose but it may affect other disaccharides such as sucrose or maltose (38). At times, it also may affect all carbohydrates, including monosaccharides such as fructose (23-25). The frequent occurrence of lactose intolerance in diarrheal disease may be due to the fact that lactase is the most superficial of the brush border oligosaccharidases, its activity is rate limited, and its concentrations are considerably lower than the other brush border enzymes (39-41). In addition, it may be the target enzyme for viral enteritis (37).

Malabsorption of carbohydrates may result in a cycle of events leading to intolerance (Fig. 3). The major cause of trouble is the presence of osmotically active carbohydrate and fermentative products within the lumen of the bowel. The osmotic pressure of the unabsorbed carbohydrate results in secretion of fluid and electrolytes into the small intestine and colon until osmotic equilibrium is reached (9). A part of the carbohydrate is excreted in the feces unaltered while a small portion may be absorbed by diffusion across the intestinal mucosa and subsequently excreted in the urine. However, the greater portion is hydrolyzed by intestinal bacteria in the lower segments of the intestine to smaller carbohydrate molecules and to other fermentative products. These include short-chain organic acids such as lactic acid and large quantities of hydrogen gas (42). The concentration of carbohydrate within the luminal contents is thus reduced and the pH decreases. The low molecular-weight organic acids produced are poorly absorbed by the colon and they further increase the osmotic pressure within the lumen. In addition, they interfere with the colonic absorption of water and electrolytes. Furthermore, intestinal motility may

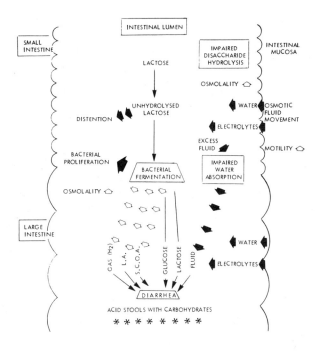

FIGURE 3   Pathogenesis of lactose intolerance. (From Ref. 41. Reprinted with permission.)

be enhanced by the increased intraluminal volume (9), thus contributing to the production of diarrhea. The elimination of carbohydrates from the diet, on the other hand, will often break the cycle with improvement of the stools (44).

CLINICAL FEATURES OF CARBOHYDRATE INTOLERANCE

Carbohydrate intolerance may prolong diarrhea following gastroenteritis. Infants with diarrhea who were able to tolerate lactose usually have a short illness, whereas those who were not able to tolerate this disaccharide have a more prolonged diarrhea (33). Diarrhea may persist for more than 3 weeks if lactose is not removed from the diet. Carbohydrate intolerance can aggravate the loss of water and electrolytes in diarrhea and contribute to other specific metabolic problems. The consumption of cow's milk in various forms by children with diarrhea has been associated with hypernatremia and prominent losses of extracellular sodium and chloride and intracellular potassium (43). Unabsorbed carbohydrates in the intestine may also potentiate a large water and electrolyte loss since the volume excreted may be about three times that of the isotonic solution of the disaccharide (9).

Metabolic acidosis is often a complicating feature of diarrhea. Malabsorption of carbohydrates may also play an important role in the development of this complication (45). There are several mechanisms whereby carbohydrate intolerance may lead to metabolic acidosis. Those include (1) the presence of large quantities of organic acids within the intestinal lumen, which stimulate the secretion of large amounts of bicarbonate to neutralize the acid load; and (2) some of these acids may also be absorbed by the small intestine into the circulation. However, the hydrogen ion increase in body fluids in diarrhea is largely due to the bacterial carbohydrate fermentation which occurs in the colon (45). The important role of the intestine in acid-base homeostasis is apparent in premature infants who develop metabolic acidosis when given lactose (46).

The nutritional status of an infant can rapidly be jeopardized by carbohydrate intolerance. In addition to the severe energy deficiency which results from carbohydrate malabsorption, there may be increased depletion of nutrients by diarrhea. Nitrogen loss may be a prominent feature (43) and decreased nitrogen absorption is particularly correlated with the severity of diarrhea (47). It also has been suggested that the osmotic effect of unhydrolyzed lactose in the small intestine may lead to dilution of the bile acid concentration below the necessary levels for maximal absorption of fats (48). Malabsorption of a variety of vitamins and minerals leading to specific nutritional deficiencies has been reported.

The presence in the small bowel of free carbohydrates and of metabolic by-products of carbohydrate fermentation may facilitate colonization and proliferation of enteric microorganisms. The disturbed small-intestinal function might deteriorate further, because this leads to additional factors which injure the small intestine, i.e., deconjugated bile salts, hydroxy fatty acids, short-chain organic acids, and alcohol. If diarrhea persists, there is further deterioration of intestinal absorption and intolerance to other disaccharides, in addition to lactose, and even intolerance to monosaccharides may develop (25, 33). Such patients then may fail to respond to lactose elimination from the diet and would continue having diarrhea and carbohydrate intolerance until all carbohydrates are eliminated from the diet. The intensification of intestinal malabsorption usually occurs in infants who have lactose intolerance for 2-3 weeks before dietary therapy is initiated (25, 33). Transient secondary monosaccharide intolerance following gastroenteritis occurred in 3.6% of all mildly lactose intolerant and in 16.6% of all severely lactose intolerant patients (25, 33).

Continued nutrient losses and dietary intolerance may impair an infant's ability to recover from the initial illness and increase susceptibility to other conditions. Pneumatosis intestinalis may result from carbohydrate intolerance since unabsorbed carbohydrates constitute an important source of gas in the intestine. The quantity of lactose that is contained in 30 ml of milk may produce 50 ml of gas in normal people (42). Under abnormal circumstances, the bowel flora may increase the hydrogen production over 100-fold. If the production of gas in the intestinal lumen exceeds the ability of the bowel to expel it, there will be resulting distention of the gut with increasing pressure. When this is severe, it may lead to ischemia and necrosis of the intestinal mucosa, thus providing access of the gas to the tissue space, resulting in pneumatosis intestinalis. Indeed, this complication often occurs in infants with lactose intolerance secondary to diarrheal disease (24) and in neonatal hypoxia (49, 50).

Protein intolerance is frequently associated with carbohydrate intolerance in children with gastroenteritis (51). Under certain conditions of pathophysiologic stress the normal barriers to intestinal transport of macromolecules may be functionally and structurally altered, leading to an increased leakage of intact proteins across the intestinal epithelium (52) (see Fig. 3). In diarrheal disease there are several alterations which may promote an increased passage of macromolecules across the intestine, including luminal hyperosmolar gradients, cellular disruption, increased levels of deconjugated bile salts, and lactose intolerance (53). One may therefore hypothesize that a child with diarrhea may become sensitive to food proteins; however, the reverse may also occur. Protein-sensitive enteropathy may lead to diarrhea (54, 55).

HOST MECHANISMS IN DEFENSE AGAINST DIARRHEA

The alterations which may lead to diarrhea have to be viewed in relationship to the host mechanisms in defense against disease. Table 2 depicts some of the factors which may play a role in determining whether diarrhea occurs as a result of a given pathogenic agent. Even the most pathogenic agent will not produce disease if

TABLE 2   Host Mechanisms in Defense Against Diarrhea

1. Dose exposure

2. General host factors
     Age
     Nutrition
     Health status
     Medication

3. Local host factors
     Breast milk
     Gastric acidity
     Motility
     Diarrhea
     Antibodies
     Bacterial flora

the patient is not exposed to a sufficient dose. Gastrointestinal microorganisms must multiply before infection and may be pathogenic only in excessive amounts. Even the classic enteropathogens may not infect if the dose is small. For example, the minimal infective dose for Shigella is 10^1, Salmonella 10^5, E. coli 10^8 and V. cholerae 10^8 (56, 57).

General host factors such as age and nutritional status are of considerable importance; newborn infants seem more susceptible to enteric infections. Diarrheal disease is a particularly important problem in malnourished children (58, 59). They suffer an increased incidence and severity of diarrhea and this disease may cause or contribute greatly to the aggravation of their nutritional status. The prevalent poor sanitary conditions in developing countries may expose the child to an excess of bacteria, while the marginal nutritional status decreases the host capacity to respond to enteric infection. Previous treatment with antibiotics and/or other medications also may facilitate the development of enteric infections as a result of overgrowth of bacteria not susceptible to antibiotic treatment.

The benefits of human milk are related to decreased contamination as well as general and local protective factors which have been reviewed in detail, elsewhere (60-63). Several studies performed as long as five decades ago, revealed some of the alarming hazards of cow's milk feeding (64, 65). It was shown that breast-feeding is better and preferable to bottle-feeding under nearly all conditions. This is particularly important in developing societies.

Local gastrointestinal factors are also of great consequence in allowing intestinal microflora to induce diarrheal disease. Although the organisms must be swallowed before infection, they may never reach the small bowel as viable bacteria because of their vulnerability to gastric acidity. This observation has been supported by the increased incidence and seriousness of salmonellosis and cholera infections which occurred when there was reduced acidity (66, 67). The same phenomenon also may help explain the increased rate of diarrheal disease in malnourished children who show a diminished gastric acid secretory capacity. In addition, the cleansing role of intestinal motility plays a part in determining pathogenicity and in maintaining a relative lack of bacteria in the upper segment of the bowel of normal children. Diarrhea itself may be a protective mechanism, limiting the time of contact between the infecting organism and the intestinal epithelium. Interference with diarrhea by the pharmacological agents frequently employed in its treatment may cause a more severe disease by increasing the time exposure of the intestinal epithelial cell to the infective microorganism (68). Other important factors are intestinal antibodies (secretory IgA) which may prevent adherence of the organism to the mucosa (69) or may interfere with the multiplication of the ingested organism (70) and bacterial flora, which seem to elicit a strong homeostatic influence on potential pathogenic organisms either by competition for space and nutrients, or by elaborating antibacterial catabolites (71, 72).

CLINICAL ASSESSMENT OF DIARRHEA

The evaluation of the patient with diarrhea should include an assessment of the stools in relation to the cause of the disease as well as to tolerance to foodstuffs. Examination of the stools should include analysis of fecal leukocytes, pH, and carbohydrate excretion, in addition to the customary cultures. This will allow a more accurate assessment of the type of process that may be involved in the cause of the diarrhea as well as provide tools for rational decisions regarding treatment of these patients. Diagnosis of bacterial diarrhea using the clinical features mentioned previously is often difficult (73). The fecal leukocytes may provide a rapid diagnosis of the possible infective process, which will later be confirmed by the classical cultural isolation of the microorganisms (74). Leukocyte analysis provides immediate clues regarding bacterial or nonbacterial causes. It may even shed light on the possible types of organisms and whether antibiotic treatment may or may not be used (75). A patient with diarrhea with marked leukorrhea and a high proportion of neutrophils in the stool may require antibiotics for treatment before cultural isolation of the bacterial infection. It must be emphasized that this test should not be used alone to indicate appropriateness of antibiotic therapy, since fecal leukocytes may be found in patients with bacterial infection, i.e., most cases of salmonellosis, where antibiotic therapy may be contraindicated (76). However, the absence of fecal leukocytes may be a rapid and reliable way to identify patients with viral or nonspecific diarrhea for whom antibiotic therapy is not indicated. In addition, the quantitative and qualitative type of the cell may be suggestive of other causes of diarrhea. For example, the presence of eosinophils in stools may give clues to a possible allergic manifestation.

Fecal leukocytes in the stools may be assayed by the methylene blue wet mount preparation (72). Stool specimens or rectal swabs from the patient are examined by placing a small fleck of mucus, or stool liquid when no mucus is present, on a clean glass slide and mixing it thoroughly with two drops of Loffler methylene blue stain (77). The slide is then cover-slipped and examined microscopically after waiting 2-3 minutes for good nuclear staining. Counting the average number of nuclei of the leukocytes may be done by approximating the average cell number to that of erythrocytes. Only those cells clearly identifiable should be counted, and a large number of degenerated cells that cannot be identified should be ignored.

Sugar malabsorption of all types is clinically characterized by watery, sour-smelling diarrheal stools that have an acid pH and contain carbohydrates and organic acids, especially lactic acid. Weight loss, failure to thrive, dehydration, and electrolyte loss may be present. These symptoms improve when the offending carbohydrate is eliminated from the diet. Various investigators place reliance on different criteria for diagnosis of the capacity of patients to tolerate carbohydrates. These vary from simple clinical observations following empirical dietary changes, to the performance of sugar tolerance tests, measurements of disaccharidase activity of the intestinal mucosa, metabolic balance studies with quantitation of organic acid and carbohydrate excretion, and determination of intestinal absorptive rates for specific carbohydrates by transintestinal intubation.

The diagnosis of carbohydrate intolerance also can be made by simple semiquantitative methods that measure the presence of reducing substances, glucose, and the pH of the stools (33, 34). These techniques are now widely employed; however, a very important source of error is commonly introduced by testing for these variables in nonfresh stool specimens. Within minutes after excretion, there is exogenous bacterial fermentation, the stool pH and glucose concentrations rapidly drop, and lactic acid rapidly increases (44). Thus the stool has to be tested immediately after it is excreted. A simple electronic device to signal each bowel movement is useful to ensure fresh stool testing. An alternative would involve retrieving the stool sample by rectal digital examination, and the feces tested immediately.

The best clinical indices of carbohydrate intolerances in infants with diarrhea are: the presence of carbohydrates in the stools in concentrations above 0.25% reducing substances (1+ glucose), and the presence of stools with a pH of less than 6.

It is important that patients with diarrhea be followed by stool testing throughout the time that they have abnormal stools. Most fecal samples analyzed at random with these simple bedside methods have a pH of 6.0 or more and contain concentrations of carbohydrates below clinical significance. Thus to assess the capacity of infants and children to tolerate carbohydrates, two to three fresh liquid stools should be checked daily throughout the illness in relation to a known dietary intake.

These simple bedside tests also should be done following specific oral loads of monosaccharides or disaccharides. A severe lactose intolerance is considered to be present when the patient excretes many stools with carbohydrates and with an acid pH, while on milk formula. Mild intolerance is considered when fewer than 30% of the stools are positive for these measurements. The specimens should be fresh and only the liquid portion of the stool should be tested. Tests on formed stools are without value, as are those obtained during periods of fasting.

pH OF STOOLS (Also see Chap. 20)

Special paper strips, designed primarily for testing urine samples, can be used to test the pH. A pH less than 6 is indicative of carbohydrate malabsorption and its fermentation by bacteria in the bowel. The pH normally may be low in the early neonatal period.

REDUCING SUBSTANCES IN STOOLS (Also see Chap. 20)

These measurements are carried out the same way as testing urine for glucose. One part of fluid stool is diluted with two parts water and a Clinitest tablet is placed in the test tube. A color change indicative of 0.25% or more of reducing substances is abnormal. If sucrose malabsorption is suspected, the test should be modified by boiling the stools with 1N hydrochloric acid before testing.

GLUCOSE IN STOOLS (Also see Chap. 20)

Glucose in stools can be tested by the glucose oxidase (Clinistix) method. If no glucose is present, but the test for reducing substances is positive, then the intolerance is most likely due to disaccharides only.

OTHER TESTS (Also see Chap. 20)

The response to a carbohydrate oral load is frequently employed as a test to assess the capacity to tolerate specific disaccharides or monosaccharides after recovery from diarrhea (78). The rise in blood sugar after carbohydrate ingestion is frequently the sole criterium of impaired hydrolysis. However, up to 30% of healthy subjects may have a flat lactose tolerance test, and patients with a normal intestinal lactase activity may have no elevation in blood sugar following lactose loads. Moreover, the blood sugar level after carbohydrate ingestion varies according to the site where the blood is obtained, i.e., capillary vs venous. The response of infants to a carbohydrate oral load after recovery from diarrhea was variable, and blood sugar rise in response to the tolerance test was not correlated with the stool pattern (78). Therefore, it is preferable to assess carbohydrate tolerance in patients on the basis of the presence of diarrhea, acid stools, and/or excretion of carbohydrates in relation to the carbohydrate intake.

The breath hydrogen is useful for most cases of carbohydrate intolerance and may also be of value in infectious diarrheas (79). This is a noninvasive procedure that requires no blood samples and is more sensitive than other measures.

THERAPEUTIC CONSIDERATIONS

The prevention of diarrhea is still a challenge that concerns everyone. Improvement in economic levels, nutrition, and sanitation are of paramount importance. Proper handwashing, refrigeration, and cooking are basic public health measures, as are improvements in socioeconomic and environmental standards, e.g., safe water supply and control of flies. For certain groups at high risk of developing specific enteric infections, it may shortly be feasible to control diarrhea through use of an oral vaccine. It is unlikely, however, that immunological approaches will offer the solution in the widespread control of diarrheal diseases that are due to a myriad of bacteria, viral, and protozoal etiologies among the general population.

The natural history of infectious diarrheal disease varies considerably within each specific etiologic group, so that the effectiveness of antibiotics against these diarrheal diseases can only be demonstrated by well-controlled, double-blind treatment studies. However, even the "proven" drugs have limited value because antibiotic-resistant organisms continue to emerge and will eventually nullify the effect of the drug therapy currently available. Studies have shown that ampicillin is effective against Shigella (80) and neomycin or colistin (orally) against E. coli (81). On the other hand, antibiotics are not indicated in most cases infected with Salmonella (76) and in nonspecific gastroenteritis.

Nonspecific antidiarrheal drugs (opium preparations, Lomotil, etc.) are not recommended in children. Drug efficacy studies are very limited and poorly controlled, and the studies that are available indicate that these drugs are either ineffective or may even prolong the illness (68). Antispasmodic and nonspecific antidiarrheal agents are of little value. Other medicines which are intended to modify the physical appearance of the stool do not decrease water and electrolyte losses and may provide a false sense of security, since the stools appear improved, e.g., Kaopectate. Maintenance of fluid and electrolyte balance and dietary treatment remains the central vital factor in the successful treatment of diarrheal disorders. The reader is referred elsewhere for the considerations regarding oral fluid electrolytes in diarrheal disease (82). Since lactose intolerance is a frequent occurrence in patients who are fed cow's milk formulas, the administration of a feeding preparation, which contains carbohydrates other than lactose as a source of calories, is recommended (83). Infants with a short diarrheal course usually tolerate other disaccharides and may, therefore, be given a lactose-free, disaccharide-containing diet. Those patients who have had a prolonged diarrheal course usually have a generalized disaccharide intolerance and therefore may be treated with a disaccharide-free, glucose-containing formula. Now that these proprietary preparations are commercially available they may be routinely employed in all infants hospitalized for severe diarrheal disease as a starting formula, provided glucose is not given in a concentration above 5% (84). The use of carbohydrate-free formulas should be reserved for those patients who continue to have diarrhea and glucose intolerance. Carbohydrate-free feedings are not without danger; hypoglycemia may ensue as a severe complication during the acute stage or after recovery. Utmost care should be exercised to provide parenteral glucose to these infants throughout the time they are not fed carbohydrates.

The capacity to tolerate all carbohydrates is rapidly recovered after the diarrhea ceases. An increased number of more complex carbohydrates, e.g., Polycose, may be given to the patient soon afterward. After glucose is tolerated, disaccharides may be introduced, at first starch, followed by sucrose, and finally lactose. Even patients with severe forms of carbohydrate intolerance following gastroenteritis tolerate lactose within a few weeks of the acute stage of the illness. An attempt should be made to diagnose other diseases if carbohydrate intolerance persists. The elimination of dietary lactose for prolonged periods may in itself perpetuate alterations in carbohydrate absorption or other nutritional alterations (42, 85, 86).

It is also prudent to eliminate food proteins, particularly cow's milk protein, during diarrheal disease (51). Substitutes of potentially antigenic protein with protein hydrolysates appear satisfactory. Most commercially available milk formulas in which the carbohydrate is modified, also modify the protein to the more hydrolyzed preparation (84).

These dietary recommendations should be limited to infants receiving cow's milk formulas. Infants fed human milk need not have a change in their dietary habits and breast-feeding should be encouraged even during diarrheal disease.

REFERENCES

1. Elliot, K.: Acute Diarrhea in Childhood. K. Elliot and J. Knight (eds.), Ciba Foundation Symposium 42 (new series) Elsevier/Excerpta Medica, 1976, p. 1.

2. Mclaren, D.S.: The great protein fiasco. Lancet 11:93, 1974.

3. Waterlow, J.C. and P.R. Payne: Review article: The protein gap. Nature 258:113, 1975.

4. Lifshitz, F.: Diarrheal disorders. in Clinical Disorders in Pediatric Gastroenterology and Nutrition. F. Lifshitz (ed.). Marcel Dekker, New York, 1980, pp. 267-276.

5. Cohen, S.A., K.M. Hendricks, R.K. Mathis, S. Lorriane, and W.A. Walker: Chronic nonspecific diarrhea. Dietary relationship. Pediatrics 64:4027, 1979.

6. Curran, P.F., and S.G. Schultz: Transport across membranes: General principles. in Handbook of Physiology, Sec. 6 Alimentary Canal, Vol. III. F.S. Code (ed.). Am Physiol Soc, Washington, 1968, p. 1217.

7. Davenport, H.W.: Physiology of the Digestive Tract, 3rd ed. Year Book Medical Publishers, Chicago, 1971, p. 171.

8. Field, M., J.S. Fordtram, and S.G. Schultz: Secretory Diarrhea. Am Physiol Soc, Williams & Wilkins Co., Baltimore, 1980.

9. Launialia, K.: The effect of unabsorbed sucrose and mannitol in the small intestinal flow rate and mean transit time. Scand J Gastroenterol 39:665, 1968.

10. Dupont, H.C., S.B. Formal, R.B. Hornick, M.J. Snyder, J.P. Libonati, D.G. Sheahan, E.H. Labrec, and J.P. Kalas: Pathogenesis of Escherichia coli diarrhea. N Engl J Med 285:1, 1971.

11.   Alekseen, P.A., M.I. Berman, and R.A. Korneeva: Clinical and pathohistological picture of S. typhimurium infection in children. J Microbiol Epidemiol Immunol 31:111, 1960.

12.   Powell, D.W., G.R. Plotkin, R.M. Maenza, L.I. Solberg, D.H. Catlin, and S.B. Formal: Experimental diarrhea. I. Intestinal water and electrolyte transport in rat salmonella enterocolitis. Gastroenterology 60:1053, 1971.

13.   Rout, W.R., B. Formals, R.A. Giannella, and G.J. Dammin: Pathophysiology of shigella diarrhea in the Rhesus monkey: Intestinal transport, morphological and bacteriological studies. Gastroenterology 68:270, 1975.

14.   Midtvedt, T.: Microbial bile acid transportation. Am J Clin Nutr 27:1341, 1974.

15.   Binder, H.J.: Fecal fatty acids—mediators of diarrhea? Gastroenterology 65:847, 1973.

16.   Chernov, A.J., W.F. Doe, and D. Compertz: Intrajejunal volatile fatty acids in the stagnant loop syndrome. Gut 13:103, 1972.

17.   Slipstein, F.A., L.V. Holdeman, J.J. Corcino, and W.E.C. Moore: Enterotoxigenic intestinal bacteria in tropical sprue. Ann Intern Med 79:632, 1973.

18.   Baraona, E., R.C. Pirola, and C.S. Lieber: Small intestinal damage and changes in cell population produced by ethanol ingestion in the rat. Gastroenterology 66:226, 1974.

19.   Gracey, M., V. Burke, J.A. Thomasa, and D.C. Stone: Effect of microorganisms isolated from the upper gut of malnourished children on intestinal sugar absorption in vivo. Am J Clin Nutr 28:891, 1975.

20.   Burke, V., and C.M. Anderson: Sugar intolerance as a cause of protracted diarrhea following surgery of the gastrointestinal tract in neonates. Aust Paediatr J 2:219, 1966.

21.   Coello-Ramirez, P., and F. Lifshitz: Enteric microflora and carbohydrate intolerance in infants with diarrhea. Pediatrics 49:233, 1972.

22.   Ramos-Alvarez, M., and J. Olarte: Diarrheal disease of children: Occurrence of enteropathogenic viruses and bacteria. Am J Dis Child 107:218, 1964.

23.   Burke, V., and D.M. Danks: Monosaccharide malabsorption in young infants. Lancet 1:1177, 1966.

24.   Coello-Ramirez, P., G. Gutierrez-Topete, and F. Lifshitz: Pneumatosis intestinalis. Am J Dis Child 120:3, 1970.

25.   Lifshitz, F., P. Coello-Ramirez, and G. Gutierrez-Topete: Monosaccharide intolerance and hypoglycemia in infants with diarrhea. I. Clinical course of 23 infants. J Pediatr 77:595, 1970.

26.   Bishop, R.F., G.P. Davidson, I.H. Holmes, and B.J. Ruck: Virus particles in epithelial cells of duodenal mucosa from children with acute nonbacterial

gastroenteritis. Lancet 2:1281, 1973.

27.   Agus, S.G., R. Dolin, R.G. Wyatt, A.J. Tousimis, and R.S. Northrup: Acute infectious non-bacterial gastroenteritis, intestinal histopathology. Ann Intern Med 79:18, 1973.

28.   Flewett, T.H., A.S. Bryden, H. Davies, G.N. Woode, J.C. Bridger, and J.M. Derrick: Relation between viruses from acute gastroenteritis of children and newborn calves. Lancet 2:61, 1974.

29.   Davidson, G.P., I. Goller, R.F. Bishop, R.W. Townley, I.H. Holmes, and B.J. Ruck: Immunofluorescence in duodenal mucosa of children with acute enteritis due to a new virus. J Clin Pathol 28:263, 1975.

30.   McClung, H.J., D.G. Butler, B. Kerzner, D.G. Gla, and J.R. Hamilton: Transmissible gastroenteritis. Mucosal ion transport in acute viral enteritis. Gastroenterology 70:1091, 1976.

31.   Banwell, J.G., and H. Sherr: Effect of bacterial enterotoxins on the gastrointestinal tract. Gastroenterology 65:847, 1973.

32.   Gorbach, S.L., B.H. Kean, D.G. Evans, D.J. Evans, Jr., and D. Bessudo: Traveler's diarrhea and toxigenic Escherichia coli. N Engl J Med 292:933, 1975.

33.   Lifshitz, F., P. Coello-Ramirez, G. Gutierrez-Topete, and M.C. Cornado-Cornet: Carbohydrate intolerance in infants with diarrhea. J Pediatr 79:760, 1971.

34.   Lifshitz, F., and G.H. Holman: Disaccharidase deficiencies with steatorrhea. J Pediatr 64:34, 1969.

35.   Sunshine, P., and N. Kretchmer: Studies of small intestine during development. III. Infantile diarrhea associated with intolerance to disaccharides. Pediatrics 34:38, 1969.

36.   Johnson, J.D., N. Kretchmer, and F.J. Simoons: Lactose malabsorption: Its biology and history. Adv Pediatr 21:197, 1974.

37.   Holmes, I.H., R.D. Schnagi, S.M. Rodger, B.J. Ruck, I.D. Gust, R.F. Bishop, and G.L. Barnes: Is lactase the receptor and uncoating enzyme for infantile enteritis (rota) viruses? Lancet 1:1387, 1976.

38.   Lifshitz, F.: Carbohydrate problems in pediatric gastroenterology. Clin Gastroenterol 6:415, 1977.

39.   Crane, R.K.: Absorption of sugars. Handb Physiol 3:1323, 1963.

40.   Gray, G.M.: Carbohydrate digestion and absorption. Role of the small intestine. N Engl J Med 292:1225, 1975.

41.   Pergolizzi, R., F. Lifshitz, S. Teichberg, and R.A. Wapnir: Interaction between dietary carbohydrates and intestinal disaccharidase in experimental diarrhea. Am J Clin Nutr 30:482, 1977.

42.   Ingelfinger, F.J.: Malabsorption: The clinical background. Fed Proc 26: 1388, 1967.

43.   Darrow, D.C.: The retention of electrolytes during recovery from severe dehydration due to diarrhea. J Pediatr 28:515, 1946.

44.   Lifshitz, F.: Clinical studies in diarrheal disease and malnutrition associated with carbohydrate intolerance. Proc. IV Int'l Cong. in Nutrition 1972, A. Chavez, H. Bourges, and S. Basta (eds.). S. Karger, Switzerland, 1975, pp. 173-181.

45.   Lugo-de-Rivera, C., H. Rodriguez, and R. Torres-Pineda: Studies on the mechanism of sugar malabsorption in infantile infectious diarrhea. Am J Clin Nutr 25:1248, 1972.

46.   Lifshitz, F., S. Diaz-Bensussen, V. Martinez-Garza, F. Abdo-Bassols, and E. Diaz del Castillo: The influence of disaccharides on the development of systemic acidosis in the premature infant. Pediatr Res 5:213, 1971.

47.   Bowie, M.D.: Effect of lactose-induced diarrhea on absorption of nitrogen and fat. Arch Dis Child 50:363, 1975.

48.   Ringrose, R.E., J.B. Thompson, and J.D. Walsh: Lactose malabsorption and steatorrhea. Digest Dis 17:533, 1972.

49.   Akesode, F., F. Lifshitz, and K.M. Hoffman: Transient monosaccharide. Pediatrics 51:891, 1973.

50.   Book, L.S., J.J. Herbst, and A.L. Jung: Carbohydrate malabsorption in necrotizing enterocolitis. Pediatrics 57:201, 1976.

51.   Iyngkaran, N., and Z. Abidin: Intolerance to food proteins. in Pediatric Nutrition. Infant Feedings - Deficiencies - Diseases. F. Lifshitz (ed.). Marcel Dekker, New York, 1982, p. 449.

52.   Fagundes-Neto, U., S. Teichberg, M.A. Bayne, B. Morton, and F. Lifshitz: Bile salt enhanced rat jejunal absorption of a macromolecular tracer. Lab Invest 44:18, 1981.

53.   Teichberg, S.: Penetration of epithelial barriers by macromolecules: The intestinal mucosa. in Clinical Disorders in Pediatric Gastroenterology and Nutrition. F. Lifshitz (ed.). Marcel Dekker, New York, 1980, p. 185.

54.   Stintzing, G., and R. Zetterstrom: Cow's milk allergy. Incidence and pathogenic role of early response to cow's milk formula. Acta Paediatr Scand 68:383, 1979.

55.   Lubos, M.C., J.W. Gerrard, and D.J. Buchan: Disaccharidase activities in milk sensitive and celiac patients. J Pediatr 70:325, 1967.

56.   Levine, M.M., H.L. DuPont, S. Formal, R.B. Hornick, A. Takeuchi, E.J. Gangarosa, M.J. Snyder, and J.P. Libonati: Pathogenesis of Shigella dysenteriae, I. (Shiga) dysentery. J Infect Dis 127:261, 1963.

57.   DuPont, H.L.: Pathogenesis of enteric diarrhea and gut immune mechanisms in defense against enteric infection. Proc. XIV Int'l Congress of Pediatr.

Buenos Aires, Argentina, Oct. 1974, p. 96.

58. Gordon, J. E., M. Behar, and N. S. Scrimshaw: Acute diarrheal disease in less developed countries. I. An epidemiological basis for control. Bull WHO 31:1, 1964.

59. Gordon, J. E.: Diarrheal disease of early childhood—worldwide scope of the problem. Part 1. Factors determining host susceptibility and response to neonatal gastroenteritis. Ann NY Acad Sci 176:9, 1971.

60. Jelliffe, D. B., and E. F. P. Jelliffe: Human Milk in the Modern World. Oxford University Press, Oxford, 1978.

61. Mata, L.: Breast feedings, diarrheal disease and malnutrition in less developed countries. in Pediatric Nutrition. Infant Feedings - Deficiencies - Diseases. F. Lifshitz (ed.). Marcel Dekker, New York, 1982, p. 355.

62. Mata, L., S. Murillo, P. Jimenez, M. A. Allen, B. Garcia: Child feedings in less developed countries: induced breast feedings in a transitional society. in Pediatric Nutrition. Infant Feedings - Deficiencies - Diseases. F. Lifshitz, (ed.). Marcel Dekker, New York, 1982, pp. 35-53.

63. Oski, F. A.: The non-nutritional benefits of human milk. in Pediatric Nutrition. Infant Feedings - Deficiencies - Diseases. F. Lifshitz, (ed.). Marcel Dekker, New York, 1982, p. 55.

64. Faber, H. K., and F. L. Sutton: A statistical comparison of breast fed and bottle fed babies during the first year. Am J Dis Child 40:1163, 1930.

65. Glazier, M. M.: Comparing the breast fed and the bottle fed infant. N Engl J Med 230:626, 1930.

66. Giannella, R. A., S. A. Broitman, and N. Zamcheck: Salmonella enteritis. I. Role of reduced gastric secretion in pathogenesis. Am J Dig Dis 26:1000, 1971.

67. Waddell, W. R., and L. J. Kunz: Association of salmonella enteritis with operation on the stomach. N Engl J Med 255:555, 1956.

68. DuPont, H. L., and R. B. Hornick: Adverse effect of Lomotil therapy in shigellosis. JAMA 226:1525, 1973.

69. Freter, R., S. P. De, A. Mondal, D. L. Shrivastava, and F. W. Sunderman Jr.: Coproantibody and serum antibody in cholera patients. J Infect Dis 115:83, 1963.

70. DuPont, H. L., R. B. Hornick, M. J. Snyder, J. P. Libonati, S. B. Formal, and E. J. Gangarosa: Immunity in shigellosis. II. Protection induced by oral live vaccine or primary infection. J Infect Dis 125:12, 1972.

71. Freter, R.: Interactions between mechanisms controlling the intestinal microflora. Am J Clin Nutr 27:1409, 1974.

72. Wolin, M. J.: Metabolic interactions among intestinal microorganisms. Am J Clin Nutr 27:1320, 1974.

73. Knox, J.D.E., A.R. Laurence, G. MacNaughton, and A.A. Robertson: Diagnosis of diarrhea in general practice, bacteriologic "self-help." Lancet 2:1392, 1967.

74. Harris, J.C., H.L. DuPont, and R.B. Hornick: Fecal leukocytes in diarrheal illness. Ann Intern Med 76:697, 1972.

75. Nelson, J.D., and K.C. Haltalin: Accuracy of diagnosis of bacterial diarrheal disease by clinical features. J Pediatr 78:519, 1971.

76. Aserkoff, B., and J.V. Bennett: Effect of antibiotic therapy in acute salmonellosis on the fecal excretion of salmonellae. N Engl J Med 281:636, 1969.

77. Harris, A.H., and M.B. Coleman: Diagnostic Procedures and Reagents, 4th ed. American Public Health Assoc., Inc., New York, 1963, p. 43.

78. Lifshitz, F., P. Coello-Ramirez, G. Gutierrez-Topete, and M.C. Cornado-Cornet: Carbohydrate oral loads after recovery from diarrhea. J Pediatr 79:612, 1971.

79. Lifschitz, C.: Breath hydrogen testing in infants with diarrhea. in Carbohydrate Intolerance in Infancy. F. Lifshitz (ed.). Marcel Dekker, New York, 1982, pp. 31-42.

80. Maltalm, K.C., J.K. Nelson, R. Ring, II., M. Sladoje, and L.V. Minton: Double-blind treatment study of shigellosis comparing ampicillin, sulfadiazine and placebo. J Pediatr 70:970, 1967.

81. Nelson, J.D.: Duration of neomycin therapy for enteropathogenic Escherichia coli diarrheal disease. Pediatrics 48:248, 1971.

82. Finberg, L.: Water and electrolyte alterations in clinical disorders and malnutrition. in Pediatric Nutrition. Infant Feedings - Deficiencies - Diseases. F. Lifshitz (ed.). Marcel Dekker, New York, 1982, pp. 427-437.

83. Lifshitz, F.: Current therapy of the malabsorption syndrome and intestinal disaccharidase deficiencies. in Current Pediatric Therapy, 6th ed. S. Gellis and B.M. Kagan (eds.). W.B. Saunders Co., Philadelphia, 1973, p. 236.

84. Cook, D., and H. Sarett: Design of infant formulas for meeting normal and special needs. in Clinical Disorders in Pediatric Nutrition, F. Lifshitz (ed.). Marcel Dekker, New York (in press).

85. Hyman, C.J., J. Reiter, J. Rodnan, and A.L. Drash: Parenteral and oral alimentation in the treatment of non-specific protracted diarrheal syndrome in infancy. J Pediatr 78:17, 1971.

86. Deren, J.J., S.A. Broitman, and N. Zamcheck: Effect of diet upon intestinal disaccharidases and disaccharide absorption. J Clin Invest 46:186, 1967.

15

THE MALABSORPTION SYNDROME

Fima Lifshitz, M. D. and Ulysses Fagundes-Neto, M. D.

INTRODUCTION

Malabsorption of nutrients may be of serious consequence to a growing child. Any gastrointestinal disorder with consequent malabsorption can lead to malnutrition in any age group or socioeconomic bracket. Indeed, the most frequent form of malnutrition in the United States is found in children who have chronic diarrhea and malabsorption. On the other hand, in developing countries, chronic diarrhea and malabsorption are almost always part of the syndrome of primary malnutrition.

The malabsorption syndrome is characterized by failure to thrive, weight loss, and passage of abnormal stools. A precise diagnosis of the pathophysiological alterations associated with the malabsorption syndrome is essential for rational treatment.

The purpose of this chapter is to review the most important causes of the malabsorption syndrome in children, as well as to give an orientation for the diagnostic and therapeutic approach in a child with malabsorption.

ETIOLOGY

There are many conditions which may produce malabsorption in children. Tables 1-3 list some of the most frequent diseases and disorders that form part of the malabsorption syndrome. We have classified them according to pathophysiological mechanisms, as described below.

PATHOPHYSIOLOGY

In the past, the term malabsorption and steatorrhea were used synonymously because the first well-recognized diseases causing malabsorption (celiac disease and cystic fibrosis) characteristically presented with elevated fecal fat. In the last two decades, however, as a result of progress in the understanding of the physiology and pathophysiology of the digestive absorptive process, it became well-established that other nutrients may be affected in malabsorption caused by a variety of processes.

TABLE 1   Disorders of Inadequate Digestion

1. Pancreatic insufficiency
   a. Cystic fibrosis
   b. Shwachman syndrome
   c. Enterokinase deficiency
   d. Amylase, lipase, and trypsinogen deficiency
   e. Others

2. Acid hypersecretion (Zollinger-Ellison syndrome)

3. Altered bile salt metabolism including intestinal resection
   a. Bile salt insufficiency
   b. Short-gut syndrome
   c. Intestinal stasis syndrome

TABLE 2   Conditions Associated with Intestinal Stasis Syndrome

1. Diarrheal disease
2. Tropical sprue
3. Protein-energy malnutrition
4. Hypogammaglobulinemias
5. Gastric achlorhydria and/or hypochlorhydria
6. Scleroderma and other peristaltic alterations
7. Regional enteritis
8. Intestinal tuberculosis
9. Abdominal and gastrointestinal surgery
10. Afferent loop dysfunction following gastrojejunostomy
11. Gastrojejunocolic fistula
12. Partial obstruction due to adhesions

TABLE 3   Disorders of Inadequate Intestinal Mucosa Cell Transport

1. Generalized defects
   a. Celiac disease: gluten-sensitive enteropathy
   b. Transient gluten intolerance
   c. Tropical sprue
   d. Giardiasis and other infestations
   e. Protein hypersensitivity: cow's milk, soy, and multiple intolerances
   f. Unusual causes: Whipple disease, radiation, or drugs

2. Selective defects
   a. Specific amino acid malabsorption
   b. Carbohydrate malabsorption
      1. Primary oligodisaccharidase deficiencies
      2. Primary intestinal glucose transport alterations
      3. Ontogenetic lactase deficiency
      4. Secondary carbohydrate malabsorption
   c. Abetalipoproteinemia
   d. Acrodermatitis enteropathica
   e. Congenital chloridorrhea (congenital alkalosis with diarrhea)
   f. Vitamin B_{12} and folate malabsorption

There is a frequent tendency to separate malabsorption syndromes by the alterations in protein, carbohydrate, fat, and/or minerals. However, most often the malabsorption syndrome combines alterations in the absorption of all nutrients of the diet. Therefore, we will discuss the pathophysiology of each entity by the alterations which precipitate the disease. Tables 1-3 list the mechanisms leading to intestinal malabsorption in the different entities which may produce this syndrome.

DISORDERS OF INADEQUATE DIGESTION

PANCREATIC EXOCRINE INSUFFICIENCY (See also Chap. 19)

Cystic Fibrosis

Cystic fibrosis is the most frequent manifestation of pancreatic insufficiency (approximately 95% of the cases) in childhood. It is the most prevalent potentially lethal disorder in the white United States population, affecting 1:1500 to 1:2000 Caucasian live births (1).

This autosomal recessive disease is characterized by altered function of the mucous and exocrine glands, being the best example of lipolytic pancreatic insufficiency.

The basic defect in cystic fibrosis remains unknown, and no single unifying concept that provides an explanation for the abnormalities of exocrine gland secretions, has been found. For a long time, the hallmark for cystic fibrosis was pancreatic achylia, but now it is well established that up to 20% of the patients have normal pancreatic function or show only discrete deficiency (2) with normal growth in stature and weight. In these cases the respiratory tract and other glands are affected and the patients may not need pancreatic enzymatic replacement therapy.

The clinical features of the disease are variable depending on the age group considered. In 90% of the cases the symptomatology is present by the first year of life, and by 2 years of age more than 75% of the affected children have pulmonary symptoms (3). During the child's first 6 months, pulmonary involvement dominates the clinical picture with recurrent episodes of bronchitis and pulmonary infections in 20% of the cases. Most patients, however, suffer from both pancreatic and pulmonary disorders.

The early symptoms of cystic fibrosis may be present at birth with intestinal obstruction due to meconium ileus. The clinical manifestation of obstruction usually appears within the first 48 hours of life. Meconium ileus may be present in up to 20% of patients, so a delayed meconium passage in the newborn must be suggestive of cystic fibrosis. The patients also may present with poor growth in spite of attempts to provide an increased caloric intake in the diet. The onset of puberty may be greatly delayed and girls may have irregular menses with frequently missed periods.

The gastrointestinal symptoms are variable depending on the extension of the pancreatic lesion, but the most characteristic signs are the passage of bulky, foul, fatty diarrheic stools associated with failure to thrive, despite a good intake.

Cirrhosis of the liver of unknown origin occurs approximately in 4-6% of the patients, and occasionally may be the initial clinical manifestation (4). Intestinal intussusception and rectal prolapse are rare complications reported in these children. Recurrent rectal prolapse is more commonly noted in untreated or poorly treated patients.

As a general rule moderate to massive steatorrhea, up to 50-60 g/day depending upon the degree of pancreatic dysfunction, with a normal D-xylose absorption test is highly suggestive of cystic fibrosis. There also may be hypoproteinemic edema because of protein malabsorption, particularly when soy protein diets are offered to these patients. Metabolic alkalosis also may occur. A hemorrhagic diathesis caused by vitamin K deficiency may be seen. Lactase deficiency with respective lactose intolerance was reported with a high incidence in cystic fibrosis patients, but subsequently it could not be confirmed (5).

The diagnosis of cystic fibrosis is best established by a sweat chloride test of over 60 mEq/L. The indications for a sweat test are the following (6): growth failure, chronic diarrhea or abnormal stools, malabsorption, rectal prolapse, recurrent episodes of abdominal pain and fecal impaction, chronic cough, recurrent pneumonia, or recurrent episodes of asthmatic bronchitis, bronchrolitis, nasal polyps, or x-ray evidence of chronic obstructive disease. In addition, patients who have idiopathic hypoproteinemia, cirrhosis and portal hypertension, or pancreatitis, as well as patients with heat stroke, metabolic acidosis, or alkalosis, and infants with salty taste, should be given a sweat test. Also, siblings of known patients with cystic fibrosis and the offspring of mothers with cystic fibrosis should be tested.

There are a few conditions, however, other than cystic fibrosis in which sweat electrolytes may be elevated. They are: untreated adrenal insufficiency, hypothyroidism, glycogen storage disease, vasopressin (Pitressin)-resistant nephrogenic diabetes insipidus, fucosidosis, mucopolysaccharidosis, hyperhydrotic ectodermal dysplasia and sensorineural deafness, malnutrition, and advancing age.

It should be kept in mind that infants in the first month of life are notoriously difficult to "sweat." Therefore, spurious results are not infrequent, particularly if the laboratory that performs the sweat test is not experienced.

Shwachman Syndrome

This syndrome, although rare, is considered to be the major disorder of pancreatic exocrine function in childhood excluding cystic fibrosis (7).

This is a familial syndrome characterized by pancreatic insufficiency, neutropenia, severe stunting growth, eczema, and susceptibility to infections.

The common symptoms of this disease are failure to thrive, steatorrhea, and nonwatery diarrhea, generally present since birth, although in some patients it can appear any time during the first year of life. Leukopenia with severe neutropenia usually occurs either as a constant or a cyclic manifestation, which favors recurrent infections. Otitis media, pneumonia, mastoiditis, meningitis, and septicemia have been reported (8). Anemia and thrombocytopenia also may be present, all resulting from bone marrow hypoplasia. Metaphyseal dysostosis of the hips and knees, and lesions of the ribs and other bones also have been reported (9).

The pancreatic dysfunction is characterized by markedly reduced or absent proteolytic enzymes, lipase, and amylase activities in the duodenal fluid. Pancreas stimulation with secretin-pancreozymin shows reduced pancreatic enzyme secretion and bicarbonate concentrations although the volume of secretion is normal.

It is important to emphasize that the sweat chloride test is always normal in children with this disorder.

Enterokinase Deficiency

There are two forms of enterokinase deficiency reported, namely, the congenital and the secondary forms. Congenital enterokinase deficiency was first described by Hadorn et al. in 1969 in a 4-month-old infant with a history of diarrhea since birth, failure to thrive, and severe malnutrition, hypoalbuminemic edema, anemia, and steatorrhea (10). Pancreatic enzymes at the time of diagnosis, while the patient was severely malnourished, showed low levels of amylase, lipase, and proteolytic activity. The addition of pancreatic extract to the diet improved the patient's general condition and further studies at 7 and 12 months of age showed normal levels of lipase and amylase activity, but still very little proteolytic activity was in evidence.

Trypsin, chymotrypsin, and carboxypeptidase A activity was undetectable in the patient's duodenal fluid, and enterokinase activity was extremely low. The addition of human enterokinase resulted in the appearance of normal or even higher than normal levels of proteolytic enzymes, and incubation of the juice under the same conditions, but without added enterokinase, showed no activation. Withdrawal of pancreatic extract resulted in recurrence of diarrhea and clinical deterioration. Jejunal histology and repeated sweat tests were always normal.

Some other patients with congenital enterokinase deficiency have been reported, and most of them presented with steatorrhea at the time of diagnosis (11). This feature has been attributed to a generalized enzyme deficiency secondary to protein malnutrition that disappears with improvement of the poor nutritional condition.

Recently, Lebenthal et al. have described secondary enterokinase deficiency resulting from intestinal morphological abnormalities (12). Infants with chronic diarrhea and severe malnutrition showed alterations of the small-bowel morphology and very low levels of intestinal mucosal and duodenal juice enterokinase activity. After treatment with total parenteral nutrition, the enzymatic levels improved, reaching normal concentration with complete clinical recovery. On the other hand, untreated celiac patients revealed essentially normal levels of enterokinase activity. Since both patients with chronic diarrhea and malnutrition and those with celiac disease may have marked histological alterations in the small-intestine, the enterokinase activity may be a good enzymatic marker to distinguish between these two abnormalities. The difference in concentrations of enterokinase activity in these two groups of patients may be explained by differences in intestinal cell turnover. These differences also suggest that enterokinase may not be a brush border enzyme, but a mucosal enzyme, which is made in the Brunner glands, as postulated by Takano's hypothesis (13). According to this author, in celiac disease the goblet cell population remains unaffected while in chronic diarrhea it is decreased, thus leading to secondary enterokinase deficiency.

Isolated Amylase, Lipase, and Trypsinogen Deficiency

These enzyme deficiencies are rare. Amylase deficiency may occur as a primary manifestation but it is more often found as a physiological problem resulting from feedings with a high starch content to the premature baby. Diarrhea is the major symptom and is alleviated by lightening the starch load. Lipase deficiency is a very rare familial disease that causes steatorrhea. The duodenal fluid contains normal tryptic and amylase activities but there is an absent lipase. Trypsinogen deficiency is a rare disease with symptoms similar to those of enterokinase deficiency. This entity was diagnosed before knowledge of the existence of enterokinase deficiency, and there is a possibility that both are the same disorders.

Other Pancreatic Disorders

There are other rare primary pancreatic disorders (see Chap. 19) leading to an inadequate digestion. Hereditary pancreatitis which begins in childhood is transmitted as a non-sex-linked autosomal-dominant trait. Another entity is chronic painless pancreatitis which also may lead to malabsorption, diabetes, and malnutrition with calcification of the pancreas; the cause of this disorder has not been determined. In addition, any other cause of chronic or acute relapsing pancreatitis may lead to pancreatic insufficiency.

Treatment of Pancreatic Exocrine Insufficiency Disorders

Inadequate digestion because of pancreatic insufficiency may be treated by the oral administration of pancreatic enzymes.   Patients with pancreatic exocrine insufficiency of any sort, as well as those with specific processes such as cystic fibrosis, trypsinogen deficiency, enterokinase deficiency, and lipase deficiency, are candidates for replacement therapy.   There are several products available for pancreatic replacement. Pancrelipase (Cotazym), 300 mg capsules, has lipolytic activity; each capsule may digest 17 g of dietary fat.   Pancreatin (Viokase), powder, 1. 5 g/teaspoon; or 325 mg tablets, has good lipase activity and protein hydrolysis.   It is less expensive than other products.   All of these products have an unpleasant odor and taste.   Generally, the extract is fed at the beginning of the meal to ensure intake.   The powder must be added to the food just before its administration to minimize its decomposition in vitro; for the same reason it is not wise to combine it with warm foods.   The required dosage of these preparations varies from patient to patient.   Adequate replacement is judged by the character and the decrease in the frequency of the stools.   Infants usually require $\frac{1}{4}$-$\frac{1}{2}$ teaspoon with each feeding; children from 5-10 years of age require two to four tablets per meal.   Since lipase is inactivated by a pH of less than 4. 5, it may be helpful to administer these preparations with sodium bicarbonate (0. 2 g/kg/day). Overdosage of pancreatic extracts induces constipation.   Patients with pancreatic exocrine insufficiency and bone marrow failure may require additional blood transfusions and corticosteroid therapy.   In all instances the diet should be supplemented with medium-chain triglycerides.

ACID HYPERSECRETION (See also Chap. 13)

Zollinger-Ellison Syndrome

This is an uncommon disease in children.   It is due to a gastrinoma in which a pancreatic tumor (delta cell) produces an excess of gastrin.   In this condition there is diarrhea and there may be steatorrhea, nausea, vomiting, and abdominal pain as well.   The high plasma levels of gastrin and gastric acid may be the cause of acid-induced injury and of multiple gastric and intestinal ulcers found in these patients.   The inactivation of pancreatic enzymes by excess gastric acid secretion accounts for the malabsorption present in these patients.   High acidity within the intestinal lumen also leads to micellar deficiency, further inhibiting fat absorption.   Alteration in pH results in decreased glucose transport as well as inactivation of intestinal disaccharidases.   A limited ability to absorb and reesterify fatty acids also occurs in these patients.

Radiographically, multiple peptic ulcers are seen as well as thickening of gastric and duodenal folds.   There is no distinctive jejunal pathological pattern in this syndrome although acute inflammation and microulcers provide diagnostic clues when present.   Marked acid hypersecretion associated with Zollinger-Ellison syndrome is preferably managed by resection of the tumor; however, since an isolated obvious tumor is rare, total gastrectomy is preferred by most surgeons, although many of these patients will respond to cimetidine.

ALTERED BILE SALT METABOLISM
INCLUDING INTESTINAL RESECTION

Bile Salt Insufficiency

Insufficient production of conjugated bile salt, diminished bile salt pool or deconjugation of bile salts in the upper intestine may decrease solubilization of lipids and result in steatorrhea due to subnormal concentrations of conjugated bile salts necessary for micelle formation. Insufficient bile occurs in liver disease, extra-hepatic biliary tract obstruction or atresia, and with inborn errors of bile salt metabolism. All may lead to malabsorption in various degrees that involves alterations in the absorption of fat and fat soluble vitamins. These could result in steatorrhea and/or in other problems such as rickets. When decreased conjugated bile salts cause steatorrhea, replacement therapy may be feasible. Congenital or acquired bile salt deficiency might be treated by conjugated bile salt preparations; i. e. , dehydrocholic acid (Decholin tablets) 0. 25-0. 75 g three times a day. The dose should be increased gradually to this level because of the possibility that diarrhea might be induced. When bile salts are lost, hepatic synthesis may be capable of keeping the bile salt pool at nearly normal levels. The fat digestion and absorption is only moderately impaired. This kind of malabsorption can be alleviated by feedings of cholestyramine (a bile-salt-binding resin). However, if hepatic synthesis of bile salt is not capable of maintaining the bile salt pool, maldigestion and malabsorption of long-chain triglycerides occur with severe excretion of fat in the stools. This kind of malabsorption cannot be controlled by adsorption of bile salt alone but by a combination of adsorption of bile salts with cholestyramine and substitution of medium-chain triglycerides for long-chain rats in the diet. Cholestyramine resin (USP) (Cuemid powder, Questran, 2-4 g four times a day) may be given mixed in orange juice or milk formula. It should be kept in mind that this preparation interferes with the absorption of vitamins A, D, and K and other nutrients and may produce hyperchloremic acidosis. Malabsorption of fat might be worsened by cholestyramine if the dose exceeds 12 g/day.

Short-Gut Syndrome

The short-gut syndrome is a consequence of abnormal small-intestine function due to extensive intestinal resection. The digestive absorptive surface area provided by the small bowel is equivalent to 2×10^6 cm^2. This constitutes a larger area than that which is necessary to maintain a good state of nutrition. Therefore, man can tolerate intestinal resection relatively safely. A resection of up to 40% of the total length is usually well tolerated, but the duodenum, the distal half of the ileum, and the ileocecal sphincter must remain intact; otherwise, serious functional problems such as diarrhea and malabsorption can result. Resections of 70% or more are usually life-threatening.

In the pediatric age group, most of resections occur in the neonatal period as a consequence of intestinal malformations such as intestinal malrotation, jejunal atresia, meconium ileus, volvulus, bands, intestinal duplications, etc. Intussusception and regional ileitis are the most common causes of intestinal resection in older children. In developing countries intestinal obstruction due to parasites (ascaris bolus) also may be a frequent cause.

As was pointed out previously, some of the consequences of malabsorption due to intestinal resection depend on what part of the gut is removed. Duodenal and upper jejunum resection may lead to nutrient malabsorption including water, electrolytes, fat, protein, carbohydrate, and vitamins. Fluid loss is usually greatest in the first few days, but soon after adaptative mechanisms take place which facilitate efficient digestion and absorption. These include increased absorption, particularly of carbohydrate, as a result of intestinal cell hyperplasia and leads to a steady state during which there is no residual disease.

Gastric hypersecretion is the most common complication occurring as a consequence of massive intestinal resection. The exact mechanism is unknown though it may be due to the removal of an inhibiting intestinal factor. It may cause serious peptic ulcer disease as well as other alterations leading to malabsorption as described previously. Occasionally, the problem is further complicated by the appearance of pancreatitis. Hypersecretion may be limited to the postoperative

period or persist for months.   Thus vagotomy and pyloroplasty or gastroenteros-
tomy should not be considered as a primary therapy in such patients because hypersecretion is usually self-limited and the decreased gastric emptying time
following surgery may worsen steatorrhea.   To combat excessive duodenal acidity,
effective antacids should be used in adequate dosages, i. e. , sodium bicarbonate,
0. 2 g/kg/day, or magnesium-aluminum hydroxide (Maalox, tablets or oral suspension).   More recently, an effective antacid, cimetidine, has been useful
in reducing gastric acidity, both basal and after food.   This is beneficial in pathological hypersecretory conditions such as the Zollinger-Ellison syndrome and it
may be useful in the short-gut syndrome.   However, there is limited experience
with this drug in infancy; doses of 20-40 mg/kg have been used.

Resection of the distal portion of the ileum also may cause serious diarrhea and
steatorrhea due to an alteration in bile salt metabolism.   In the normal person the
bile salts are almost completely reabsorbed in the ileum and little reaches the colon.   After ileal resection there is a decrease in the bile salt pool, with excessive
amounts passed into the colon.   A decreased bile salt pool leads to fat malabsorption, and an increased bile salt concentration in the colon provokes water secretion by an irritative mechanism.   Bile salts have a strong laxative effect in the colon. Resection of the distal ileum may also induce vitamin B_{12} malabsorption, since
the specific transport mechanism for intrinsic factor-mediated vitamin B_{12} absorption is localized to the ileal absorptive cells.   Cholestyramine, an insoluble
anion exchange resin with a molecular weight of about 1 million, binds cholate and
increases bile salt excretion in stools.   When this drug is given in large doses, a
similar problem to the one of ileal resection occurs by virtue of the interrupted
enterohepatic circulation.

Feeding in these patients may be initiated with a dilute glucose electrolyte solution.   If the infant has frequent watery bowel movements while taking this solution, it is unlikely that he will be successfully fed by mouth.   The use of parenteral
hyperalimentation in this type of patient should be considered.   However, if dilute
glucose and electrolytes are tolerated, frequent feedings of   small amounts of formula may be offered.   It is advisable to begin feedings with a simple hyposmolar
formula containing low concentrations of glucose, protein hydrolysate, and medium-chain triglycerides.   A full caloric supply should not be attempted by mouth
until diarrhea has subsided.   Intravenous hyperalimentation can be employed to
meet the caloric requirements. After this diet is tolerated, it may be changed to
an isosmolar formula with glucose, or glucose polymers, and later to a more complex formula which contains disaccharides and even lactose as a source of carbohydrate.   Medium-chain triglycerides should be continued in the diet.

Intestinal Stasis Syndrome

This syndrome also has been referred to as the blind loop syndrome, or stagnant
loop syndrome.   Any small-intestine abnormality that predisposes to stasis of intestinal contents or allows its contamination may lead to small-bowel bacterial
overgrowth and to the intestinal stasis syndrome (14).   Surgical removal of the
ileocecal valve results in removal of the protective barrier of the small bowel
against invasion by colonic bacteria and may thus lead to intestinal contamination.
Whatever the cause of bacterial overgrowth in the upper gut malabsorption results,
being particularly severe for fat and vitamin B_{12}.

A large number of disorders have been associated with proliferation of enteric
microorganisms.   This bacterial contamination may be responsible for many of
the alterations found in this disorder.   Some of the most frequent diseases in children are listed in Table 2.

The pathophysiological mechanisms of bacterial overgrowth may vary in each of
the previously mentioned entities; however, in all of them bacterial contamination

plays an important role in the symptomatology of the disease and in the intestinal malabsorption (15). A major pathophysiological mechanism for steatorrhea in bacterial overgrowth is the diminished concentrations of conjugated bile salts and the corresponding increase in free bile acids in the lumen of the upper small intestine (16). Another factor is damage to the intestinal epithelial cells which results from direct bacterial effects with tissue invasion and disruption of the enterocyte, or from the injurious factors generated from the metabolism of bacteria upon foodstuffs and host secretions, i. e. , deconjugated bile salts, hydroxy fatty acids, and alcohol (15). Other factors may include competition with the host for space and nutrients.

Histologically, the mucosa of patients with bacterial overgrowth varies from a mild to rarely severe abnormality. The abnormal mucosa is patchy. However, despite the histological abnormality, failure of adequate micellar concentration because of low levels of conjugated bile salts (below 2. 5 mM) is the major factor in the steatorrhea of intestinal stasis syndromes. On the other hand, deconjugated bile salts damage intestinal mucosa causing morphological derangements, leading to water secretion and impairing glucose absorption by the enterocyte (17).

The diagnosis of the intestinal stasis syndrome is difficult to confirm because bacterial anaerobic cultures and measurements of bile salts in duodenal fluid are not easily available in clinical settings. A Shilling test may reveal a pernicious anemia-like type of urinary excretion of vitamin B_{12}, and no increase in uptake occurs after intrinsic factor is given. Folate levels are normal in contrast with tropical spruelike infections of the small bowel. Breath hydrogen testing after oral carbohydrate administration also may be diagnostic.

When bile salt metabolism is altered by bacterial overgrowth resulting in deconjugation of bile salts, cholestyramine is not effective. In these instances the therapy should be directed toward controlling bacterial overgrowth. Excision of a fistula or resection of blind loops due to multiple stricture might be curative. When corrective surgery is not possible, oral administration of specific antimicrobials should be given after appropriate cultures are obtained. These preparations might be rotated on a schedule as indicated by bacterial and antibiotic sensitivity studies. The culture of intestinal fluid by transintestinal tubes may be very helpful. Chronic stasis in the small intestine with bacterial overgrowth in scleroderma and diabetic neuropathy requires continuous administration of broad-spectrum antimicrobials.

DISORDERS OF INADEQUATE INTESTINAL MUCOSA CELL TRANSPORT

GENERALIZED DEFECTS

Celiac Disease: Gluten-Sensitive Enteropathy

This is a hereditary type of malabsorption inherited as a mendelian-dominant gene of incomplete penetrance. It is due to a permanent inability to tolerate dietary gluten and it is characterized by clinical and/or laboratory manifestations of intestinal dysfunction after introduction of wheat and rye gluten in the diet with total or subtotal villous atrophy of the mucosa of the duodenum and proximal jejunum (Fig. 1a, b). These patients show a dramatic clinical and histological improvement after withdrawal of gluten from the diet, with clinical and/or laboratory and histological relapse after reintroduction of this dietary compound (18).

Celiac disease was first described by Gee in 1888, and for many years this term included a variety of disorders of childhood in which chronic diarrhea, steatorrhea, and malnutrition were the presenting symptoms (19-21). The steatorrhea of celiac

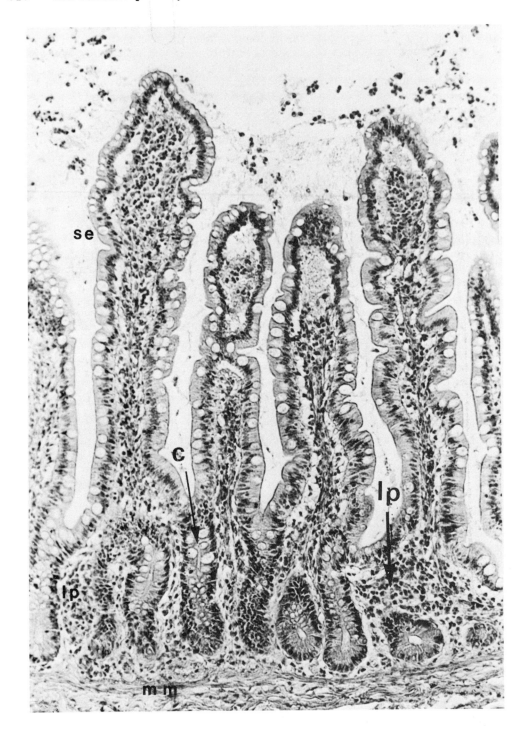

FIGURE 1a   Normal jejunum. Finger-like villi, three times as long as crypts:
(Se) surface epithelium with columnar cells containing basally located ovoid nuclei;
(lp) lamina propria; (C) crypt; (mm) muscularis mucosa. Hematoxylin-eosin stain.
Original magnification x 121. (Courtesy of Dr. E. Kahn.)

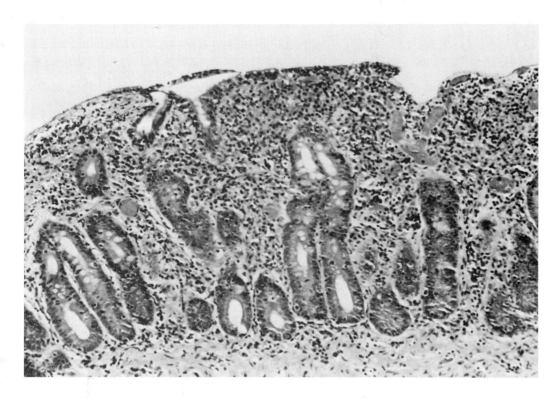

FIGURE 1b   Biopsy of jejunum revealing subtotal villus atrophy. Flat mucosa
without villi, with crypt hyperplasia and increased mononuclear infiltration of the
lamina propria.   Epithelial cells are more cuboidal and nuclei are rounder and hap-
hazardly placed.   Goblet cells are decreased in number. Hematoxylin-eosin stain.
Original magnification x 306. (Courtesy of Dr. E. Kahn.)

disease was not clearly differentiated from that of pancreatic insufficiency until
1938, when Andersen separated cystic fibrosis as a distinct entity from celiac disease (20).

Etiology

The etiology of celiac disease was unknown until 1950 when the Dutch pediatrician
Dicke first suggested that removal of gluten from the diet of these patients reversed the malabsorption (22). Weijers and Van de Kamer a few years later pointed out
that gliadin (the protein molecule of gluten), and more specifically an acidic peptide bound to glutamine, is the toxic fraction that provokes deleterious effects on
the intestinal mucosa of susceptible individuals (21).   Furthermore, in 1962, Rubin et al. showed that exposure of normal-appearing ileum of celiac patients to
gluten was followed rapidly by loss of villi and appearance of the characteristic lesion (23).   This experiment suggested that gluten exposure precedes the altered
intestinal morphology in celiac disease.   The mechanism of malabsorption in celiac
disease is primarily related to the marked reduction in intestinal mucosal surface
area.   All these morphological alterations are perfectly reversible when a celiac
child is put under a rigorous gluten-free diet (24).

Morphology

The characteristic intestinal lesion of celiac disease, namely, total villous atrophy with crypt enlargement with cuboidal changes of the absorbing cell and lymphocytic infiltration was thought to be specific. However, it is well known that in other clinical entities there also may be a flat lesion of the intestinal mucosa. Included are protein hypersensitivity (protein cow's milk intolerance and protein soybean intolerance), acute bacterial and nonbacterial diarrhea, intestinal stasis syndrome, tropical sprue, and severe protein-energy malnutrition (kwashiorkor). As mentioned previously, enterokinase activity may be a biochemical marker to differentiate among some of the entities which produce mucosal atrophy. There are some other diseases that also may show total villous atrophy. However, they almost always have other histological features differentiating them from the characteristic lesion of celiac disease. Specifically they are: hypogammaglobulinemia (virtual absence of IgA-producing plasma cells), Whipple disease (lamina propria stuffed with periodic acid-Schiff-positive macrophages), Zollinger-Ellison syndrome, eosinophilic gastroenteritis (spotty infiltration with eosinophils), and primary intestinal lymphoma (malignant cells in many biopsies).

Gluten-sensitive enteropathy affects primarily the mucosa of the small intestine; the submucosa, muscularis mucosa, and serosa are not involved. In active celiac disease the intestinal cell turnover is greatly increased and the number of crypt cells in mitosis is strikingly increased. In severe cases the villi become flat and the crypts markedly elongated in an apparent attempt to compensate for the lost cells. The enterocytes lose their normal cylindrical shape becoming cuboidal in appearance and the nuclei lose their basal polarity. The lamina propria shows an evident cellular increase, especially in plasma cells and lymphocytes; these last cells migrate out of the lamina propria and infiltrate between the enterocytes reaching the intestinal lumen.

Pathophysiology

Two possible mechanisms have been postulated to explain the intestinal alterations seen in celiac patients: (1) an inborn error of metabolism which results in the accumulation of undigested toxic gluten peptides with subsequent mucosal damage because of deficiency or absence of specific peptidases, (2) an immunological reaction to the acidic peptides contained in gliadin is responsible for the intestinal damage. Increased serum IgA concentration, an increased number of IgM- and IgG-containing cells in the small bowel, associated with an elevated number of antigluten antibodies shown by immunofluorescence, have all been reported in celiac patients, with a further increase with a gluten challenge. Carswell and Ferguson reported a significantly higher incidence of precipitins to gluten as well as to other food proteins in the serum of patients with celiac disease in comparison with non-celiac patients (25). However, the role of these antigluten antibodies in the pathogenesis of the disease is not clear. Antigluten antibody may attach to the cell but it does not require complement and does not produce an injury in itself. The high incidence of HLA-8 in these patients suggests a genetic predisposition. Furthermore IgA deficiency also predisposes to this disease.

Incidence

The precise incidence of celiac disease is unknown because a large number of patients have asymptomatic disease. Transient gluten intolerance also may confuse the statistics. Rolles et al. reported that the incidence of asymptomatic celiac disease among the patient's first-degree relatives is 5. 5% (26). Nevertheless, celiac disease seems to be more common in certain European countries than in the

United States. The estimated incidence of celiac disease in some European countries is: England, 1:3000 births; West Scotland, 1:1850 births; Glasgow, 1:1100
births; very common in the west of Ireland, 1:300 births; Switzerland, 1:1890
births; and Sweden, 1:6500 births.

Onset

The age of onset of the disease is variable and it seems to have a direct relation
with the time when gluten is first fed. Young and Pringle showed that in 110 celiac
children the interval between the age of gluten introduction to the diet and the onset
of symptoms was between 3-6 months (27). It was never less than 1 month and
sometimes it was over 1 year. In Hamilton and colleagues series in Toronto,
42 children had a mean age of onset of symptoms of 19 months, with a range up to
7 years (28). In all of the children, wheat gluten had been introduced into the diet
between 1-5 months of age.

Recently, Anderson et al. stressed the dramatic reduction in the mean age of
presentation of the disease which has occurred in these last few years (18). For-
merly, in the early 1950s, the mean age of onset of disease was 43.6 months. In
contrast, nowadays, the mean age is 9.3 months. It is interesting to note that
there has been a corresponding drop in the mean age of introduction of gluten-containing cereals into the diet, i.e., from 9.4 to 3.4 months.

Clinical picture

The classical clinical picture of the disease is characterized by an insidious onset
of symptoms associated with failure to thrive. The main complaint is chronic
diarrhea with soft, pale, bulky, and offensive stools, and the infant becomes irritable, apathetic, pale, and anorexic. There is muscle wasting, generalized hypotonia and abdominal distension. However, the general clinical experience shows
that the presentation in most patients differs. Hamilton et al. reported that 12 of
42 children had no diarrhea, 12 were not irritable, and 18 were not anorexic (28).
Vomiting was present in 24 cases and definite abdominal pain in 8. Symptoms
noted most frequently were chronic diarrhea and failure to thrive. Constipation
and fecal impaction may also occur. The classical features of celiac disease may
not appear until the third to sixth decade of life.

The physical features of the patients with celiac disease depend, to some extent,
on the duration and severity of the disease. The most important are: malnutrition
with body weight deficits, finger clubbing, peripheral edema, intestinal bleeding as
a consequence of vitamin K deficiency, hypocalcemic and/or hypomagnesemic tetany, iron deficiency anemia, and rickets. Many patients with celiac disease may
present with only one of these major manifestations of malabsorption.

Laboratory data

It is now recognized that 10-25% of celiac children may not have a raised fecal fat
at the time of diagnosis, and that the D-xylose test using the urine collection technique is not reliable. Whole blood folate levels were proposed as a very consistent
method for diagnosis of active celiac disease (29). Levels below 60 ng/ml were
considered indicative of disease. However, it has been demonstrated that red cell
folate may be occasionally normal in celiac patients and there may be low levels in
nonceliac patients (30). Frequently there is elevation of serum IgA and depression
of IgM along with increased numbers of IgA containing plasma cells in the intestinal
biopsy. Vitamin B_{12} absorption is usually normal but may be depressed if the disease is extensive and involves the ileum. Roentgenologically, there are no specific
findings although there are some characteristic changes, i.e., an altered bowel
pattern with dilatation of the proximal loops and coarsening of the jejunal folds.

Differential diagnosis

Nowadays the differential diagnosis of celiac disease from cystic fibrosis is easy because the widespread use of sweat tests allows a clear differentation. However, cystic fibrosis and celiac disease have been described coexisting in the same patients. An effort should be made to differentiate celiac disease from those entities which also manifest a flat intestinal mucosa, namely, food protein hypersensitivity, infectious enteritis, tropical sprue, and protein-energy malnutrition. Transient gluten intolerance and asymptomatic celiac disease are also often a cause of confusion. The symptomatic response to a gluten-free diet and the subsequent growth pattern are both important parameters used to help confirm the diagnosis. Nevertheless, a therapeutic trial of a gluten-free diet is never justified in a child who has malabsorption if a peroral jejunal biopsy is not performed, particularly since there may be nonspecific improvement with gluten-free diets in other malabsorptive syndromes. This may encourage the physician to subject the patient to a rigorous difficult regimen for a prolonged period without justification.

Evolution of the disease

The intestinal mucosal abnormalities may be expected to return to normal after treatment in celiac disease. The time taken for complete restoration of normal morphology varies, and might take 1-2 years. The gluten withdrawal from the diet must be for life. Barr et al. demonstrated that the catch-up features after institution of a gluten-free diet is faster in terms of the weight reaching normal levels after 6 months to 1 year of treatment (31). Height and bone age were not normal until after 2 years of treatment. Sheldon reported a relapse rate of 75% in his patients after treatments had been abandoned (32). Moreover, there is strong evidence for development of malignant lymphoma and other malignancies of the gastrointestinal tract in adults as a consequence of prolonged exposure to dietary gluten.

Treatment

Most cases of celiac disease (childhood and adult) respond to elimination of gluten from the diet. This regimen must be lifelong. It is of utmost importance that the dietary exclusion of gluten and its components be as strict as possible. Frequently, neither the physician nor the patient is alert to the possibility that gluten is present in commercial preparations in the form of "fillers" or "additives." Such factors are frequently involved in the "failure of gluten-free diets."

Most investigators agree that the improvement in patients with celiac disease is related to the degree to which gluten is eliminated from the diet. Improvement can be observed clinically by reduction in diarrhea and steatorrhea, by weight gain, and by loss of abdominal distention. These symptoms usually are alleviated in a few days. At the same time, tests of intestinal absorption show a progressive return to normal. When a series of jejunal mucosal biopsies are performed, it is possible to demonstrate a marked improvement in the mucosal structure with the villi often showing an almost normal appearance; however, such a pronounced degree of improvement may take up to six months.

If gluten is readministered to a patient with celiac disease, who has been on a gluten-free diet, a variable response may be observed. In some, a return of symptoms may be induced almost immediately or in a matter of days; in others the malabsorption might be delayed, with symptoms being either mild or subtle.

However, when objective observations are made, changes may be observed quite early. Biochemical documentation of increased fecal fat excretion and of changes in the proximal jejunal mucosa as early as 1 day after administrating gluten can be documented. Histological deteriorations may take from 3 to 6 months.

In most published reports, good response to the use of a gluten-free diet has been observed in almost all patients with celiac disease. When dietary treatment fails, at least three factors should be considered: the dietary restriction may have been inadequate, the patient may have an intestinal villous atrophy due to a disorder other than celiac disease, or there may be other complicating features.

One should be reluctant to consider dietary therapy a failure unless the patient has been hospitalized and the response to treatment has been observed under the close supervision of the physician and the dietitian. As pointed out previously, there are several possible errors in the diagnosis of celiac disease. A group of patients with severe malabsorption, extensive atrophy of the jejunal mucosa, and few or no Paneth cells, who failed to respond to gluten-free diets has also been described. A "true" failure of gluten-free diet in celiacs rarely occurs. Initially the response to gluten withdrawal may be limited by the secondary malnutrition and pancreatic insufficiency. Subsequently, the superimposition of a malignant process such as lymphoma may account for failure to respond to a gluten-free diet.

Oats were originally considered to be deleterious to the patient with celiac disease, but recent observations have not supported this belief. Oats might be included in the diet of these patients without observing adverse effects clinically, biochemically, or morphologically.

Before the use of gluten-free diets, corticosteroids were used to treat celiac disease and led to a reasonable degree of clinical improvement. However, usually this does not correct the steatorrhea to the extent observed after dietary therapy, and the mucosal biopsy tends to remain abnormal. In patients who are treated initially with steroids and in whom a response is achieved, gluten restriction almost always results in further improvement.

Elimination of milk from the diet has enhanced the degree of clinical improvement in patients with celiac disease. The possibility that they may have lactose intolerance secondary to mucosal atrophy with secondary lactase deficiency should be kept in mind. Lactose-free diets, however, usually are not necessary in the treatment of these patients unless there is diarrhea and carbohydrate intolerance (24).

Transient Gluten Intolerance

Transient gluten intolerance has to be distinguished from celiac disease. Children with the latter will require a life-long gluten-free diet, whereas patients with transient gluten intolerance will need such dietary restriction for a shorter period. Recently, Walker-Smith and McNeish et al. reported on two infants with intestinal malabsorption and flat mucosa due to gluten intolerance that showed total recovery on a gluten-free diet (33, 34). Later gluten challenges were done several times and the intestinal mucosa remained normal. Despite all of the evidence of transient gluten intolerance in these patients, they must be closely followed since histological abnormalities of the upper small intestine may not appear for months after gluten reintroduction. Schmerling has suggested that the delay may be as long as 2 years (35). The age of the patient, the duration of previous therapy, and the dose of gluten all may be factors determining the time of frank mucosal relapse.

Tropical Sprue

Tropical sprue is a chronic syndrome characterized by diarrhea, steatorrhea, weight loss, weakness, and eventually severe macrocytic anemia and malnutrition. It occurs in widespread areas throughout the tropical and subtropical zones of the world. This syndrome may involve several diseases and is particularly likely to affect persons from temperate zones traveling to areas where the disease is endemic, with symptoms developing even several years after the visit. Hence, tropical sprue has been considered an overt manifestation of a disease that may be present more frequently in a subclinical form (36).

The major clinical features of this syndrome are due to intestinal malabsorption of fat, carbohydrates, vitamin B_{12}, and folic acid. This malabsorption of multiple nutrients is best explained by the presence of diffuse intestinal mucosal lesions (37). These are similar to those of celiac disease, thus the latter must be excluded before diagnosis can be established. However, the lesions are usually milder in tropical sprue. Of interest is that many control populations in the tropics have the same intestinal lesions as those of patients with tropical sprue (38, 39). Furthermore, the disease may be present in patients with chronic diarrhea with or without steatorrhea (40).

The etiology of this disease is unknown. Occasional epidemics and a favorable response to antibiotic therapy (tetracycline 50 mg/kg/day for 2 weeks) by these patients suggests that it may be an infectious disease (41-44), but efforts to isolate an etiologic agent have been unsuccessful (45). A favorable response also has been reported to follow folic acid therapy (15 mg/day for 2 weeks, followed by 5 mg daily for 5 months), particularly in newly symptomatic patients (43). After a prolonged treatment with antibiotics, folic acid and supplemental vitamin B_{12} (20 μ g intramuscularly daily for 1 week) may be required to reverse the intestinal lesions (42-44). It has been known for several years that these patients have disaccharidase deficiencies, and nutritional restriction of poorly tolerated carbohydrates may be of help in children with tropical sprue (46).

Giardiasis and Other Parasitoses

Among the human intestinal parasites, Giardia lamblia is the only one which definitely has been proved to cause malabsorption. The other intestinal parasitoses such as strongyloidiasis, necatoriasis, ancylostomiasis, ascariasis, etc. , may cause gastrointestinal symptoms, but their role as causative agents of malabsorption syndrome has not been clearly ascertained.

The incidence of G. lamblia infection in the United States varies from 1% in a group of government personnel to as high as 9% in eastern Kentucky (47), the average prevalence being 7. 4% (48). The attack rate in Americans who traveled to Leningrad during 1969-1973 has been calculated to be 23%. In Vietnam giardiasis was diagnosed in 36% of servicemen hospitalized for chronic diarrhea.

G. lamblia resides in the upper part of the small intestine of man in an optimal pH environment between 6 and 7. The parasite exists in two forms: trophozoites and cysts. The active form is the trophozoite, which is piriform in shape, measuring 12-15 x 5-15 x 2-4 μ m. The trophozoites are usually seen in duodenal aspirates and in diarrheal stools, but not in formed feces (Figs. 2a, b, c). The cysts are thick walled and oval measuring 8-12 x 7-10 μ m. The stools of infected individuals usually contain the cyst forms, which are the infective stage of the parasite. Cysts remain viable in water for longer than 3 months and have been shown to be infective after storage in tap water for 16 days.

Infection is spread either by direct fecal-oral contamination or by transmission of cysts in food or water. When ingested, the cyst divides into two trophozoites in the upper gastrointestinal tract. Experimental studies in mice have shown that after innoculation of cysts of giardia into the jejunum, there is a progressive reduction in the villus to crypt ratio of the intestinal morphology (49). This abnormality reaches the climax 7 days after inoculation.

The mechanisms of malabsorption in giardiasis remain obscure. The total parasite load may be important as well as the secondary disturbances in intestinal

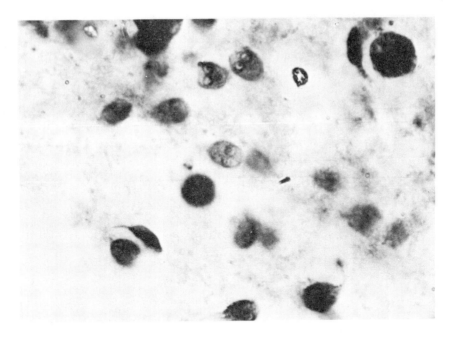

FIGURE 2a   Giardia lamblia trophozoites in a 7-year-old boy with deficiency of immunoglobulins A and G. Duodenal fluid aspirate with iron-hematoxylin stain. Note paired nuclei, axostyle, and flagella in some organisms. Original magnification x 800. (Courtesy of Dr. T. Sun.)

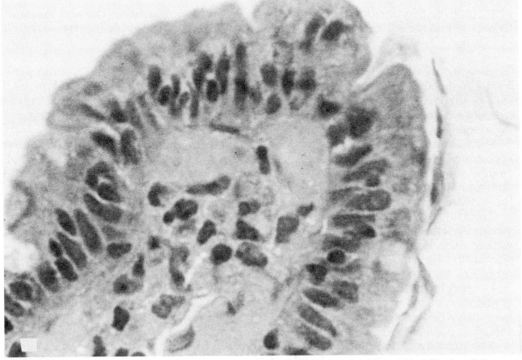

FIGURE 2b   Same patient. Peroral jejunal biopsy, revealing Giardia lamblia trophozoites covering the surface of a villus. Original magnification x 800.

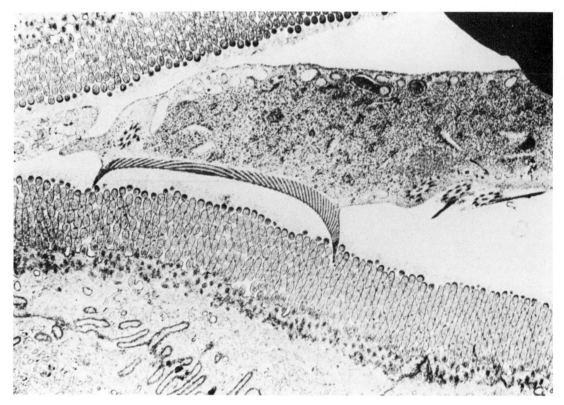

FIGURE 2c   Same patient.   Electron micrograph demonstrating Giardia lamblia trophozoite large sucking disc covering microvilli of a jejunal enterocyte.

function induced by the parasite.   The role of tissue invasion by giardiasis in producing malabsorption is difficult to assess (see Figs 2b, c).   However, the presence of circulating antibodies to the parasite in subjects with malabsorption may indicate that mucosal invasion plays an important pathophysiological role during the disease.

Manifestations of infection with G. lamblia may range from asymptomatic to severe chronic malabsorption.   The percentage of symptomatic patients was as high as 55% in an epidemic, whereas in a group of patients examined for gastrointestinal complaints it was 80%.   However, the prevalence of symptomatology in surveys for endemic giardiasis appears to be far lower (48).

The majority of symptomatic patients present with persistent diarrhea accompanied by flatulence and abdominal pain.   The diarrhea is described as bulky, greasy, and foul smelling.   Other associated symptoms have included weight loss, alternating diarrhea and constipation, anorexia, and bloating, but vomiting and fever are seldom observed.

In experimental infections of prison volunteers, it was found that spontaneous eradication of the parasite was the rule, but clinical experience indicates that patients may be infected and symptomatic for several years.   It is likely that immunological mechanisms may be involved in the process of eradication (50).

The parasitological diagnosis is usually made by stool examination (51).   However, cysts may be seen in up to 50% of stools from patients who are asymptomatic, and may only be seen in half of the stools from subjects with severe malabsorption. In 15% of the patients the diagnosis can only be established by examining duodenal aspirates. These aspirates were positive in 100% of the symptomatic patients (52).

In patients with G. lamblia infection, there may be a response to quinacrine therapy (6 mg/kg/day for 5 days; maximum 300 mg/day), or the response to metronidazole (Flagyl, 250-750 mg/day according to age, for 10 days) is highly successful. In smaller children, 10-20 mg/kg/day is used. A second treatment might be administered after 1 week of rest if G. lamblia persists. Quinacrine treatment is contraindicated in patients with psoriasis, and in patients with a past psychiatric history since it may lead to toxic psychosis. Metronidazole may be carcinogenic and mutagenic, thus its use should be restricted.

Protein Hypersensitivity

Cow's milk protein-sensitive enteropathy

Adverse reactions to milk have been known since Hippocrates who recorded that milk could cause vomiting and urticaria. Finkelstein in 1905, described cow's milk as a cause of death in infancy (53), and Von Pirquet in 1906, introduced the concept of milk allergy (54). While there is evidence that cow's milk protein may produce an immune reaction leading to intestinal injury, the mechanisms remain unclear. In these patients there are gastrointestinal symptoms and diarrhea with or without extragastrointestinal disease of various types and degrees (55). Cow's milk protein sensitive enteropathy (CMPSE) refers specifically to the intestinal pathology and malabsorption induced by cow's milk protein (56).

Incidence. The reported incidence of milk protein hypersensitivity ranges widely from 0. 5-7. 5% in the general population, and up to 21% in infants referred for "allergic studies" (57). The CMPSE also has a high association with other atopic conditions and familial clusterings of allergy (58). It also has been associated with a decrease in breast-feeding and early introduction of cow's milk in infancy (59), immunological abnormalities such as IgA deficiency (60), and diarrheal disease (61).

Pathogenesis. An infant may ingest 15-20 g/day of milk protein and there are as many as 20 different proteins in cow's milk. The five main proteins which may be highly immunogenic and capable of stimulating a systemic antibody response are bovine serum albumin, bovine serum globulin, casein, alpha-lactoglobulin, and beta-lactoglobulins. The latter is the cause of allergic reactions in up to 82% of these patients (62). The beta-lactoglobulin protein fraction is not present in breast milk. Cow's milk is generally richer in protein than breast milk, containing three times the amount present in human milk. Some of the "humanized" milk formulas are less allergenic than unmodified cow's milk because they have a reduced amount of protein and they contain denatured antigenic components as a result of the manufacturing process, but they also contain beta-lactoglobulin.

For CMPSE to occur there must be passage of antigens, which evoke a systemic pathologic response to a susceptible host, into the organism. Under normal circumstances, cow's milk protein antigen does not get absorbed to any significant extent owing to the gastrointestinal barrier and the digestive processes, including gastric acidity and proteolytic and lysosomal enzymes which degrade the antigens. The normal peristaltic activity facilitates the exclusion of the antigens from the gastrointestinal tract. In addition, the local S-IgA immune mechanisms of the host also neutralize the antigens. In this process there is increased local S-IgA response which is associated with increased serum IgA levels (63). Furthermore, some antigens may be cleared by a S-IgA-mediated process in the liver (64). Failure of the digestive and the S-IgA mechanisms to exclude small amounts of antigen results in systemic immunization with luminal (IgG, IgA, and IgE)and cell-mediated (protein sensitized lymphocytes) responses. This may be seen without any disease process. In other words, the presence of circulating antibodies may be a normal event. However, in the susceptible host, reexposure with the antigenic proteins leads to binding to the enterocyte rendering it the target for killer T cells, or type I reagenic or type III Arthus reaction which results in CMPSE with structural and functional damage of the small bowel.

A CMPSE may occur in infants suffering from a variety of disorders that may facilitate the exposure to the protein antigen. Included are patients with intestinal mucosal damage of any type as seen in acute gastroenteritis (61), celiac disease (65), malnutrition and other gastrointestinal disorders (66, 67). It may also occur in young infants who have an immature intestinal mucosa which is permeable for these antigens during the first weeks of life (59), and in children with immune deficiency disorders such as IgA deficiency (60). However, whenever CMPSE occurs, there probably is an underlying genetic predisposition and the acquired illness may be the precipitating factor which facilitates the development of the disease. A similar association of environmental injury and genetic predisposition to disease occurs in other conditions, e. g. , diabetes mellitus (68).

In infants with intestinal malabsorption it is often difficult to ascertain whether CMPSE is the primary event leading to intestinal mucosal damage, with diarrhea occurring as a consequence of this alteration, or a secondary process resulting from intestinal damage from other causes which lead to increased permeability to protein antigens and sensitization of a susceptible host (69). Milk protein hypersensitivity also may be associated with carbohydrate intolerance in infants with gastroenteritis (55). The CMPSE may be the result or the cause of carbohydrate intolerance as discussed elsewhere (70). Despite the uncertainties as to the exact relationships between CMPSE, carbohydrate intolerance malabsorption, and diarrheal disease, it is clear that the jejunal mucosa of young infants, as well as children with diarrhea, is sensitive for a period of time to antigenic protein such as cow's milk, soy, and gluten.

Clinical Manifestations and Diagnosis. The clinical manifestations of protein hypersensitivity and cow's milk protein-sensitive enteropathy are varied. Affected infants may present gastrointestinal manifestations with chronic diarrhea and malabsorption and/or extragastrointestinal manifestations pertaining to the skin, respiratory tract, central nervous system, or others, separately or in several different combinations (55). Similarly, there is an absence of a pattern and there may be no reproducibility in the signs or symptoms of the disease. There is also a variation in the duration and onset of the symptoms with exposure to the offending antigen, with symptoms varying from anaphylactic reactions to mild, nonspecific complaints.

The absence of a specific clinical presentation has led to the use of a strict criteria to establish the diagnosis of milk protein allergy, as suggested by Goldman et al. (71): (1) Disappearance of symptoms after cow's milk withdrawal from the diet; (2) symptoms reappearing within 48 hours following a challenge with cow's milk; (3) three such challenges positive and similar as to onset, duration, and clinical features; and (4) disappearance of symptoms after each challenge reaction.

The criteria, while basically sound, are not practical and have many drawbacks. First, most mothers are reluctant to subject their infants to repeated hazardous milk challenges particularly when the first milk challenge is positive. Reactions to milk challenge can occur as early as 0. 5 hour to as late as 28 days (72, 73), and initial symptoms are not always reproducible in character, onset, or duration at subsequent challenges. Because of these difficulties many clinicians have accepted a single positive milk challenge as diagnostic of CMPSE (74).

The use of per oral intestinal biopsy in the diagnosis of CMPSE just before and 24 hours after milk provocation can be extremely useful in providing a definitive diagnosis (75, 76). On this basis, Iyngkaran et al. proposed a combined clinical and histological criteria for the diagnosis of CMPSE (72): (1) clinical disease (diarrhea with or without vomiting) while receiving cow's milk protein; (2) clinical improvement on a diet free of cow's milk protein; (3) normal or mildly abnormal histology of the jejunal mucosa when taken 6-8 weeks after symptoms subside, and (4) histological relapse, with or without clinical relapse, after reexposure to cow's milk protein. The major drawback of this criteria is the need for jejunal biopsy.

There are other methods which attempt to make the diagnosis by simple means. Included are: the 1-hour blood xylose test following milk challenge (77), the serial evaluation of blood leukocytes after exposure to the offending foodstuff (74), and various immunological methods (78, 79). However, all of the preceding methods are not very reliable and are fraught with false-negative and false-positive results. Therefore, it is obvious that as yet there are no simple reliable means for the diagnosis of CMPSE.

Soy protein and multiple protein enteropathies

A significant proporation of infants who have intolerance to one food protein have or develop intolerance to several other proteins in the course of time. Infants with CMPSE have been shown to commonly have associated intolerance to soy, wheat, and egg protein (56, 80, 81). It is imperative to recognize this phenomenon because of its important therapeutic implications. The approach to diagnosis of these food proteins (e. g. , soy, egg, and wheat protein) rests along lines similar to that of CMPSE.

Gastrointestinal and anaphylactic reactions following soy protein ingestion have been recognized since the early 1960s (82, 83). Since then soy protein intolerance has become well documented (69, 74, 83, 84). The pathogenesis of soy protein intolerance is not established. Immune mechanisms are probably involved. As in CMPSE, soy protein intolerance may be primary or secondary (69). The pathological and enzymological findings of the small-bowel mucosa of infants with soy protein intolerance are closely similar to that in CMPSE, and consist of nonspecific villous atrophy with mucosal enzyme depletion. While various workers have reported that 30-50% of infants with CMPSE have associated soy protein intolerance the exact incidence of this malady is unknown. Clinical reactions to soy protein may be of the immediate or delayed type (84, 85), and include vomiting, diarrhea, fever, lethargy, tachypnea, metabolic acidosis, and cyanosis (86). Nongastrointestinal manifestations such as eczema, rhinorrhea, bronchiolitis, and asthma also have been described (56).

The use of soybean preparations has been advocated for prophylaxis against CMPSE in infants potentially at risk (84, 87). However, the antigenicity of soy protein is at least equal to that of other proteins used in milk formulas (88). Additionally, soy protein intolerance may be expected in a susceptible host who is being fed a formula with this protein, and similarly CMPSE may not occur in infants who are fed cow's milk.

Management of Food Protein Intolerance

The management can be considered along three avenues: exclusion diets, drug therapy, and hyposensitization, or a combination of these. Exclusion diets are the oldest and most successful approach to therapy. While they are easy to institute in cases with intolerance to one food protein, they are difficult to plan and comply with in cases of multiple food protein intolerance, particularly when some of the offending proteins cannot be identified. In the latter situations oral cromolyn sodium (disodium cromoglycate) which otherwise has a limited application in the management of food protein intolerance may have an important role to play. Desensitization has been tried with variable success in individual patients but again has limited scope on a wider scale.

Unusual Causes of Malabsorption

Whipple disease

This disease is caused by a microorganism which causes a systemic and an intestinal reaction. The principal findings are diarrhea, abdominal distress, steatorrhea, and malabsorption in addition to fever, lymphadenopathy, and pleurisy. In rare instances, there is endocarditis and central neurological system symptoms. Arthritis is common although joint effusions are rare (89).

A rod-shaped bacterium is the cause of Whipple disease, which is characterized by the appearance of fat- and glycoprotein-filled macrophages in the lamina propria of the intestine and many other organs, particularly in lymphoid tissues. The intestinal mucosa is edematous with variable alterations in villous architecture causing malabsorption. Electron microscopic examination of the intestinal mucosa can confirm the presence of the bacilli and establish the diagnosis (90). Adrenocorticosteroids and penicillin or tetracycline have changed the prognosis of this illness which was once considered to be fatal (91). Withdrawal of therapy is almost always associated with a recurrence of the disease in a period of weeks to months. The mild malabsorption which results from constrictive pericarditis is corrected by pericardiolysis.

Radiation

Radiation suppresses the intestinal cell proliferation in the crypts with consequent denudation of the mucosa because of a decreased rate of population of the intestinal epithelial cells. Radiation results in an inflammatory, ulcerating type of lesion when given in a dose of 5000 rads (92) or more. Since the number of conditions for which radiation therapy is given has increased, a higher incidence of damaged gut leading to intestinal malabsorption has occurred. The clinical picture is variable; symptoms may appear during radiation therapy or may not appear until months or years after completion. Early in this disease the involvement of the rectum may give a picture that resembles ulcerative colitis. Later on, crampy abdominal pain, diarrhea, malabsorption of fat, and intestinal obstruction due to stricture formation may follow some months after completion of the therapy. The lymphatic obstruction produced by radiation also may contribute to the malabsorption (93).

Drugs

Malabsorption of nutrients may be produced by a number of pharmacological agents used by physicians. These may produce morphological damage to the mucosa of the small intestine, interference with the mucosal enzymes' activity, precipitation of micellar substances such as fatty acids and bile acids, and alterations of the physical chemistry of dietary nutrients. Any of these abnormalities may result in generalized intestinal malabsorption which is usually dose plus time related to the drug. Among the most commonly used drugs causing malabsorption are neomycin, colchicine, cholestyramine, biguanides, antacids, ethanol, oral contraceptives, para-aminosalicylic acid, and laxatives (94).

SELECTIVE ABSORPTION DEFECTS

Specific Amino Acid Malabsorption

A number of specific metabolic disorders have been associated with abnormalities of intestinal transport. These have been reviewed in detail elsewhere (95). Included are cystinuria, hyperdibasic aminoaciduria, Hartnup disease, tryptophan malabsorption, phenylketonuria, methionine malabsorption, iminoglycosuria, and Lowe syndrome. These diseases manifest specific intestinal transport alterations involving one or several amino acids. In addition, there may be alterations in the transport of these compounds in other tissues, e.g., kidney tubule. It is beyond the scope of this chapter to review the specific complications of each of these diseases; suffice it to say that they are inherited defects of amino acid transport which may manifest alterations due to the amino acid malabsorption of one or a group of amino acids. These can manifest themselves in several degrees of aminoaciduria and/or hyperaminoacidemia. The alteration found may also result from the bacterial metabolism of an unabsorbed amino acid in the gut (95).

Amino acid metabolic disorders require specific mixtures of proteins to provide the required restriction of dietary intake of one or more amino acids. Since these disorders occur in rare instances, specific dietary preparations are commercially available. For example, a low phenylalanine diet, provided by Lofenalac, or Product 80056 (Mead Johnson) contains all essential vitamins, minerals, and calories in the form of fat and carbohydrate and is made for use with the appropriate amino acid mixture.

Carbohydrate Malabsorption (Also see Chap. 14)

There are three types of carbohydrate malabsorption syndromes : (1) primary, (2) secondary, and (3) ontogenetic. The primary or congenital carbohydrate malabsorption syndromes are rare. Primary deficiencies have been described for each of the intestinal surface oligosaccharidases, namely, lactase, sucrase-isomaltase, and trehalase deficiencies. In addition, primary alterations in the capacity of the intestine to transport glucose are known to occur, namely glucose-galactose malabsorption. These entities may manifest themselves very early in life or may have a late onset in adults. The late onset of any one of the previously mentioned primary carbohydrate malabsorption syndromes is of interest (96-98). The usual view is that these are genetically controlled diseases which are first manifested in adult life.

The patients with primary carbohydrate malabsorption have a virtual absence of hydrolytic activity for a single disaccharide, or an absence of the intestinal capacity to transport lactose and galactose. However, they have no other abnormality of intestinal function or structure. The precise biochemical defect responsible for the absence of enzymatic activity has not been characterized in any primary deficiency state. There may be a complete deletion of the enzyme protein, or there may be an abnormal biologically inactive molecule.

Primary oligodisaccharidase deficiencies

Congenital lactose malabsorption is a rare disorder. There are very few patients with direct biopsy proof of low-intestinal lactase activity. The mode of inheritance has not been clarified. In the literature there are more males than females described with lactase deficiency, and three pairs of siblings also have been reported. Sucrase-isomaltase deficiency is an inherited autosomal-recessive disorder, which is more common than other disaccharidase deficiencies (99). This entity may be due to an abnormal sucrase protein (100). which is quite prevalent among Greenland Eskimos, with an incidence of up to 10% (101). Children with this disease seem to tolerate dextrins because of the low osmotic force of these high-molecular-weight sugars. Trehalase deficiency also has been reported in a patient who had diarrhea after ingestion of mushrooms (102). However, there may be other patients with this alteration who have no symptoms since the intake of trehalose is minimal in the Western diet. Isolated maltase deficiency probably does not exist because of the existence of several brush border enzymes with maltase activity.

Primary intestinal glucose transport alterations

A primary inability to absorb the products of disaccharide hydrolysis also may occur. Glucose-galactose malabsorption is a hereditary autosomal-recessive disorder of actively transported monosaccharides affecting the intestine and kidney tubules. It may result from an abnormality in the membrane-binding sites for these carbohydrates (103). Kinetic analysis of the absorption of glucose has indicated that there is a reduced transport capacity (V_{max}) and a normal affinity for the carbohydrate (K_m). These patients develop diarrhea and glycosuria as soon as milk feedings are begun. On the other hand, fructose is absorbed at normal rates and can, therefore, be utilized to supply carbohydrates in the diet.

Ontogenetic lactase deficiency

The ontogenetic type of carbohydrate malabsorption has been comprehensively studied by Kretchmer (104, 105). This term describes the lactose malabsorption which occurs during the time that lactase activity is normally low. This is seen in both the immediate neonatal period and beyond 3-5 years of age in many ethnic groups. Newborn babies do not absorb lactose well until the first week of life, whereas in premature infants, a normal response to lactose loading is not observed until 2-3 weeks of life (106). Lactose malabsorption in newborn children usually is not associated with diarrhea; however, in preterm infants, there is metabolic acidosis following lactose loading (107). The improvement in the neonatal period is independent of lactose ingestion and may be due to the maturity of the microvilli that is achieved after birth.

The striking regional and ethnic, or racial, incidence of lactose malabsorption usually becomes apparent after 3-5 years of age. Conversely, individuals who are destined to be able to tolerate lactose continue to digest and absorb this carbohydrate throughout life. Several hypotheses attempt to account for changes in the capacity to absorb lactose. The inductive hypothesis correlates lactase deficiency with decreased consumption of milk after weaning (108). The inhibitory proposal emphasizes the capacity of certain sugars and drugs to inhibit lactase activity and hence to decrease lactose tolerance with age. The adaptive theory relates the increased incidence of enteric disease to those groups with nonspecific small-bowel injury and reduced lactase activity. The recent observation that lactase is the target enzyme for enteric rotaviruses fits with this theory (109). In addition, adaptation of the individual to intestinal stress may vary. The dependence of intestinal oligosaccharidases on dietary carbohydrate substrate susceptibility was enhanced during diarrhea induced by hyperosmotic loads (110). Finally, the most widely accepted ontogenetic thesis relates the persistence of lactase activity into adulthood to an adaptive human evolutionary trait of certain ethnic or racial groups (104, 105). The ability of humans to tolerate lactose after age 5 may result from a mutation, since this enzymatic activity normally decreases after weaning in mammals. Persistence of the infantile level of lactase activity throughout adult life is thus the exception and may represent an evolutionary adaptive process which provided selective advantage when humans were first exposed to increased lactose intake. The ability to tolerate lactose was thereafter inherited as a dominant characteristic, which helped in the natural selection process of the lactose digesters in some specific groups, particularly, Anglo-Saxons and some African tribes.

Secondary carbohydrate malabsorption (See also Chap. 14)

Secondary or acquired generalized carbohydrate malabsorption syndromes are associated with a number of intestinal and extraintestinal diseases which produce a
depression of the small intestinal oligosaccharidases from mucosal damage. The
lesions may be expected to affect all the oligosaccharidases as well as alter intestinal glucose transport. At times, they may even interfere with intestinal permeability, leading to impaired fructose transport. Lactose malabsorption is the
most frequent alteration encountered. However, it often may be complicated by
malabsorption of sucrose and other disaccharides, including maltose. When the
alteration is more severe there also may be malabsorption of all monosaccharides including fructose. The most frequent cause of secondary lactose malabsorption is diarrheal disease (111).

Abeta- and/or Hypobetalipoproteinemia
(Bassen-Kornzweig Syndrome)

This disorder of fat absorption is due to an autosomal recessive defect in the formation of very low density lipoprotein (VLDL) and chylomicrons in the absorptive
cell. The primary abnormality appears to be the absence of apolipoprotein B within the enterocyte (112). This causes hypolipidemia, modest steatorrhea, and the
accumulation of triglycerides in the epithelial cells which is evident in the "frosted-
cake" appearance of small bowel biopsies.
    Diarrhea and malabsorption of fat is noted early and the infants are often treated
as gluten-sensitive enteropathy despite their poor response to an exclusion diet.
Irregular erythrocytes with spiny projections, acanthocytes, are noted in half of
the patients, and after 5 years of age degenerative retinal and cerebellar changes
occur. The exact etiology for all three abnormalities is still unclear. The serum
cholesterol is usually less than 80 mg/dl and the plasma triglycerides less than
20 mg/dl. Although the ocular and neurological manifestations are usually irreversible, the other clinical features respond to a low-fat diet with supplemental
medium chain triglycerides (112).

Acrodermatitis Enteropathica

Acrodermatitis enteropathica is a rare autosomal recessive disorder associated
with zinc deficiency, presumably due to a defect in zinc absorption (113). It is
characterized by chronic diarrhea, failure to thrive, dermatitis, and neuropsychi-
atric symptoms. The cutaneous eruption often precedes the diarrhea, and pre-
dominates over the peripheral aspects of the extremities and around the mouth,
anus, and genital areas. It consists of vesicobullous and exzematoid lesions, which
are usually symmetrical and chronically appear hyperkeratotic and psoriatic. Alopecia, conjunctivitis, blepharitis, glossitis, nail abnormalities, and bacterial and
candida infections may be found. Steatorrhea and carbohydrate intolerance occasionally can be demonstrated. It never occurs in purely breast-feeding infants,
and most cases are over 6 months of age.
    Daily, possibly lifetime, oral therapy with zinc compounds is indicated, i.e.,
50 mg zinc sulfate or 150 mg zinc gluconate daily. Serial studies of plasma zinc
levels should be done to individualize the dosage. Some patients never develop
hypozincemia (114). Diiodohydroxyquin is no longer recommended treatment in
view of its potential ophthalmotoxicity.

Congenital Chloridorrhea (Congenital Alkalosis with Diarrhea)

A defect in intestinal absorption of chloride is associated with chronic diarrhea and
is inherited in an autosomal recessive fashion. Usually, the infant is premature,

does not pass meconium, has very watery diarrhea and there is a maternal history of hydramnios (119). The result is a primary diarrheal disorder associated with hypochloremic alkalosis. Sodium absorption is normal; however, intraluminal chloride cannot be exchanged for bicarbonate, resulting in stool chloride losses exceeding 50 m Eq/L and measuring more than the sodium and potassium ions combined. Many of the patients are of Finnish origin. Aggressive therapy maintaining normal fluid and electrolytes results in relatively normal growth and development with few or no complications, such as renal disease which develops in untreated patients. The infant may be given oral supplements of sodium chloride and potassium chloride solutions, roughly in a ratio of 2:1. The amount of potassium ion is increased after the second year of life, i.e., to a ratio of 1:1 (116).

Vitamin B_{12} Malabsorption

This is a rare hereditary disorder which is believed to be due to an impaired transport of vitamin B_{12} within the ileal epithelial cell (117). The onset of the disease is usually after the second year of life and neurologic sequellae are unusual.

Another rare familial disorder is associated with a congenital absence of intrinsic factor. The stomach is normal in structure and function, and antibodies to intrinsic factor are absent.

Folic Acid Malabsorption

This rare absorptive disorder is characterized by an impaired folic acid loading test, low levels of serum folate, and bone marrow maturation arrest (118). Diarrhea and poor weight gain may be associated findings in early infancy. Patients usually respond to large doses of oral folic acid, i.e., 10-100 mg/day, although parenteral administration may be necessary.

REFERENCES

1. D'Sant'Agnese, P.A., and R.C. Talamo: Medical progress: Pathogenesis and physiopathology of cystic fibrosis of the pancreas. N Eng J Med 227:1287, 1343, 1399, 1967.

2. Shwachman, H.: Gastrointestinal manifestations of cystic fibrosis. Pediatr Clin N Amer 22:787-805, 1975.

3. Lebenthal, E., and H. Shwachman: The pancreas—development, adaptation and malfunction in infancy and childhood. Clin Gastroenterol 6:397, 413, 1977.

4. Oppenheimer, E.H., and J.R. Esterly: Hepatic changes in young infants with cystic fibrosis: Possible relation to focal biliary cirrhosis. J Pediatr 86: 6839, 1975.

5. Antonowicz, I., E. Lebenthal, and H. Shwachman: Activities in small intestinal mucosa in patients with cystic fibrosis. J Pediatr 92:214-219, 1978.

6. Shwachman, H., and R.J. Grand: Gastrointestinal Disease. W. B. Saunders Co., Philadelphia, 1973, p. 1206.

7. Shwachman, H., L.K. Diamond, F.A. Oski, and K.T. Khaw: The syndrome of pancreatic insufficiency and bone marrow dysfunction. J Pediatr 65:645, 1964.

8. Shwachman, H., and D. Holsdam: Some clinical observations on the Shwachman syndrome (pancreatic insufficiency and bone marrow hypoplasia). Birth Defects Part XIV. 8:469, 1972.

9. Giedion, A., A. Prader, B. Hadorn, D.H. Shmerling, and S. Auricchio: Metaphysare dysostose und angeborene pankreas insufficizienz. Fortsch Geb Roentgenstr Nuklearmed 108:517, 1968.

10. Hadorn, B., J.B. Tarlow, J.K. Lloyd, and O.H. Wolff: Intestinal enterokinase deficiency. Lancet 1:812-813, 1969.

11. Tarlow, J.B., B. Hadorn, M.W. Arthurton, and J.K. Lloyd: Intestinal enterokinase deficiency: A newly recognized disorder of protein digestion. Arch Dis Child 45:651, 1970.

12. Lebenthal, E., I. Antonowicz, and H. Shwachman: Enterokinase and trypsin activities in pancreatic insufficiency and diseases of the small intestine. Gastroenterology 70:508-512, 1976.

13. Takano, K., T. Suzuki, and K. Yasuda: Immunohistochemical localization of enterokinase in the porcine intestine. Okajimas Folia Anat Jap 48:15, 1971.

14. Gorbach, S.G.: Intestinal microflora. Gastroenterology 60:1110-1129, 1971.

15. Lifshitz, F.: Enteric flora in childhood disease—diarrhea. Am J Clin Nutr 30:1811, 1977.

16. Ament, M.E., S.S. Shimoda, D.R. Saunders, and C.E. Rubin: Pathogenesis of steatorrhea in three cases of small intestinal stasis syndrome. Gastroenterology 63:728-747, 1972.

17. Gracey, M., V. Burke, A. Oshin, J. Barker, and E.F. Glasgow: Bacteria, bile salts, and intestinal monosaccharide malabsorption. Gut 12:683, 1971.

18. Anderson, C.M., M. Gracey, and V. Burke: Coeliac disease. Some still controversial aspects. Arch Dis Child 47:292-298, 1972.

19. Gee, S.: On the celiac affection. St Bartholomew's Hosp Rep 24:17, 1888.

20. Anderson, D.H.: Cystic fibrosis of pancreas and its relation to celiac disease. Am J Dis Child 56:344-399, 1938.

21. Weijers, H.A., J.H. Van de Kamer, and W.K. Dicke: Celiac disease. Adv Pediatr 9:277-318, 1957.

22. Dicke, W.K.: Coeliac disease: Investigation of the harmful effects of certain types of cereal on patients with coeliac disease. Thesis, Univ. of Utrecht. 1950, pp. 1-114.

23. Rubin, C., L.L. Brandborg, A.L. Flick, P. Phelps, C. Parmenter, and S. Vanniel: Studies of celiac sprue. III. The effect of repeated wheat instillation into the proximal ileum of patients on a gluten-free diet. Gastroenterology 43:621, 1962.

24. Lifshitz, F., A.P. Katz, and G.H. Holman: Intestinal disaccharidase deficiencies in gluten-sensitive enteropathy. Am J Dig Dis 10:47-57, 1965.

25. Carswell, F., and A. Ferguson: Food antibodies in serum—a screening test for coeliac disease. Arch Dis Child 47:594, 1972.

26. Rolles, C.J., and A. McNeish: Standardized approach to gluten challenge in diagnosing childhood coeliac disease. Br Med J 1:1309-1311, 1976.

27. Young, W.F., and E.M. Pringle: 110 children with coeliac disease, 1950-1969. Arch Dis Child 46:421, 1971.

28. Hamilton, J.R., M.J. Lynch, and B.J. Reilly: Active coeliac disease in childhood. Clinical and laboratory findings of forty-two cases. Quart J Med 38:135-158, 1969.

29. McNeish, A.S. and M.L.N. Willoughby: Whole-blood folate as a screening test for coeliac disease in childhood. Lancet 1:442-443, 1969.

30. Cook, D.M., N. Evans, A. Lloyd, and J.S. Stewart: Normal serum and red cell folate levels in a child with coeliac disease. Lancet 1:571-572, 1970.

31. Barr, D.G.D., D.H. Shmerling, and A. Prader: Catch-up growth in malnutrition, studied in celiac disease after institution of gluten-free diet. Pediatr Res 6:521-527, 1972.

32. Sheldon, W.: Prognosis in early adult life of coeliac children treated with a gluten-free diet. Br Med J 2:401-404, 1969.

33. Walker-Smith, J.: Transient gluten intolerance. Arch Dis Child 45:523, 1970.

34. McNeish, A.S., C.J. Rolles, and L.J.H. Arthur: Criteria for diagnosis of temporary gluten intolerance. Arch Dis Child 51:275-278, 1976.

35. Shmerling, D.H.: An analysis of controlled relapses in gluten-induced coeliac disease. Acta Paediatr Scand 58:311, 1969.

36. Layrisse, M., N. Blumenfeld, L. Carbonell, J. Desenne, and M. Roche: Intestinal absorption tests and biopsy of the jejunum in subjects with heavy hookworm infection. Am J Trop Med Hyg 13:297, 1964.

37. Manson-Bahr, P.H.: A Report on Researches on Sprue in Ceylon. 1912-1914. Cambridge University Press, London, 1915.

38. Baker, S.J., M. Ignatius, V.I. Mathan, S.K. Vaish, and C.C. Chacko: Intestinal biopsy in tropical sprue. in Intestinal Biopsy, Ciba Foundation Study Group No. 14. G.E.W. Wolstenholme and M.P. Cameron (eds.). Little, Brown and Co., Boston, 1962, p. 84.

39. Lindenbaum, J., A.K.M. Jamiul Alam, and T.H. Kent: Subclinical small-intestinal disease in East Pakistan. Br Med J 2:1616, 1966.

40. Jeejeebhoy, K.N., H.G. Desai, J.M. Noronha, F.P. Anita, and D.V. Parekh: Idiopathic tropical diarrhea with or without steatorrhea. Tropical malabsorption syndrome. Gastroenterology 51:333, 1966.

41. Baker, S.J., V.I. Mathan, and I. Joseph: Epidemic tropical sprue. Am J Dig Dis 7:959, 1962.

42. Sheehy, T.W., G. Baggs, E. Perez-Santiago, and M.H. Floch: Prognosis of tropical sprue. A study of the effect of folic acid on the intestinal aspects of acute and chronic sprue. Ann Intern Med 57:892, 1962.

43. Sheehy, T.W., W.C. Cohen, D.K. Wallace, and L.J. Legters: Tropical sprue in North Americans. JAMA 194:1069, 1965.

44. Klipstein, F.A.: Tropical sprue in New York City. Gastroenterology 47: 457, 1964.

45. Bayless, T.M., A. Rotger-Guardiola, and M.S. Wheby: Tropical sprue: Viral cultures of rectal swabs. Gastroenterology 51:32, 1966.

46. Fagundes-Neto, U., and T. Viaro: Tropical enteropathy and the nutritional status. in Pediatric Nutrition: Infant Feedings - Deficiencies - Diseases. F. Lifshitz (ed.). Marcel Dekker, New York, 1982, p. 438.

47. Brady, P.G., and J.C. Wolfe: Waterborne giardiasis. Ann Intern Med 81, 498-499, 1974.

48. Mahmoud, A.A.F., and K.S. Warren: Algorithm in the diagnosis and management of exotic diseases. II. Giardiasis. J Inf Dis 131:621-624, 1975.

49. Thomson, I.C.R., D.P. Stevens, A.A.F. Mahmoud, and K.S. Warren: Giardiasis in the mouse: An animal model. Gastroenterology 71:57-61, 1976.

50. Rendtorff, R.C.: Experimental transmission of human intestinal protozoan parasites: Giardia lamblia cysts given in capsules. Am J Hyg 59:209, 1954.

51. Wright, J.G., A.M. Tomkins, and D.A. Ridley: Giardiasis: Clinical and therapeutic aspects. Gut 18:343-350, 1977.

52. Kamath, K.R., and R. Murugash: A comparative study of four methods for detecting Giardia lamblia in children with diarrheal disease and malabsorption. Gastroenterology 66:16-21, 1974.

53. Finkelstein, H.: Kuhmilch als Ursache Akuter Ernahrungstoerungen bei Saenglingen. Monatschr Kinderheilkd 4:64, 1905. Quoted by Dees, S.C.: Allergy to cow's milk. Pediatr Clin N Am 6:882, 1959.

54. Von Pirquet, C.: Allergie Munch Med Wochenscher 53:1457, 1906.

55. Iyngkaran, N., and Z. Abidin: Intolerance to food proteins. in Pediatric Nutrition. Infant Feedings - Deficiencies - Diseases. F. Lifshitz (ed.). Marcel Dekker, New York, 1982, p. 449.

56. Gerrard, J.W., J.W.A. Mackenzie, and N. Goluboff et al.: Cow's milk allergy: Prevalence and manifestations in an unselected series of newborns. Acta Paediatr Scand 234 (suppl):1, 1973.

57. Bachman, K.D., and S.C. Dees: Milk allergy I. Observations on incidence and symptoms in "well" babies. Pediatrics 20:393, 1957.

58. Bachman, K.D., and S.C. Dees: Milk allergy II. Observations on incidence and symptoms of allergy to milk in allergic infants. Pediatrics 20:400, 1957.

59. Stintzing, G., and R. Zetterstrom: Cow's milk allergy, incidence and pathogenetic role of early exposure to cow's milk formula. Acta Paediatr Scand 68:383, 1979.

60. Koivikko, A.: IgA deficiency and infantile atopy. Lancet 2: 668, 1973.

61. Lebenthal, E.: Cow's milk protein allergy. Pediatr Clin N Am 22:827, 1975.

62. Eastham, E.J., and W.A. Walker: Effects of cow's milk on the gastrointestinal tract: A persistent dilemma for the pediatrician. Pediatrics 60:477, 1977.

63. Gunther, M., R. Aschaffenburg, R.N. Matthews, W.E. Parish, and R.R.A. Coombs: The level of antibodies to the proteins of cow's milk in the serum of normal human infants. Immunology 3:296, 1960.

64. Renston, R.H., D.G. Maloney, A.L. Jones, G.T. Hradek, K.Y. Wong, and I.D. Goldfine: Bile secretory apparatus: Evidence for a vesicular transport mechanism for proteins in the rat, using horseradish peroxidase and ^{125}I insulin. Gastroenterology 78:1373, 1980.

65. Ashkenazi, A., Z.T. Handzel, D. Idar, M. Ofarim, and S. Levin: An immunologic assay for diagnosis of celiac disease. Lancet 1:627-629, 1978.

66. Worthington, B.S., E.S. Boatman, and G.E. Kenny: Intestinal absorption of intact proteins in normal and protein deficient rats. Am J Clin Nutr 27:276, 1974.

67. Gruskey, F.L., and R.E. Cooke: The gastrointestinal absorption of unaltered protein in normal infants and in infants recovering from diarrhea. Pediatrics 16:763-770, 1955.

68. Freinkel, N.: On the etiology of diabetes mellitus. in Diabetes Mellitus Vol. V. H. Rifkin and P. Raskin (eds.). Robert J. Brady Co., Bowie, MD., 1981, pp. 1-6.

69. Goel, K., F. Lifshitz, E. Kahn, and S. Teichberg: Monosaccharide intolerance and soy protein hypersensitivity in an infant with diarrhea. J Pediatr 93: 617-619, 1978.

70. Iyngkaran, N., K. Davis, M.J. Robinson, C.G. Boey, E. Sumithran, M. Yadav, S.K. Lam, and S.D. Puthucheary: Cow's milk protein sensitive enteropathy: An important contributing cause of secondary sugar intolerance in young infants with acute infective enteritis. Arch Dis Child 54:39, 1979.

71. Goldman, A.S., D.W. Anderson Jr., W.A. Sellers, et al.: Milk allergy. I. Oral challenge with milk and isolated milk proteins in allergic children. Pediatrics 32:455, 1963.

72. Iyngkaran, N., M.J. Robinson, K. Prathap, E. Sumithran, S. Yadav: Cow's milk protein sensitive enteropathy: Combined clinical and histological criteria for diagnosis. Arch Dis Child 53:20, 1978.

73. Iyngkaran, N., Z. Abdin, K. Davis, C.G. Boey, K. Prathap, M. Yadav, S.K. Lam, and S.D. Puthucheary: Acquired carbohydrate intolerance and cow's milk protein sensitive enteropathy in young infants. J Pediatr 95:373, 1979.

74. Powell, G.K.: Milk and soy-induced enterocolitis of infancy. J Pediatr 95: 553–560, 1978.

75. Kuitunen, P., J.K. Visakorpi, and N. Hallman: Histopathology of duodenum mucosa in malabsorption. Syndrome induced by cow's milk. Ann Paediatr 205:54, 1965.

76. Shiner, M., J. Balland, and M.E. Smith: The small intestinal mucosa in cow's milk allergy. Lancet 1:136, 1975.

77. Morin, C.L., J.P. Buts, A. Weber, C.C. Roy, and P. Brochu: One hour blood xylose test in diagnosis of cow's milk protein intolerance. Lancet 1: 1102–1104, 1979.

78. LaRose, C., P. Delorme, M. Richter, and B. Rose: Immunologic studies on milk and egg allergy. J Allergy 33:306, 1962.

79. Johnstone, D.E.: Study of the significance of food antigen precipitins in sera of food sensitive and normal children. Ann Allergy 21:206, 1963.

80. Kuitunen, P., J.K. Visakorpi, E. Savilahti, and P. Pelkonen: Malabsorption syndrome with cow's milk intolerance, clinical findings and course in 54 cases. Arch Dis Child 50:351, 1975.

81. Ford, R.P.K., and D.M. Fergusson: Egg and cow's milk allergy in children. Arch Dis Child 55:608, 1980.

82. Cook, C.D.: Probable gsstrointestinal reaction to soybean. N Engl J Med 262:1076, 1960.

83. Mortimer, E.Z.: Anaphylaxis following ingestion of soybean. J Pediatr 58: 90, 1961.

84. Hill, L.W., and H.C. Stuart: A soy-bean food preparation for feeding infants with milk allergy. JAMA 93:986, 1929.

85. Mendoza, S., and J. Meyers. Soybean sensitivity. Pediatrics 46:771, 1970.

86. Ament, M.E., and C.E. Rubin: Soy protein—another cause of the flat intestinal lesion. Gastroenterology 62:277, 1972.

87. Glaser, J., and D.C. Johnstone: Prophylaxis of allergy in the newborn. JAMA 1953:620, 1953.

88. Eastham, E.J., T. Lichauco, M.I. Grady, and W.A. Walker: Antigenicity of infant formulas: Role of immature intestine on protein permeability. J Pediatr 93:561, 1978.

89. Maizel, H., J.M. Ruffin, and W.O. Dobbins III: Whipple's disease: Review of 19 patients from one hospital and review of literature since 1950. Medicine 49:175, 1970.

90. Trier, J.S., P.C. Phelps, S. Eidelman, and C.E. Rubin: Whipple's disease: Light and electron microscope correlation of jejunal mucosal histology with antibiotic treatment and clinical status. Gastroenterology 48:684, 1965.

91. Sleisenger, M.H., and L.L. Brandborg: Malabsorption, Vol. XIII, in the series, Major Problems in Internal Medicine. L.H. Smith (ed.). W.B. Saunders Co., Philadelphia, 1977, pp. 174-180.

92. Decosse, J.J., R.S. Rhodes, W.B. Wentz, J.W. Reagan, H.J. Dworken, and W.D. Holden: The natural history and management of radiation-induced injury of the gastrointestinal tract. Ann Surg 170, 369-384, 1969.

93. Sleisenger, M.H., and L.L. Brandborg: Malabsorption, Vol. XIII in the series, Major Problems in Internal Medicine. L.H. Smith (ed.). W.B. Saunders Co., Philadelphia, 1977, pp. 209-212.

94. Sleisenger, M.H., and L.L. Brandborg: Malabsorption, Vol. XIII in the series, Major Problems in Internal Medicine. L.H. Smith (ed.). W.B. Saunders Co., Philadelphia, 1977, pp. 249-253.

95. Wapnir, R.A.: Genetic factors in the absorption of protein breakdown products. in Clinical Disorders in Pediatric Gastroenterology and Nutrition. F. Lifshitz (ed.). Marcel Dekker, New York, 1980, pp. 215-228.

96. Neale, G., M. Clark, and B. Levin: Intestinal sucrase deficiency presenting as sucrose intolerance in adult life. Br. Med J 2:1223-1225, 1965.

97. Welsh, J.D.: Isolated lactase deficiency in humans: Report on 100 patients. Medicine 49:257-277, 1970.

98. Phillips, S.F., and D.B. McGill: Glucose-galactose malabsorption in an adult; Perfusion studies of sugar, electrolyte and water transport. Dig Dis 18:1017-1024, 1973.

99. Ament, M.E., D.R. Perera, and L.J. Esther: Sucrease-isomaltase deficiency a frequently misdiagnosed disease. J Pediatr 83:721-727, 1973.

100. Preiser, H., D. Menard, R.K. Crane, and J.J. Cerda: Deletion of enzyme protein from the brush border membrane in sucrase-isomaltase deficiency. Biochim Biophys Acta 363:279-282, 1974.

101. McNair, A., E.G. Hyer, S. Jarnum, and L. Orrid: Sucrose malabsorption in Greenland. Br Med J 2:19-21, 1972.

102. Bergoz, R.: Trehalose malabsorption causing intolerance to mushrooms. Report of a probable case. Gastroenterology 60:909-912, 1963.

103. Elsas, L.J., R.E. Hillman, J.H. Patterson, and L.E. Rosenberg: Renal and intestinal hexose transport in familial glucose-galactose malabsorption. J Clin Invest 49:576-585, 1970.

104. Kretchmer, N.: Lactose and lactase. Sci Am 277:70-78, 1972.

105. Johnson, J.D., N. Kretchmer, and F.J. Simoons: Lactose malabsorption - its biology and history. Adv Pediatr 21:197-237, 1974.

106. Boellner, S.W., A.G. Beard, and T.C. Panos: Impairment of intestinal hydrolysis of lactose in newborn infants. Pediatrics 36:542-550, 1965.

107. Lifshitz, F., S. Diaz-Benussen, V. Martinez-Garza, F. Abdo-Bassols, and E. Diaz del Castillo: The influence of disaccharides on the development of systemic acidosis in the premature infant. Pediatr Res 5:213-235, 1971.

108. Bolin, T.D., and A.E. Davis: Primary lactase deficiency. Genetic or acquired? Am J Dig Dis 15:679-692, 1970.

109. Holmes, I.H., R.D. Schnagi, S. Rodger, B.J. Ruck, I.D. Gust, R.F. Bishop, and G.L. Barnes: Is lactase the receptor and uncoating enzyme for infantile enteritis (rota) viruses? Lancet 1:1387-1388, 1976.

110. Pergolizzi, R., F. Lifshitz, S. Teichberg, and R.A. Wapnir: Interaction between dietary carbohydrates and intestinal disaccharidase in experimental diarrhea. Am J Clin Nutr 30:482-489, 1977.

111. Lifshitz, F., P. Coello-Ramirez, G. Gutierrez-Topete, and M.C. Cornado-Cornet: Carbohydrate intolerance in infants with diarrhea. J Pediatr 79:760, 1971.

112. Gotto, A.M., R.I. Levy, K. John, and D.S. Frederickson: On the protein defect in a-beta lipoproteinemia. N Engl J Med 284:813, 1974.

113. Lombeck, I., H.G. Schnippering, F. Ritzl, et al.: Absorption of zinc in acrodermatitis enteropathica. Lancet 7:855, 1975.

114. Krieger, I., and G.W. Evans: Acrodermatitis enteropathica without hypozincemia: Therapeutic effect of a pancreatic enzyme preparation due to a zinc-binding ligand. J Pediatr 96:32, 1980.

115. Lanniala, K., J. Perheentupa, A. Pasternack, and N. Hallimans: Familial chloride diarrhea-chloride malabsorption. Mod Probl Paediat 11:137, 1968.

116. Norio, R., J. Perheentupa, K. Lanniala, et al.: Congenital chloride diarrhea, an autosomal recessive disease. Genetic study of 14 Finnish and 12 other families. Clin Genet 2:182, 1971.

117. Mackenzie, J.L., R. Donaldson, J.S. Trier, et al.: Ileal mucosa in familial selective vitamins B_{12} malabsorption. N Engl J Med 286:1021, 1972.

118. Lanzkowsky, P.: Congenital malabsorption of folate. Am J Med 48:580, 1970.

16

INFLAMMATORY BOWEL DISEASE

Fredric Daum, M. D. and Harvey Aiges, M. D.

INTRODUCTION

Of all the organic noninfectious chronic gastrointestinal disorders seen by the pediatric gastroenterologist, the idiopathic chronic inflammatory intestinal diseases, nonspecific ulcerative colitis and Crohn disease, are by far the most common and perplexing. Despite the endemic nature of these illnesses, especially Crohn disease, little is known about their underlying causes and pathophysiology. Controversy also flourishes with regard to pharmacological treatment, operative indications, and the specific nature of the surgical intervention.

Historically, simple ulcerative colitis first appeared in the medical literature in 1875 (1) and Helmholtz was the first to describe ulcerative colitis in children in 1923 (2). Chronic ileitis was described in less precise terms in the 1700s, but it was Crohn, Ginsberg, and Oppenheimer who first described patients in 1932 with terminal ileitis in clinical and pathological terms as we understand them today (3, 4). Two years later, after three patients were reported who had only jejunal involvement, it was suggested that a more applicable term would be regional enteritis. At about the same time it was noted that the right colon also might be involved. It was not until 1960 that an attempt was made to distinguish Crohn disease of the colon from inflammation due to ulcerative colitis (5, 6). It is now appreciated that Crohn disease may involve the entire alimentary tract from esophagus to anus.

EPIDEMIOLOGY AND PATHOGENESIS

Recently, the first pediatric epidemiologic study was made that focused specifically on 105 families of children with inflammatory bowel disease (IBD) compared to those of a control population (7). The results of this study indicate there is an increased incidence of ulcerative colitis and Crohn disease in families of higher socioeconomic status and a high incidence of inflammatory bowel disease among Jewish children (62%) as compared with other ethnic groups. There was also a 25% incidence of IBD among first- and second-degree relatives of these patients, a higher incidence than has been reported in studies in families of adult patients with IBD (10-14%) (8, 9). Finally, no correlation with birth order, place of residence, or level of parental education was noted.

The discovery of a genetic marker for inflammatory bowel disease unfortunately has eluded investigators. The distribution of the ABO blood groups does not differ from expectations in ulcerative colitis or Crohn disease, nor has the correlation between either disease and a particular histocompatibility locus antigen (HLA) been noted. However, ankylosing spondylitis, a familial disorder associated with the HLA-B27 in 80-90% of the cases, occurs with increased frequency in patients with IBD. These patients will have an incidence of HLA-B27 positivity similar to those with ankylosing spondylitis alone.

Currently, there is neither evidence to demonstrate that children with IBD have psychological profiles different from those of control subjects, nor do they appear to experience unique psychological precipitating factors before the onset of illness.

Several etiologies for IBD have been proposed, and these have been recently summarized in a comprehensive review (10). Included are immunologic factors, infectious agents, psychosomatic factors, food allergies, vascular disturbances, and recently, prostaglandins as mediator of intestinal inflammation.

The role of immune mechanisms in tissue injury causing host susceptibility, or as mediators for other etiological factors has been studied extensively. Unfortunately, no conclusions are apparent in terms of tissue damage. Circulating anti-colon antibodies have been found in these patients, but they are nonspecific, bear no relationship to disease activity, and have never been recorded to cause any cytopathogenic effects in tissue culture. Circulating immune complexes have not been demonstrated regardless of the activity of the disease or the type of extraintestinal complications. IgE-mediated hypersensitivity reactions have been studied with conflicting results. The therapeutic use of cromolyn sodium (disodium cromoglycate) has only anecdotal support. Finally, studies of lymphocyte-mediated reactions, including T cell toxicity and K cell activity, have not been revealing.

In terms of susceptibility, depressed cell-mediated immunity, particularly in Crohn disease, has been demonstrated by a number of investigators. The findings are believed to be secondary abnormalities. An IgA deficiency has been found in ulcerative colitis patients with a frequency greater than expected for a normal population. The significance of this association has yet to be determined.

Although enteric bacterial flora, viruses, and mycobacteria all have been implicated in the etiology of inflammatory bowel disease, data are conflicting, and efforts continue to further elucidate the role of these agents. A recent flurry of interest in ultrafiltrable agents was unable to conclude what type of transmissible agent was involved, if any.

Knowledge of the psychosomatic aspects of inflammatory bowel disease remains limited and is predicated on either anecdotal or uncontrolled studies. Currently, it is doubtful that the inflammatory process itself is the result of stress alone or specific predisposing personality traits. Many authors claim that the "typical" child is passive and dependent with an above-average intelligence. However, it is generally accepted that symptoms such as abdominal pain, diarrhea, and anorexia are often exacerbated by psychosocial factors.

The effects of diet in the etiology and pathophysiology of inflammatory bowel disease also remain uncertain. To date, there are no conclusive data to implicate cow's milk protein or any of the other traditional dietary foodstuffs. Lactose intolerance is probably a secondary phenomenon. However, the association of inflammatory bowel disease and the relatively recent addition of food additives to our diet remains an interesting hypothesis because the increased incidence of Crohn disease corresponds with the more prevalent use of these substances by the food industry.

Finally, recent gastrointestinal literature has been replete with studies suggesting that prostaglandins may be important in the pathogenesis of ulcerative colitis. Increased concentrations of these endogenous hormones have been noted in the stool, urine, and colonic venous blood of adults with ulcerative colitis (11).

Sulfasalazine (salicylazosulfapyridine) has been noted to inhibit the in vitro synthesis of prostaglandin E by rectal mucosa (12).

CLINICAL FEATURES (Table 1)

The clinical aspects of IBD in children have been exhaustively reviewed (13-15).

Approximately 50% of patients with IBD have symptoms at age 10 years or less. Of those with Crohn disease, about 30% will have only ileal disease, 55% ileal and colonic involvement, and about 15% pathology confined to the colon. Therefore, 85% of these children will have involvement of the ileum. Symptoms in ulcerative colitis and in Crohn disease are similar and, on an individual basis, often do not distinguish one entity from the other. Abdominal pain is the most common complaint and often awakens the patient from sleep. It is crampy, usually in the lower abdomen, and is often associated with fecal urgency. Diarrhea is the next most frequent symptom. It often is associated with gross or occult blood, pus, and mucus in the stools. Blood per rectum is more commonly seen with ulcerative colitis because the mucosa is primarily involved. Other common manifestations of inflammatory bowel disease are anorexia, weight loss, and low-grade fever. About 10% of the children with IBD will have significant anemia with hematocrits of less than 30%. Even without obvious blood loss, the erythrocytes appear hypochromic and microcytic, suggestive of iron deficiency. However, the iron-binding capacity is usually normal or low, and iron often is present in the bone marrow. This suggests that iron is deposited in the reticuloendothelial system and is not being used for normal red blood cell production. Abnormalities of peripheral red blood cells suggestive of folate or vitamin B_{12} deficiency are quite uncommon (16). Ten to 50% of patients with Crohn disease will have significant hypoalbuminemia with less than 3 g% of serum albumin. In comparison, about 30% of patients with ulcerative colitis will have significantly abnormal serum albumin concentrations. Commonly, these patients have pitting edema of the lower extremities. Growth and sexual retardation are not uncommon and have been described in 20-30% of the patients with inflammatory bowel disease, particularly Crohn disease (17). It is noteworthy that approximately 10% of the patients with Crohn disease may appear to have "acute appendicitis" when they first develop symptomatology. This is a feature of acute ileitis which has been well described in adults with Crohn disease (18, 19), where about half of these patients develop clinical features of chronic disease at a later date. Colonic carcinoma is a feared complication of ulcerative colitis (20-22), but is an uncommon problem even in the busiest pediatric

TABLE 1   Clinical Features of Inflammatory Bowel Disease

Symptoms or Signs	Percent of Patients
Abdominal pain, diarrhea, guaiac (+) stools	70-80
Anorexia, weight loss, fever	70-80
Anemia	10
Edema (hypoalbuminemia)	10-50
Growth and sexual retardation	20-30
Pseudo-appendicitis	10
Carcinoma	0

(Reprinted with permission, Ref. 13.)

gastrointestinal services. The child who develops the disease before the age of 10 years   and has universal colitis appears to be at greatest risk. The problem does not usually surface until the second decade of the disease.

Extraintestinal manifestations are a considerable problem for children with IBD. Of the 60 cases of extraintestinal disease recorded in one series, 55 were associated with Crohn disease and only five with ulcerative colitis (Table 2). Fifty percent of children with Crohn disease will have perianal lesions including fistulas, abscesses or fissures with involvement of either the small or large bowel or both. Perianal fistulas do not appear to arise from direct communication with the bowel but rather from the anal crypts (23). Twenty percent have either arthralgia or arthritis involving knees, ankles, and elbows (24, 25) which may be indistinguishable from rheumatoid arthritis. Arthropathy may be the presenting manifestation with abdominal complaints occurring at a later date. Atypical initial presentations of Crohn disease with minimal to absent gastrointestinal complaints include arthritis, growth failure, fever of unknown origin, and chronic anemia. Rashes are seen in about 7% of the patients with erythema nodosum being most common. Pyoderma gangrenosum may be seen with either Crohn disease or ulcerative colitis, but is extremely uncommon. Mouth sores occur in approximately 7% of the patients (26). Except for the fact that these sores are painless, they are indistinguishable from the lesions of aphthous stomatitis. Nephrolithiasis occurs in 1-2% of cases and is associated with severe diarrhea or more commonly in patients with an ileostomy. In situations where significant ileal resection have occurred, calcium oxalate stones are common.

Uveitis is a complication of inflammatory bowel disease in children which, until recently, had not been well appreciated. In one study, a 30% incidence of subclinical uveitis in children with Crohn disease was demonstrated (27). In those children with ulcerative colitis, no uveitis was noted. However, acute symptomatic uveitis would appear to be quite uncommon in this age group. Vascular lesions are uncommon in children with inflammatory bowel disease, but phlebitis and cutaneous polyarteritis nodosa have been associated with Crohn disease (28). Hepatobiliary disease including chronic active hepatitis, sclerosing cholangitis, and cholelithiasis (29) have been reported occasionally and actually may precede the onset of overt intestinal disease. Ankylosing spondylitis is very uncommon in children.

TABLE 2   Extraintestinal Manifestations of Inflammatory Bowel Disease

Manifestation	Percent of Patients
Perianal disease	30
Joints: arthralgia or arthritis	20
Rashes	7
Mouth sores	7
Uveitis	7
Episcleritis	7
Phlebitis	1
Hepatobiliary disease	1
Ankylosing spondylitis	1

(Reprinted with permission, Ref. 13.)

DIAGNOSIS

The evaluation of IBD (Table 3) requires a thorough history and a comprehensive physical examination with special attention paid to the perianal area. A CBC and reticulocyte count may demonstrate an anemia and indicate whether or not there has been blood loss. The erythrocyte sedimentation rate would appear to be a variable but sometimes useful laboratory test. If elevated, one would think more of IBD rather than an irritable bowel syndrome in which the laboratory data are all normal. However, children with fulminant colitis often have normal erythrocyte sedimentation rates (15). Routine stool cultures and examinations for ova and parasites should be obtained to determine if there is a primary or superimposed enteric infection. Specific requests for stool cultures for <u>Yersinia enterocoletica</u> and <u>Campylobacter fetus</u> subspecies must be made as both may result in illness indistinguishable from IBD. A low serum albumin suggests that protein loss may be occurring from the inflamed mucosa, while a low serum cholesterol usually reflects loss of bile salts in the feces in the presence of significant ileal disease. The serum magnesium concentration also may be diminished if there is enteric protein loss and/or steatorrhea. An initial low serum folate suggests that the proximal small bowel may be involved while a low serum vitamin B_{12} concentration indicates widespread ileal involvement.

Barium studies are an intrinsic part of the evaluation (Figs. 1a, b), but certain pitfalls should be appreciated. In ulcerative colitis, in which only the colon is involved by definition, the initial barium enema may be normal in 25% of the children with active disease. In children with Crohn disease, the barium enema will be normal 50% of the time (30-32). Since the ileum is abnormal in 85% of children with Crohn disease, one must do a small-bowel series for a proper evaluation. In ulcerative colitis, the rectum is almost always abnormal by proctosigmoidoscopy or rectal biopsy or both. Ileal abnormalities in ulcerative colitis are due to "backwash"; these changes are rare and involve only the distal 5-10 cm of the ileum. However, it has been less clear as to how often the rectum is abnormal in Crohn disease. A biopsy (Figs 2a, b) should be done in all patients at the time of sigmoidoscopy or with a Rubin suction tube in a patient who refuses endoscopy. Proctosigmoidoscopy and biopsy are essential features of the diagnostic evaluation for

TABLE 3   Evaluation of Inflammatory Bowel Disease

History
Physical examination
CBC, sedimentation rate, reticulocyte count
Stool: culture and sensitivity, ova/parasites
Serum chemistry (albumin, cholesterol, magnesium, liver function tests)
Serum folate, vitamin B_{12}
Barium enema, small-bowel series, intravenous pyelogram
Proctosigmoidoscopy, rectal biopsy
?   Colonoscopy
Ophthalmologic examination
Growth velocity, Tanner stage, bone age
72-hr fecal fat
?   Serum and urine zinc, serum 25-hydroxyvitamin D

(Reprinted with permission, Ref. 13.)

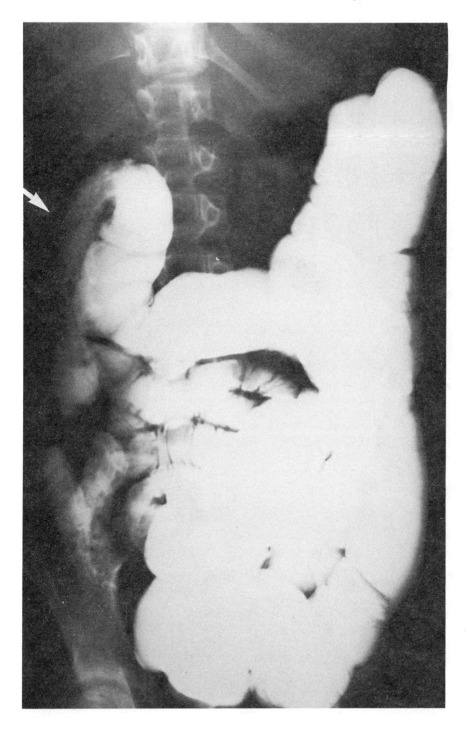

FIGURE 1a   Barium enema consistent with Crohn colitis. Deep ulcerations and
multiple filling defects indicative of inflammatory pseudopolyps are noted in the
cecum and ascending colon while the transverse colon and left colon are normal
(arrow notes diseased right colon).

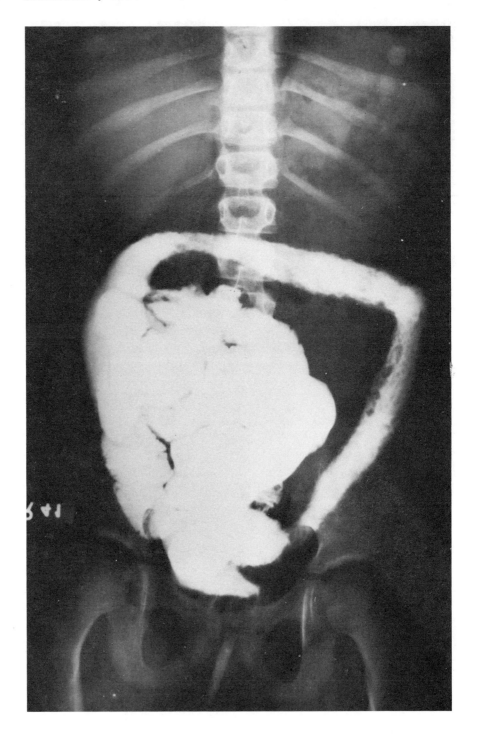

FIGURE 1b   Barium enema reveals universal mucosal colitis with loss of haustral markings, foreshortening of the colon, and fine spicules indicative of superficial ulceration.

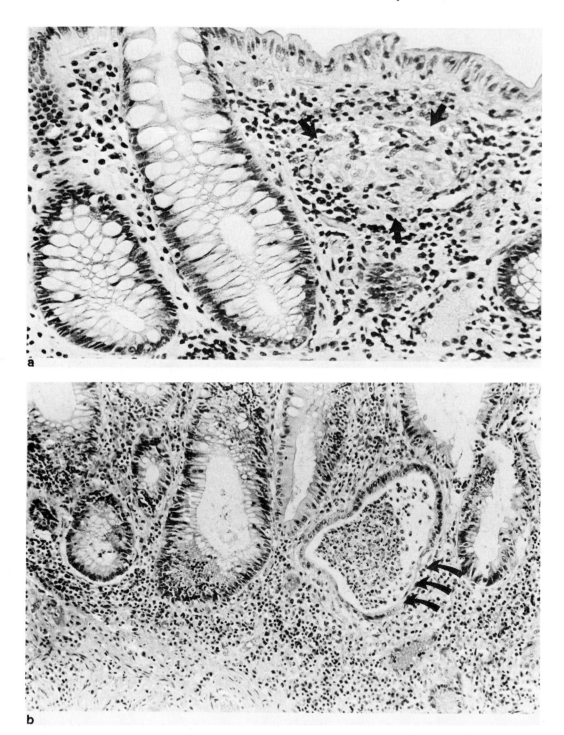

FIGURE 2   Rectal mucosa showing (a) crypt abscess (arrows pointing to lumen) with destruction of the crypt epithelium by segmented leukocytes, and (b) granuloma of Crohn disease composed of epithelial cells (arrows); hematoxylin-eosin stains.   Original magnifications a x 121, b x 900.

Crohn disease. These procedures will reveal pathology in 50% of patients with a normal colon on x-ray. The indications for colonoscopy in the child with IBD are controversial. Colonoscopy should be performed when IBD is suspected, but the diagnostic evaluation is equivocal. Colonoscopy also serves to help the surgeon define the areas before bowel surgery for IBD. An ophthalmologic evaluation including slit-lamp examination for subclinical uveitis is also indicated. Growth velocity curves, Tanner staging for sexual maturation (33), and a bone age are all useful in assessing the patient's growth and development and potential for future maturation. An abnormal 72-hour fecal fat study may suggest extensive small-bowel disease when all other studies have proved normal, and also may indicate the possible etiology, i.e., steatorrhea, for growth failure.

There is an increasing interest in mineral metabolism in IBD and its possible relationship to growth disturbance. In a recent study of zinc metabolism in children with IBD (34), the conclusions were that: (1) hypozincemia is frequent among patients with Crohn disease; (2) hypozincemia is more likely to occur with Crohn disease and short stature, weight deficit, and retarded sexual development; (3) however, not all patients with Crohn disease and retardation of growth and development have low serum or body zinc levels; and (4) there were no abnormalities of taste acuity in patients with hypozincemia.

MANAGEMENT

The pharmacological treatment of IBD is still geared primarily toward alleviation of symptoms and signs since there are no known curative agents.

In ulcerative colitis, it has been clearly shown that sulfasalazine is effective in the treatment of mild active colitis. This drug significantly diminishes the frequency of relapse in all cases (35, 36). The dose for acute disease is arbitrary but varies between 50-70 mg/kg/day. In a recent study in adults, only 2 g/day were required to prevent relapse, about half the dosage for acute disease (37). Side effects including headache, nausea, anorexia, and rashes are common with dosages exceeding 3 g/day. The patient receiving sulfasalazine should receive folate as the former interferes with the absorption of folate and may also lead to hemolysis with an increase in red cell turnover (38).

Little, if any, data are available to indicate whether sulfasalazine should be used in a patient with acute Crohn disease. Since it is metabolized to its active components, sulfapyridine and 5-aminosalicylic acid, by bacteria in the distal small bowel and colon, children with active colonic disease may respond more favorably to this drug. However, according to the National Collaborative Study, the drug would appear to be of little or no value in decreasing the incidence of relapses in adults with Crohn disease (39). High-dose, short-term, daily steroids are used to treat acute symptoms in children with both illnesses. Prednisone is commonly used in a dose of 1-2 mg/kg for 10-14 days and then tapered slowly by 2.5 mg every 3-4 days. Recently, there have been some data to suggest that day, low-dose steroids may be helpful in maintaining remission in teenagers with Crohn disease without interfering with their growth pattern (Figs. 3a, b) (40). Azathioprine and 6-mercaptopurine have been used in patients with Crohn disease with variable results. The National Collaborative Study has suggested that azathioprine used during a 4-month period was of no value in Crohn disease (39). However, in a recent report, 6-mercaptopurine used in a double-blind, cross-over control study for 1 year, or more, allowed steroid sparing in the patient previously steroid dependent (41). Anticholinergic drugs may be used to alleviate cramps and diarrhea. They should be used with caution since they may precipitate toxic megacolon. Loperamide, a relatively new drug, has alleviated diarrhea in adults with IBD but has

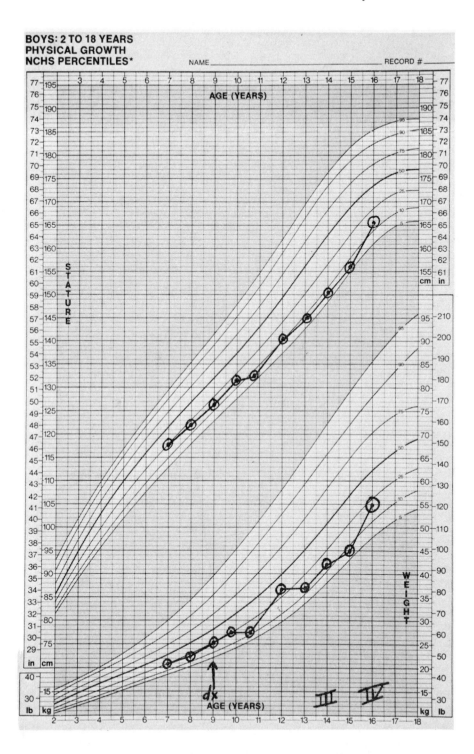

FIGURE 3a   Represents linear height and weight growth curves of a 16-year-old
male with Crohn ileocolitis showing a normal growth pattern between ages 14 and
16 despite continuous alternate day, low-dose prednisone (10-15 mg).

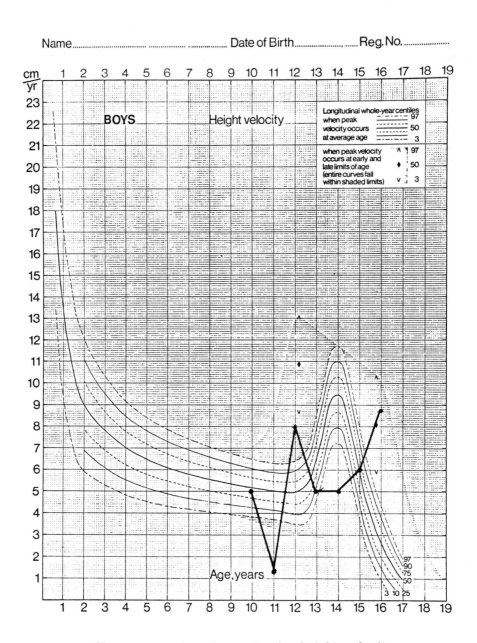

FIGURE 3b   Same patient demonstrating height-velocity curve.

not been evaluated in children under the age of 12.   Recently, motility studies have suggested that diarrhea and urgency in adult patients with ulcerative colitis is associated with an increase in colonic fast activity (42).   Elemental diets (43) and total parenteral nutrition (44) may be used alone or concomitantly to improve the nutritional status of children with IBD.   The elemental diets are costly and relatively unpalatable.   The latter is a major compliance problem in younger children. There is evidence to indicate that in Crohn disease parenteral nutrition may bring about clinical and radiographic remission by placing the bowel at relative rest (45, 46).   Total parenteral feeding may help in reversing growth arrest in patients with Crohn disease (44).   However, the salutory effect of all these therapies often appears to be temporary as most patients will eventually relapse.

Surgical intervention may be necessary because of acute catastrophic events including massive gastrointestinal bleeding, perforation, abscess, and toxic megacolon.   Steroid dependence, and growth and sexual retardation are the most common reasons for elective resection.   Surgery performed in these patients, if they have reached Tanner stage V, usually will not result in a significant "catch-up" growth (47).

The issue as to if and when to operate as prophylaxis against colonic carcinoma still remains unsettled.   Actuarial retrospective data from a select population of patients indicate that after having had ulcerative colitis for 10 years or more one is at a much higher risk for colonic carcinoma (20).   This would appear to be particularly true in the patients with universal colitis with onset in the first decade of life (48).

Surgical approaches in ulcerative colitis depend on the patient's medical status and usually consist of a subtotal colectomy with ileostomy and sigmoid mucous fistula at initial operation.   Subsequently, patients have undergone ileorectal anastomosis (49) or removal of the rectal stump with or without revision of the ileostomy.   The Kock procedure (Fig. 4), which provides a continent reservoir ileostomy beneath the abdominal wall, results in a permanent ileostomy which may be more acceptable cosmetically (50).   In ulcerative colitis, a total colectomy with either a traditional ileostomy or a Kock procedure is curative.   A subtotal colectomy, a rectal mucosectomy, and an ileal pull-through with an ileoanal anastomosis may provide another alternative surgical procedure in patients with ulcerative colitis (51).   Patients usually complain of postoperative urgency and frequent bowel movements.   A recent modification produces a distal pouch or reservoir and may obviate the bothersome sequellae (52) (Fig. 5).

The recurrence rate in patients with Crohn disease who have undergone surgery approaches 95%; and therefore, surgery is usually considered only as a palliative alternative to medical therapy.   However, acute indications for surgery in Crohn disease include abscess formation, intestinal obstruction, free perforation, and massive gastrointestinal bleeding.   Elective indications include steroid dependence, growth and sexual retardation, and the presence of an abdominal mass which may be an abscess or the result of intraabdominal fistula formation.   A diverting ileostomy is an effective means of decreasing perianal complications when medical therapy has failed.   When resection of the small bowel is warranted, it should be of a limited nature to avoid creating a short-bowel syndrome.

PROGNOSIS

ULCERATIVE COLITIS

The prognosis for patients who develop ulcerative colitis during childhood remains guarded.   Although many children are able to live relatively normal lives while receiving medical therapy, others have frequent relapses or incapacitating symptoms often requiring multiple hospitalizations.   The course of their disease results in

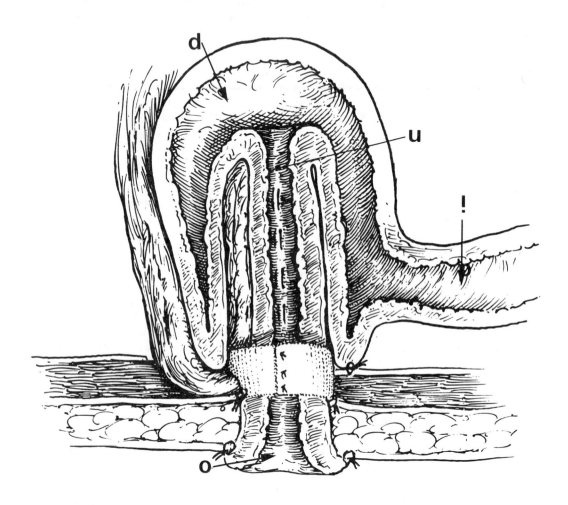

FIGURE 4   Continent ileostomy (Kock procedure) demonstrating the final position of the reservoir and the nipple-valve: (O) ostomy orifice; (P) pouch; (n) nipple-valve; and (i) distal ileum. (From ref. 50. Reprinted with permission.)

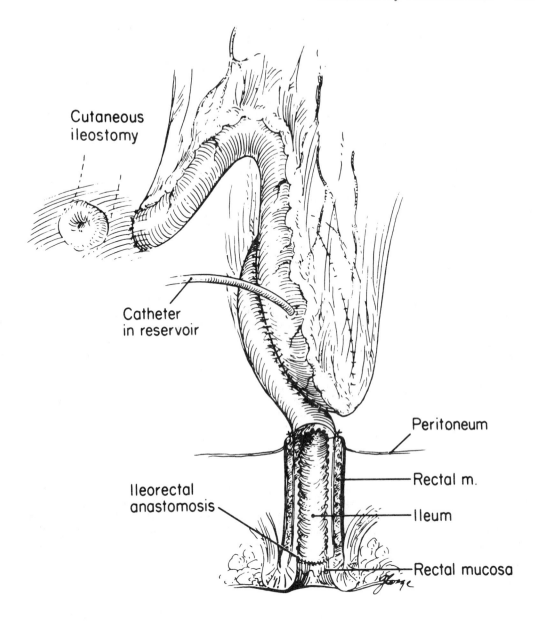

FIGURE 5   Ileal pull-through with ileoanal anastomosis and distal reservoir modification. (From ref. 52. Reprinted with permission.)

frequent absences from school and often retardation not only in their physical growth but also in their psychosocial growth and development. Moreover, the risk of adenocarcinoma of the colon, which has been noted to occur in approximately 3-5% of patients during the first 10 years of their disease, increased to 25% during the next decade and to 50% after the patient has had disease for 20 years. Adenocarcinoma of the colon associated with ulcerative colitis is a virulent lesion with early metastasis. The prognosis for a 5-year survival once the lesion has been diagnosed is less than 25%. It is still unclear as to which diagnostic studies should be performed in patients with chronic ulcerative colitis who are at high risk for developing adenocarcinoma of the colon after the first decade of illness. The absence of clinical activity does not appear to protect the patient. Presently, proctosigmoidoscopy, multiple rectal biopsies, colonic cytological washings, barium enema, and colonoscopy in one combination or another all have been suggested as diagnostic studies in these patients. It is important that both the patient and the family be educated, keeping in mind that panproctocolectomy with permanent ileostomy is a curative procedure.

CROHN DISEASE

Although the mortality of Crohn disease appears to be less than in ulcerative colitis, morbidity is significant. Patients with Crohn disease may have a chronic, indolent, unremitting course with frequent acute exacerbations of their symptoms. Complications such as growth failure, sexual retardation, abscess formation, fistulization, and malabsorption are common. Although surgical intervention may improve a patient's quality of life, the recurrence rate in this disease following surgery approaches 95% over a 10-year period. Evidence of recurrence may occur as soon as 2-4 weeks after corrective surgery—usually involving the region of the new anastomotic sites.

SUMMARY

Both ulcerative colitis and Crohn disease are chronic illnesses with periods of clinical remission and exacerbation. The two diseases share many similarities, but long-term management and prognosis may be different. However, neither illness has specifically unique features, and distinguishing between them requires careful consideration of the clinical presentation, histopathology, and radiographic data.

REFERENCES

1.   Wilkes, S., and W. Moxon: Lectures on Pathological Anatomy, 2nd ed. J & A Churchill, London, 1875.

2.   Helmholtz, H. F.: Chronic ulcerative colitis in childhood. Am J Dis Child 26:418, 1923.

3.   Crohn, B. B., L. Ginsburg, and G. D. Oppenheimer: Regional ileitis. JAMA 99:1323, 1932.

4.   Crohn, B. B., and H. D. Janowitz: Reflections on regional enteritis twenty years later. JAMA 156:1221, 1965.

5.   Lockhart-Mummery, H., and B. Morson: Crohn's disease of the large intestine and its distinction for ulcerative colitis. Gut 1:87, 1960.

6.   Lockhart-Mummery, H. E. , and B. C. Morson: Crohn's disease of the large intestine. Gut 5:493, 1964.

7.   Aiges, H. W. , J. Portnoy, F. Daum, et al. : Families of adolescents with inflammatory bowel disease: A demographic analysis. Pediatr Res 12:364, 1978.

8.   Kirsner, J. B. , and J. A. Spencer: Family occurrences of ulcerative colitis, regional enteritis, and ileocolitis. Ann Intern Med 59:133, 1963.

9.   Monk, M. , A. I. Mendeloff, C. I. Siegel, et al. : An epidemiological study of ulcerative colitis and regional enteritis among adults in Baltimore. Gastroenterology 56:847, 1969.

10. Sachar, D. G. , M. O. Auslander, and J. S. Walfish: Aetiological theories of inflammatory bowel disease. in Clinics in Gastroenterology, Vol. 9. R. G. Farmer (ed.). W. B. Saunders Co. , London, 1980, pp. 231-257.

11. Gould, S. R. , A. R. Brach, and M. E. Conolly: Increased prostaglandin production in ulcerative colitis. (letter), Lancet 2:98, 1977.

12. Sharon, P. , M. Ligunsky, D. Rachmilewitz, et al. : Role of prostaglandins in ulcerative colitis. Enhanced production during active disease and inhibition by sulfasalazine. Gastroenterology 75:638, 1978.

13. Daum, F. , and H. W. Aiges: Inflammatory bowel disease in children. in Clinical Disorders in Pediatric Gastroenterology and Nutrition. F. Lifshitz (ed.). Marcel Dekker, New York, 1980, pp. 145-157.

14. Hamilton, J. P. , G. A. Bruce, M. Abdourhamen, et al. : Inflammatory bowel disease in children and adolescents. in Advances in Pediatrics, Vol. 26. L. Bainess (ed.). Year Book Medical Publishers, Inc. , Chicago, 1979, pp. 311-341.

15. Werlin, S. L. , and R. J. Grand: Severe colitis in children and adolescents. Gastroenterology 73:828, 1977.

16. Steinberg, F. : The megaloblastic anemia of regional enteritis. N Engl J Med 264:186, 1961.

17. McCaffrey, T. D. , K. Nasor, A. M. Lawrence, et al. : Severe growth retardation in children with inflammatory bowel disease. Pediatrics 45:386, 1976.

18. Essen, S. W. B. , J. Anderson, J. M. D. Galloway, et al. : Crohn's disease initially confined to the appendix. Gastroenterology 60:853, 1971.

19. Hollings, R. M. : Crohn's disease of the appendix. Med J Aust 1:639, 1969.

20. Devroede, G. J. , W. F. Taylor, W. G. Saver, et al. : Cancer risk and life expectancy of children with ulcerative colitis. N Engl J Med 285:17, 1971.

21. Farmer, R. G. , W. A. Hawk, and R. B. Turnbull: Carcinoma associated with mucosal ulcerative colitis and with transmural colitis and enteritis. Cancer 28:289, 1971.

22.   Weedon, D. D. , R. G. Shorter, D. M. Ilstrup, et al. : Crohn's disease and
       cancer. N Engl J Med 289:1099, 1973.

23.   Lockhart-Mummery, H. E. : Anal lesion of Crohn's disease.   Clin Gastroen-
       terol 1:377, 1972.

24.   Wright, R. , K. Lumsdern, M.H. Lunt, et al.: Abnormalities of the sacroili-
       ac joints and uveitis in ulcerative colitis. Quart J Med 34:229, 1965.

25.   Brewerton, D. A. , M. Caffrey, A. Nicholls, et al. : HL-AB27 and arthropa-
       thies associated with ulcerative colitis and psoriasis.   Lancet 1:956, 1974.

26.   Dudeney, T. P. : Crohn's disease of the mouth.   Proc R Soc Med 62:1237,
       1969.

27.   Daum, F. , H. B. Gould, D. Gold, et al. : Asymptomatic transient uveitis in
       children with inflammatory bowel disease. Am J Dis Child 133:170, 1979.

28.   Kahn, E. I. , F. Daum, H. W. Aiges, et al. : Cutaneous polyarteritis nodosa
       associated with Crohn's disease. Dis Colon Rectum 23:258, 1980.

29.   Cohen, S. , M. Daplan, L. Gotleib, et al. : Liver disease and gallstones in
       regional enteritis. Gastroenterology 60:237, 1971.

30.   Gutman, F. M. : Granulomatous enterocolitis in children and adolescents. J
       Pediatr Surg 9:115, 1974.

31.   Ehrenpreis, T. H. , J. Geirup, and R. Lagercrantz: Chronic regional entero-
       colitis in children and adolescents. Acta Pediatr Scand 60:209, 1971.

32.   Miller, R. C. , and E. Larsen: Regional enteritis in infancy.   Am J Dis Child
       122:301, 1971.

33.   Tanner, J. M. , and R. H. Whitehouse: Clinical longitudinal studies for height,
       weight, height velocity, weight velocity, and stages of puberty.   Arch Dis
       Child 51:170, 1976.

34.   Nishi, Y. , F. Lifshitz, M. A. Bayne, et al. : Zinc status and its relation to
       growth retardation in children with chronic inflammatory bowel disease. Am
       J Clin Nutr 33:2613, 1980.

35.   Dick, A. P. , M. J. Grayson, R. G. Carpenter, et al. : Controlled trial of sul-
       phasalazine in treatment of ulcerative colitis.   Gut 5:437, 1964.

36.   Lennard-Jones, J. E. , A.M. Connell, J.H. Baron, et al.: Controlled trial of
       sulphasalazine in maintenance therapy for ulcerative colitis.   Lancet 1:185,
       1965.

37.   Dissanayake, A. , and S. Truelove: A controlled therapeutic trial of long term
       maintenance treatment of ulcerative colitis with sulphasalazine. Gut 14:923,
       1973.

38.   Pounder, R. E. , E. R. Craven, J. S. Henthorn, et al. : Red cell abnormalities
       associated with sulphasalazine maintenance therapy for ulcerative colitis. Gut
       16:181, 1975.

39.   Summers, R. W. , D. M. Switz, J. T. Sessions, et al. : National Cooperative Crohn's Disease Study: Results of drug treatment. Gastroenterology 77:847, 1979.

40.   Whittington, P. F. , H. V. Barnes, and T. M. Bayless. Medical management of Crohn's disease in adolescence. Gastroenterology 72:1338, 1977.

41.   Present, D. H. , B. I. Korelitz, B. Wisch, et al. : Treatment of Crohn's disease with 6-mercaptopurine. N Engl J Med 302:981, 1980.

42.   Schnape, W. J. , S. A. Matarazzo, and S. Cohen: Abnormal colonic myoelectric and motor responses to eating in ulcerative colitis. Gastroenterology 74:1097, 1978.

43.   Morin, C. L. , M. Roulet, C. C. Roy, et al. : Continuous elemental enteral alimentation in children with Crohn's disease and growth failure. Gastroenterology 79:1205, 1980.

44.   Kelts, D. G. , R. J. Grand, G. Shen, et al. : Nutritional basis of growth failure in children and adolescents with Crohn's disease. Gastroenterology 76:720, 1979.

45.   Fischer, J. E. , C. S. Foster, R. M. Abel, et al. : Hyperalimentation as primary therapy for inflammatory bowel disease. Am J Surg 125:165, 1973.

46.   Vogel, C. , T. Corwin, and A. Bave: Intravenous hyperalimentation in the treatment of inflammatory disease of the bowel. Arch Surg 108:460, 1974.

47.   Homer, D. R. , R. J. Grand, and A. H. Colodny: Growth, course and prognosis after surgery for Crohn's disease in children and adolescents. Pediatrics 59:717, 1977.

48.   Nugent, F. W. , M. C. Vendenheimer, S. Zuberi, et al. : Clinical course of ulcerative proctosigmoiditis. Am J Dig Dis 15:321, 1970.

49.   Aylett, S. O. : Three-Hundred cases of ulcerative colitis treated by total colectomy and ileorectal anastomosis. Br Med J 1:1001, 1966.

50.   Kock, N. G. : Ileostomy without external appliance. Am Surg 173:545, 1971.

51.   Telander, R. L. , and J. Perrault: Total colectomy with rectal mucosectomy and ileoanal anastomosis for chronic ulcerative colitis in children and young adults. Mayo Clin Proc 55:420, 1980.

52.   Fonkalsrud, E. W. : Total colectomy and endorectal ileal pull-through with internal ileal reservoir for ulcerative colitis. Surg Gynecol Obstet 150:1-8, 1980.

GASTROINTESTINAL TRACT TUMORS

Mervin Silverberg, M. D.

BENIGN EPITHELIAL TUMORS

Polyps are the most common tumors of the gastrointestinal tract and may be found anywhere from the stomach to the colon. The majority occur in the colon and are generally benign lesions (1). During the past two centuries an increasing variety of hereditary multiple polyposis syndromes have been described (Table 1) which appear to have extraintestinal manifestations involving skin, bones, and other tumors. In many cases, there appears to be an increased risk of carcinoma (2).

JUVENILE POLYPS (INFLAMMATORY OR RETENTION POLYPS) (Fig. 1)

Juvenile polyps are found exclusively in the colon, and are usually pedunculated and solitary. They are found mainly during the first decade of life accounting for over 90% of polyps in this age group. They are uncommon during the first year of life and unusual in adolescence (3). A number of patients have been reported (4) with extensive typical juvenile polyps of the entire gastrointestinal tract. They have the same clinical manifestations and appear to be inherited as a non-sex-linked recessive disorder.

Clinical Features

The main clinical presentation is rectal bleeding, usually involving small amounts of unmodified blood (hematochezia) and formed stools. Less commonly, cases present with profuse bleeding or chronic iron-deficiency anemia due to painless occult blood loss; pain associated with an intussusception is rare. Those low-lying polyps on long stalks may prolapse or autoamputate and appear in the stools.

FAMILIAL POLYPOSIS (5)

Familial polyposis is characterized by multiple adenomatous polyps (see Fig. 1B), anywhere from a few hundred to a few thousand, spread throughout the colon, and occasionally involving the ileum, as well. Although, as many as one-third of the patients do not have any family history, two-thirds are associated with an autosomal-dominant form of inheritance, with a variable but high degree of penetrance (over 80%).

TABLE 1   Gastrointestinal Tract Tumors

I.   Benign
  A.   Epithelial
       1. Isolated or few: juvenile (retention, inflammatory) polyps
       2. Syndromatic: multiple polyps

Basic Lesions	**Syndrome**
Juvenile polyp	a) Juvenile polyposis
Adenomatous polyp	b) Familial polyposis
	c) Gardner
	d) Turcot
Hamartomatous polyp	a) Peutz-Jeghers
	b) Cronkhite-Canada
	c) Multiple hamartomas (Cowden)

  B.   Nonepithelial
       1. Neoplastic
          a) Isolated
                 Hemangioma
                 Lymphangioma
                 Leiomyoma
                 Neurolemmoma (schwannoma)
                 Lipoma
          b) Syndromatic (multiple)

Neurofibroma	a) Neurofibromatosis
Ganglioneuroma	b) Ganglioneuromatosis

       2. Nonneoplastic
          a) Lymphoid hyperplasia
          b) Pseudopolyps
  C.   Mixed: teratoma

II. Malignant
  A.   Epithelial

1. Primary	a) Isolated	Adenocarcinoma of colon
	b) Syndromatic: (multiple)	a) Cancer family syndrome
		b) Torre-Muir syndrome
		c) Hereditary colonic cancer
		d) Hereditary gastrocolonic cancer
2. Secondary		a) Familial polyposis
		b) Juvenile polyposis
		c) Peutz-Jeghers syndrome
		d) Gardner syndrome
		e) Inflammatory bowel disease

  B.   Nonepithelial: Lymphoma

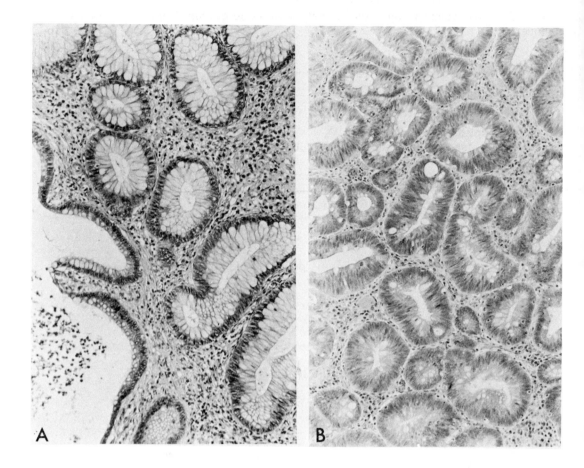

FIGURE 1   (A) Inflammatory polyp. Note the preserved crypt pattern with dilatation of the lumen and marked inflammatory infiltrate of the lamina propria. Hematoxylin-eosin stain. Original magnification x 112. 5. (B) Adenomatous polyp. Disturbed crypt pattern with picket fencing of the nuclei and absence of inflammation of the lamina propria. Hematoxylin-eosin stain. Original magnification x 112. 5. (Courtesy of Dr. Ellen Kahn.)

Clinical Features

The average age of onset of symptoms is during the early 30s, however 50% of cases are diagnosed before the age of 20, and a significant number already have malignancies by this time. Over 95% of the patients will eventually develop colorectal carcinoma if untreated, some during adolescence. Diarrhea, with or without blood loss, is the most common presentation usually associated with crampy abdominal pain. Many cases are asymptomatic, having been diagnosed during family investigations.

Treatment

Aggressive surgical intervention is indicated at the time of diagnosis in this high-risk disease. A maximum delay until the late teens may be acceptable with close observation. In most cases, a total proctocolectomy with a terminal ileostomy is indicated. When the rectum is free from polyps, a short segment of the rectum may be spared, and an ileoproctostomy is performed. The patient should be followed by a careful proctoscopic examination every 6 months.

GARDNER SYNDROME (6)

The clinical manifestations of Gardner syndrome are variable. Generally, adenomatous polyps of the large intestine are found associated with soft tissue tumors as well as with lesions of the bone. Some patients have only colonic lesions and may be confused with familial polyposis coli. However, the former are usually confined to the colon and are fewer in number. The extraintestinal lesions may precede the bowel tumors by as much as 6 years. There is a high incidence of malignant transformation of colonic polyps. The disorder is transmitted as an autosomal-dominant trait. The cutaneous lesions include epidermoid and sebaceous cysts and fibromas. Bone changes are common, consisting of osteomas, exostoses, and thickening of long bones. Dental abnormalities and tumors of the thyroid and adrenal glands are not infrequent.

TURCOT SYNDROME (7)

This is a rare syndrome involving colonic polyps as well as malignant tumors of the central nervous system. The inheritance is probably via an autosomal-recessive pathway, and there are frequent malignant changes of the colonic lesions.

PEUTZ-JEGHERS SYNDROME (8-10)

This is a dominantly inherited syndrome with nonneoplastic polyps, which may be associated with mucocutaneous pigmentation. The melanin pigmentation is found on the face, lips, buccal mucosa, palms, soles, and is usually uncommon in the preschool child (see Chap. 11). All of the areas of pigmentation, except for the buccal mucosa, may fade or disappear at puberty.

The polyps may be found throughout the intestine, but tend to occur mainly in the jejunum and ileum. They are variable sized (0. 1-3. 0 cm) hamartomas, which cause clinical features not unlike the juvenile polyp. Malignant changes, i. e. , atypia, or true invasiveness have been reported in less than 2% of these cases. In rare cases, other polyps have been reported in the nasobronchial tree and the urinary collecting system. Ovarian tumors have been noted in 5% of females (11).

CRONKHITE-CANADA SYNDROME (12)

These cases of polyposis associated with hyperpigmentation, alopecia, and onychodystrophy, occur mainly in the middle-aged adult. The polyps are hamartomatous and usually show no malignant potential.

MULTIPLE HAMARTOMA SYNDROME (COWDEN DISEASE)

This is a rare familial disorder with polyps occurring anywhere in the gastrointestinal tract. They are usually associated with multiple congenital malformations, orocutaneous hamartomas, thyroid tumors, and breast hypertrophy with fibrocystic disease and early breast cancer.

BENIGN NONEPITHELIAL TUMORS

MISCELLANEOUS TUMORS

Smooth muscle tumors are rare and usually present with upper gastrointestinal bleeding and anemia. They usually involve the stomach. Benign lesions (leiomas) outnumber malignant ones (leiomyosarcoma) by a ratio of 2:1.

Gastric teratomas are rare benign tumors found predominantly in male infants under 1 year of age. The majority of infants present with an abdominal mass, vomiting, and bleeding (13). Total excision usually is associated with a good prognosis. Similar complaints are noted in the rare gastric schwannomas. Hemangiomas (14) and lymphangiomas (15) of the gastrointestinal tract, including the esophagus, are rare lesions.

NEUROFIBROMATOSIS (16)

These tumors may be polyps or nodules involving any part of the gastrointestinal tract, particularly the stomach and jejunum. Typical skin tumors or cafe au lait spots may or may not be present. The tumors occur preponderantly in adults.

GANGLIONEUROMATOSIS

These benign tumors may be easily differentiated from neurofibromatosis, since they occur primarily in children and they are usually associated with multiple endocrine neoplasias (type 2b), particularly medullary thyroid carcinomas (17). Marfanoid habitus, "blubber lips," and lingual neuromas are present in most cases. Constipation or diarrhea or both are the most common gastrointestinal complaints.

LYMPHOID HYPERPLASIA

Submucosal hyperplasia of lymph follicles occurs with varying frequency both in normal children and in children being investigated for rectal bleeding (18). The lesions are typically nodular with occasional polypoid transformations. They occur with greater prevalence in the colon, and may reveal umbilication at the apices. Resection is indicated only with intractable bleeding or intussusception (19).

Nodular lymphoid hyperplasia of the small intestine is a distinct syndrome associated with dysgammaglobulinemia, chronic or intermittent diarrhea, and frequently giardiasis (20). Immunoglobulin A usually is deficient, both in blood and in the intestinal wall. Compensatory IgM production is commonly found. Rare cases of primary jejunal lymphomas have been reported (21) (see also Chap. 7).

MALIGNANT EPITHELIAL TUMORS

Carcinomas involving the gastrointestinal tract are rare, appear to involve primarily the adolescent age group, and the preponderance of cases occur in the colon. There are isolated reports of colorectal cancer in children under 2 years of age, but there is an unexplained surge in the incidence after puberty. A majority of cases occur in males, and black children outnumber Caucasians by more than 2:1 (22). Mucin-producing adenocarcinomas appear to be most common, particularly in the adolescent age group. Younger children tend to develop nonmucoid malignancies in an adenomatous polyp. Surgical intervention and chemotherapy are the hallmarks of treatment (23).

A number of predisposing factors are now recognized: (1) hereditary polyposis syndromes, (2) ulcerative and Crohn colitis (see Chap. 16), and (3) cancer family syndrome and other hereditary cancer syndromes. Inherited polyposis syndromes account for 1% or less of all colon cancer, while nonpolypoid hereditary cancers may account for up to 25% of the cases. The cancer family syndrome (24, 25) has been recognized for more than half a century and is characterized by an increased frequency of adenocarcinoma involving the colon and endometrium, in order of frequency. The lesions occur in young family members, and the inheritance appears to involve an autosomal-dominant factor with a high degree of penetrance. Despite the usual delay in diagnosis, awareness of the family history, and early surgical intervention may alter the typically poor prognosis.

Hereditary colonic cancer refers to the rare families who appear to have a much greater incidence of large-bowel cancer than expected. The same is true for hereditary gastrocolonic cancer; however, in these families there are primary sites involving the stomach as well as the colon. This occurs in the same individual and/or a combination of single primaries in relatives. These two syndromes may turn out to be the same.

The principal features of Torre or Muir syndrome comprise multiple skin tumors, i. e. , sebaceous adenomas, keratoacanthomas, and basal and squamous cell carcinomas occurring with polyps and adenocarcinomas, mainly of the large bowel and also of the small intestine and stomach (26). Other malignancies occurring with the multiple skin tumors, with or without the involvement of intestinal malignancies, include adenocarcinoma of the uterus, transitional cell carcinoma of the bladder or ureter, squamous cell carcinoma of the larynx, esophagus, or vulva, and cancer of the breast. The syndrome follows a dominant mode of inheritance with high penetrance and a variable expressivity, perhaps more variable in females than in males.

MALIGNANT NONEPITHELIAL TUMORS

LYMPHOMA

Lymphoma may present with intestinal obstruction, lower gastrointestinal bleeding, ileocecal intussusception, perforation, and diarrhea. The cases may be divided into reticulum cell sarcoma, lymphosarcoma, and Hodgkin disease on the basis of the histological features. Lymphosarcoma is the most common malignancy of the small intestine, usually in children over the age of 2 (27). A variety of the latter involving the upper small intestine occurs with significant frequency in adolescents of Middle Eastern origin.

REFERENCES

1.   Wennestrom, J. , E. R. Pierce, and V. A. McKusick: Hereditary benign and malignant lesions of the large bowel. Cancer 34 (suppl):850, 1974.

2.   McConnell, R. B. : Genetic aspects of gastrointestinal cancer. Clin Gastroenterol 5:483, 1976.

3.   Horrilleno, E. G. , C. Eckert, and L. V. Ackerman: Polyps of the rectum and colon in children. Cancer 10:1210, 1957.

4.   Lipper, S. , L. B. Kahn, R. S. Sandler, et al. : Multiple juvenile polyposis. Hum Pathol 12:804, 1981.

5.   Bussey, H. J. R.: Familial Polyposis. Coli. Johns Hopkins University Press, Baltimore, 1975.

6.   Schiffman, M. A.: Familial multiple polyposis. Associated with soft tissue and hard tissue tumors. JAMA 179:136, 1962.

7.   Turcot, J. , J. P. Despres, and F. St. Pierre: Malignant tumors of the central nervous system associated with familial polyposis of the colon. Dis Colon Rectum 2:465-468, 1959.

8.   Jehgers, H. , V. A. McKusick, and K. H. Katz: Generalized intestinal polyposis and melanin spots of the oral mucosa, lips and digits. N Engl J Med 241:933, 1031, 1949.

9.   Dormandy, T. L.: Gastrointestinal polyposis with mucocutaneous pigmentation (Peutz-Jeghers syndrome). N Engl J Med 256:1093, 1141, 1186, 1957.

10. Bailey, D.: Polyposis of the gastrointestinal tract: The Peutz syndrome. Br Med J 2:433, 1957.

11. Dozois, R. R. , R. D. Kempers, and D. C. Dahlin, et al.: Ovarian tumors associated with the Peutz-Jeghers syndrome. Ann Surg 172:233, 1970.

12. Johnson, G. K. , K. H. Soergel, G. T. Hensley, et al.: Cronkhite-Canada syndrome: Gastrointestinal pathophysiology and morphology. Gastroenterology 63:140, 1972.

13. Matias, I. C. and Y. C. Huang: Gastric teratoma in infancy: Report of a case and review of the world literature. Ann Surg 178:631, 1973.

14. Heald, R. J. , and J. E. Ray: Vascular malformations of the intestine. South Med J 67:33, 1974.

15. Berardi, R. S.: Lymphangioma of the large intestine: Report of a case and review of the literature. Dis Colon Rectum 17:265, 1974.

16. Hochberg, F. H. , A. B. Dasilva, J. Galdabini, et al.: Gastrointestinal involvement in von Recklinghausen's neurofibromatosis. Neurology 24:1144, 1974.

17. Carney, J. A. , V. L. W. Go, G. W. Sizemore, et al.: Alimentary tract ganglioneuromatosis. A major component of the syndrome of multiple endocrine neoplasia, type 2B. N Engl J Med 295:1287, 1976.

18. Capitanio, M. A. , and J. A. Kirkpatrick: Lymphoid hyperplasia of the colon in children. Radiology 94:323, 1970.

19. Franken, E. A. , Jr.: Lymphoid hyperplasia of the colon. Radiology 94:329, 1970.

20. Hermans, P. E. , K. A. Huizenga, H. N. Hoffman, et al.: Dysgammaglobulinemia associated with nodular lymphoid hyperplasia of the small intestine. Am J Med 40:78, 1966.

21. Matuchansky, C. , M. Morichau-Beauchant, G. Touchard, et al. : Nodular lymphoid hyperplasia of the small bowel associated with primary jejunal malignant lymphoma. Gastroenterology 78:1587, 1980.

22. Chabalko, J. J. , and J. F. Fraumeni, Jr. : Colorectal cancer in children. Epidemiological aspects. Dis Colon Rectum 18:1, 1975.

23. Donaldson, M. H. , P. Taylor, R. Rawitscher, et al. : Colon carcinoma in childhood. Pediatrics 48:307, 1971.

24. Arndt, R. D. , R. J. Kositchek, and P. D. Boasberg: Colon carcinoma and the cancer family syndrome. JAMA 237:2847, 1977.

25. Aiges, H. W. , E. Kahn, M. Silverberg, et al. : Adenocarcinoma of the colon in an adolescent with the family cancer syndrome. J Pediatr 94:632, 1979.

26. Anderson, D. E. : An inherited form of large bowel cancer. Muir's syndrome. Cancer 45:1103, 1980.

27. Mestel, A. L. : Lymphosarcoma of the small intestine in infancy and childhood. Ann Surg 149:87, 1959.

18

PROTEIN-LOSING ENTEROPATHY

Arnold Schussheim, M. D.

INTRODUCTION

Protein-losing enteropathies (PLE) represent a group of disorders jointly characterized by excessive loss of plasma proteins into the digestive tract with resultant
hypoproteinemia and edema. Any part of the gastrointestinal tract may be the
source of this protein loss. This syndrome has also been called "exudative enteropathy," "weepy gut," and "hypercatabolic hypoalbuminemia."

PATHOPHYSIOLOGY

These disorders can best be understood by using plasma albumin as a model of normal and abnormal plasma protein kinetics (Fig. 1). Serum albumin is in equilibrium with extravascular albumin with relative proportions in the two compartments
of 1:2. Complete equilibrium between the two pools is usually reached within 7
days after intravenous albumin administration. While it is well known that serum
albumin is synthesized in the liver, the main site of its catabolism is not clear.
Normally 6-10% of circulating serum albumin is degraded daily with a resultant albumin half-life of 15-23 days. About one-tenth of this degradation takes place in
the gastrointestinal tract, presumably due to loss of lymph from the apices of the
intestinal villi. This is balanced by the usual hepatic albumin synthesis of 0.2
g/kg/day. The serum albumin is exuded into the lumen and digested into its component amino acids which are mostly resorbed and thus furnish the body with a
readily available source of amino acid building blocks, even during fasting. Under certain circumstances this exudation is increased and the regenerative capacity of the liver is exceeded thus causing a fall in serum albumin levels. Hypoalbuminemia leads to a modest increase in hepatic albumin synthesis rates, which
rarely exceed twice the normal. This may be mediated by a regulatory mechanism
responding to concentrations of albumin in hepatic interstitial fluid. It is important to note that protein losses in PLE differ from renal losses of protein in that in
PLE all serum proteins are lost at the same rate, the so-called "bulk loss," irrespective of molecular size. The degree of fall of serum protein levels is generally
inversely proportional to the individual regenerative rates (half-life); thus serum
albumin and immunoglobulin-G levels are the most markedly depressed (Table 1).

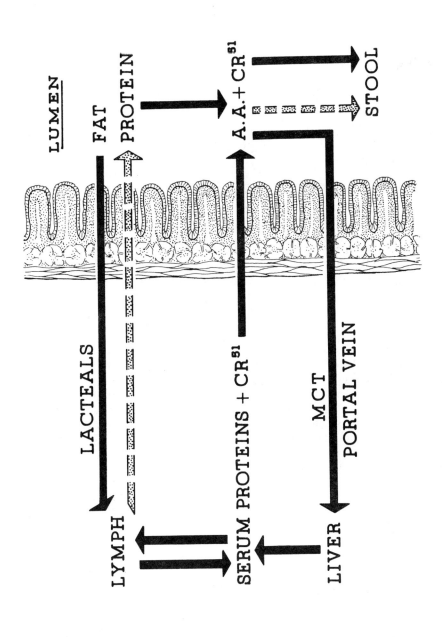

FIGURE 1   Normal and abnormal protein kinetics in the gastrointestinal tract illustrating amino acid (AA) cycles, use of ^{51}Cr as a label and pathway of medium-chain triglycerides (MCT). (From Ref. 9, reproduced with permission.)

TABLE 1   Approximate Molecular Weight and Half-Life of Serum Proteins in Relationship to Observed Serum Values in Protein-Losing Enteropathy (PLE)

Protein	Mol. Wt.	1/2 Life (Days)	PLE Serum Values
Albumin	69,000	15-23	D*
IgG	160,000	23	D
IgA	170,000	5.8	SD*
IgM	900,000	5.1	SD
Fibrinogin	340,000	3-5	V*
Insulin	5,500	4 (min)	NC*
Transferrin	90,000	12	SD
Ceruloplasmin	150,000	4	SD
Alpha$_1$-antitrypsin	50,000	3-6	SD

*D decreased; SD slightly decreased; V variable; NC no change

This prediction assumes that the endogenous anabolism and catabolism rate is unchanged. Hypogammaglobulinemia itself is a poor stimulus for compensatory increases in globulin production; however, antigenic stimulation from various sources may be an effective initiator. Factors such as malnutrition may inhibit albumin synthesis (1).

CLASSIFICATION

Protein-losing enteropathy has been described as occurring in over 80 separate conditions. These may be primary gastrointestinal disorders or systemic diseases affecting the gastrointestinal tract in various ways. One convenient categorization is noted later. Table 2 lists many of the causes of PLE, to which newer entities, such as gastroesophageal reflux, must constantly be added. A number of cases are still undiagnosed as to specific cause.

ABNORMAL, NONULCERATED INTESTINAL MUCOSA

Examples of this group include gluten-sensitive enteropathy, tropical sprue, giant rugal hypertrophy of the stomach, allergic gastroenteropathy, polyps, and amyloid disease of the bowel.

ULCERATION OF THE INTESTINAL MUCOSA

Protein loss is in excess of any accompanying red blood cell losses, and the hypoproteinemia cannot be explained by hemorrhage alone. This group includes ulcerative colitis, Crohn disease, infectious enterocolitis, tumors of the gastrointestinal tract, and the enterocolitis of Hirschsprung disease.

ABNORMALITIES OF THE INTESTINAL LYMPHATICS

Lymph is an ultrafiltrate of plasma and contains serum proteins in slightly altered proportions and decreased amounts (55-85%, in various locations). Loss of lymph protein into the intestinal tract thus represents a group of interesting and import-

TABLE 2   Some of the Known Causes of Protein-Losing Enteropathy

Agammaglobulinemia	Fistulas of gastrointestinal tract	Poisoning: sulfhydryl agents,
Allergic gastroenteropathy	Gastritis (atrophic)	arsenic
Amyloidosis of the gut	G-E reflux	Polyposis
Angioneurotic edema	Graft-vs-host reaction	Postgastrectomy syndrome
Atrial septal defect	Infectious mononucleosis	Stenosis of the small bowel
Blind loop syndrome	Inferior vena cava thrombosis	Systemic lupus erythematosus
Carcinoma: esophagus, stomach,	Intestinal lymphangiectasis	Toxemia of pregnancy
colon, small bowel	Iron deficiency anemia	Tropical sprue
Celiac disease	Kwashiorkor	Tuberculosis of gastro-
Cirrhosis	Lymphosarcoma of the bowel	intestinal tract (chronic)
Congestive heart failure	Megacolon	Ulcerative colitis
Constrictive pericarditis	Menetrier disease	Whipple disease
Crohn disease	Myocardiopathy (primary)	
Cronkhite-Canada syndrome	Nephrosis	
Dermatitis herpetiformis	Pancreatitis (chronic)	
Diverticulosis of small bowel	Parasitosis: hookworm, ameba,	
	schistosome, filaria, ascaris, trichiuris	

ant causes of PLE in children.   Primary intestinal lymphangiectasia is the prototype of this group, but constrictive pericarditis, Whipple disease, Crohn disease,
and obstruction of the lymphatic system also are to be considered.

Protein exudation may take place at all levels of the gastrointestinal tract and,
in some reports, the major localization of loss has been used as a basis for classification rather than the preceding, more physiological, outline. The mechanism
of protein loss is not clear in all cases and multiple causes and locations may be
concurrent. The classification of the pathophysiological mechanisms underlying
the losses include one or more of the following: loss via the large capillary intestinal pores, increased mucosal cell turnover, direct intraluminal rupture of lacteals, or loss in secretions of mucus or fluid. Increased permeability of tissue
membranes due to specific substances (kinins) or activated tissue plasminogen,
has been recently suggested.

CLINICAL FEATURES OF SELECTED DISORDERS

Other diseases causing PLE are discussed under their major headings in other
chapters.

COW'S MILK PROTEIN-SENSITIVE ENTEROPATHY
(ALLERGIC GASTROENTEROPATHY)

This group of patients has several different abnormalities in addition to edema   and
hypoproteinemia, including iron deficiency anemia, hypocupremia, and eosinophilia (2). Many of these patients have associated mild diarrhea, growth retardation, and clinical atopic features themselves or in family members. Bovine protein intolerance has been strongly implicated as an etiological factor, with possible
contributory factors due to iron deficiency. Peripheral blood lymphocyte counts
usually are normal; however there is frequently a significant eosinophilia. Circulating precipitant antibodies and IgA coproantibodies to cow's milk have been
demonstrated in a number of these patients, but the significance of these findings
is controversial. Guaiac-positive stools are common, and occasionally eosinophilia and large numbers of Charcot-Leyden crystals are observed in the stools.
In rare cases, hematochezia has been noted, providing a "colitis-like"picture. Radiographic studies of the intestinal tract usually are normal, or in some cases show
diffuse nonspecific mucosal edema. The exact interrelationship of this group of patients and the various deficiencies noted is not clear. Most patients improve after
exclusion of milk products; others require further bovine product restrictions and
iron administration. This disorder may be followed by gluten-sensitive enteropathy in some children at a later age.

INTESTINAL LYMPHANGIECTASIA

This may be primary, or secondary to obstructive lesions. One form of this group
of causes of PLE is found mostly in younger children and is presumably due to a a
congenital malformation of the intestinal lymphatics with dilatation of the submucosal and intravillous lacteals. Intestinal lymphangiectasia also has been noted in
association with a variety of well-defined disorders such as Noonan, Turner, and
the nephrotic syndromes. Widespread lymphatic abnormalities have been noted.
These may be asymmetric involving one or more lymphedematous extremities
(Milroy disease). Ascites, pleural, and pericardial effusions, some of which may
be chylous in nature, are common associations (3).

The exact incidence of congenital or secondary lymphangiectasia is not known, and some authors have suggested that it occurs more widely than is generally appreciated (4). There may be a genetic association in that various family members may have similar lymphatic abnormalities. Questions regarding the occurrence of PLE in relatives must be thorough. Since PLE has only recently been fully described, older cases may have been misdiagnosed as atypical liver, renal, or cardiac diseases.

The intestinal symptoms consist of diarrhea, vomiting, or abdominal pain. Gastrointestinal symptomatology may, however, be minimal, the children presenting with hypocalcemic tetany, failure to thrive, or edema. Losses of protein-rich lymph, fat, and lymphocytes lead to hypoproteinemia, edema, steatorrhea, and possible altered immune responses. A differential loss of T over B type lymphocytes has been noted. The edema is frequently variable in degree, and in the presence of hypoalbuminemia, it is both of a pitting and nonpitting (lymphedema) type.

ACUTE TRANSIENT LOSS

Hypoproteinemia of only a few weeks duration has been observed in young children. Frequently, clear-cut documentation and localization of intestinal loss is lacking. A preceding gastroenteritis is often noted, or the PLE may be related to a transient form of allergic gastroenteropathy or eosinophilic gastroenteritis. A transient form of giant gastric rugal hypertrophy (Menetrier syndrome) also has been reported. Complete recovery is the rule (5-7).

DIAGNOSIS

The mode of presentation of PLE varies greatly depending on the underlying disease (8-10). Edema and hypoproteinemia are present at some time. The hypoproteinemia is a panhypoproteinemia and not a specific loss or absence of one protein fraction. However, serum values of these proteins vary with the respective half-lives and anabolic replacement. As already mentioned, the edema is usually pitting and generally symmetrical, except when there is an accompanying disorder of the peripheral lymphatics. Even a complete absence of gastrointestinal symptoms should not rule out PLE. Tetany, retinal macular edema, and lymphopenia are more unusual initial problems.

Other causes of hypoproteinemia must be excluded and a schematic approach is outlined in Fig. 2. Hypoanabolic albuminemia is a rare inborn error of metabolism which has normal to elevated globulins. One should be aware that even in specific agammaglobulinemia there may be an accompanying PLE with secondary hypoalbuminemia. The initial surprise in the average workup of a patient with edema and hypoproteinemia comes when the urine is noted to be protein-free and the diagnosis of a nephrotic syndrome is thus reasonably eliminated. With the subsequent exclusion of chronic liver disease, PLE should be seriously considered. Some unusual causes of hypoproteinemia to be differentiated include nutritional deficiencies, pancreatic exocrine insufficiency, particularly in patients with cystic fibrosis (see Chap. 15), and enterokinase deficiency.

It is necessary to confirm the suspicion of increased enteric loss of serum proteins and to localize the pathology. A variety of tests have been used for this purpose:

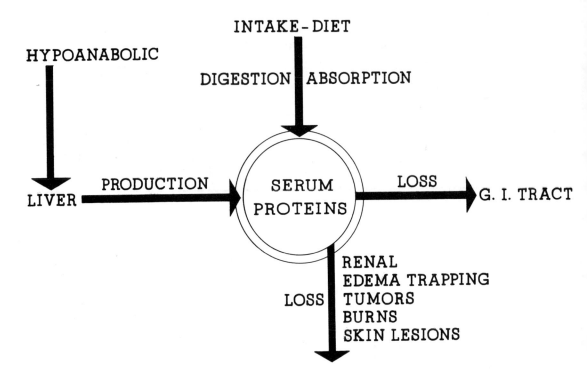

FIGURE 2   Schematic approach to the causes of hypoproteinemia. (From Ref. 9, reproduced with permission.)

ISOTOPE-LABELED PROTEIN

Large synthetic macromolecules and various serum proteins labeled with radio-active isotopes have been used as diagnostic agents. Intravenous injection and subsequent collection of stool samples for 3-4 days to document enteric loss, or to measure protein turnover rates and pools, is the most popular procedure. Chromium 51-tagged albumin is almost ideal to measure enteric loss, since the labeled complex is neither significantly absorbed from nor secreted into the intestinal lumen; it is physiologically inert. Harmless tracer amounts are injected intravenously and the stools are then collected for 96 hours. Urine must be rigorously separated, since significant amounts of the free isotope are excreted by the kidneys early in the study. Stool excretion of greater than 1% of the injected dose is considered abnormal. ^{51}Cr-labeled albumin however is not useful in measuring total body turnover or pools, since it alters its carrier protein. A more refined procedure is the measurement of the clearance of ^{51}Cr-albumin. Radioiodine labeled albumin, ^{131}I, may be used to determine the anabolic aspects and pool sizes of albumin. However, since the isotope enters the gastrointestinal tract via numerous secretions and is readily reabsorbed, it is not of value in assessing intestinal losses. Other isotopes have significant disadvantages. Polyvinyl pyrrolidine (PVP, a synthetic macromolecule) is of variable molecular weights and has been shown to be carcinogenic in animals. ^{59}Fe-dextran, ^{67}Cu-labeled ceruloplasmin, and ^{95}Nb-labeled albumin are very expensive compounds with very short half-lives.

GASTROINTESTINAL RADIOGRAPHS

Radiocontrast studies of the gastrointestinal tract often will demonstrate edematous mucosa with thick folds, which may be poorly outlined due to excessive secretions. The other radiographic features will vary with the specific etiology of the PLE.

LYMPHANGIOGRAPHY

A variety of abnormalities can be demonstrated with peripheral lymphangiography. Abnormal lymphatics in an extremity and the demonstration of reflux of the radiocontrast material into the bowel are both very suggestive of the diagnosis. This study is usually technically difficult in children under the age of 5.

MUCOSAL BIOPSY

Peroral intestinal mucosa biopsy is useful in establishing the diagnosis of intestinal lymphangiectasia; however, one must be aware of the variability of pathological findings at different times and at various sites in the gastrointestinal tract (Fig. 3). Other causes of PLE also may be diagnosed by mucosal biopsy, i. e. , celiac disease. Whipple disease, which may also have associated dilated intestinal lacteals histologically, will show the characteristics PAS-positive macrophages in a mucosal biopsy.

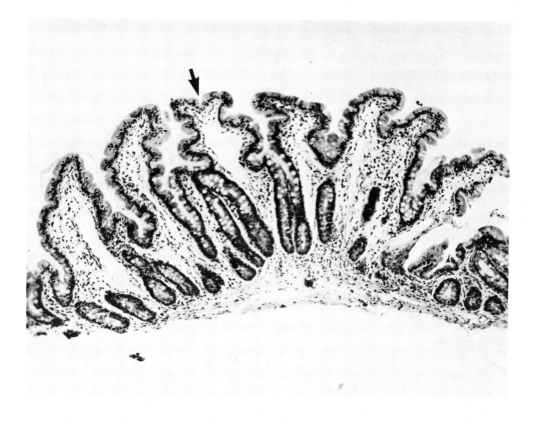

FIGURE 3   Jejunal biopsy demonstrating dilated intravillous lacteals (arrow). Hematoxylin-eosin stain.   Original magnification x 50.

STOOL PROTEIN STUDIES

Alpha$_1$-antitrypsin determination in the stool either on a random sample or by a clearance method, has recently been studied as a marker of PLE (11). Unfortunately, the results are conflicting. Measurements of stool nitrogen provide variable results and are generally not reliable in documenting PLE. Depending on the level of the gastrointestinal tract in which the exuded protein is lost, it may be digested to its amino acids which are then more or less completely resorbed. Thus there may not be any excess nitrogen loss in the stools. In some patients an interesting and often confusing association of overflow aminoaciduria has been found.

TREATMENT

It is necessary to understand that PLE is caused by a wide variety of well-defined disorders, and treatment must be directed toward the specific cause. Serum protein levels rapidly return to normal when the excessive exudation ceases, since the anabolic phase of serum protein metabolism is usually not disturbed. Frequently, the treatment is directed exclusively toward the underlying disease.

Surgery may rarely be indicated if there is a localized resectable lesion. This is relevant to polyps, other tumors, Menetrier disease, eosinophilic granuloma, localized intestinal lymphangiectasia, inflammatory bowel disease, or aganglionic megacolon. Constrictive pericarditis and selective heart disorders with chronic cardiac failure are likewise helped by surgical intervention. In rare cases, a lymph-venous anastamosis has reduced the intestinal losses.

High-protein diets and repeated protein infusions have little effect in conditions of long duration, but may help to prepare a patient for surgery. Indeed, vigorous use of protein infusions may worsen gastrointestinal symptoms as fractional protein losses are increased into the gastrointestinal tract.

NUTRITIONAL MANAGEMENT

Hypoallergenic diets are helpful in specific disorders. If the offending protein is bovine or soybean, these can be withdrawn. Iron and copper supplements are indicated when the respective transport proteins are normalized. In patients with primary or secondary lymphangiectasia, replacing most of the ingested normal long-chain triglyceride fat with medium-chain triglyceride (MCT), will reduce lymphatic flow and pressure (12). This may decrease thoracic duct flow by 50% or more, since the MCT is absorbed directly into the portal circulation. Antimicrobial agents are used in Whipple disease, and chronic inflammatory and infectious bowel diseases. Eradication of infestations by antiparasitic drugs has been useful in schistosomiasis and giardiasis. Cimetidine, an H$_2$ antagonist, has been useful in some cases of Menetrier disease. Antiplasmin agents have been used successfully in an anecdotal fashion, and requires a controlled investigation.

REFERENCES

1.   Fiftieth Ross Conference: Macromolecular Aspects of Protein Absorption and Excretion in the Mammalian Intestine. Ross Laboratories, Columbus, OH, 1964.

2.   Waldman, T. A. , R. D. Wochner, L. Laster, and R. S. Gordon: Allergic gastroenteropathy. N Engl J Med 276:761, 1967.

3. Lesser, G. T. , M. S. Bruno, and K. Enselberg: Chylous ascites. Arch Int Med 125:1073, 1970.

4. Vardy, P. A. , E. Lebenthal, and H. Shwachman: Intestinal lymphangiectasia: A reappraisal. Pediatrics 55:842, 1975.

5. Herskovic, T. , H. M. Spiro, and J. D. Gryboski: Acute transient gastrointestinal protein loss. Pediatrics 41:818, 1968.

6. Bloom, R. A. , and J. R. McQuaide: Benign hypertrophic gastropathy. Gastroenterology 19:533, 1980.

7. Stillman, A. E. , O. Sieber, U. Manthei, et al. : Transient protein-losing enteropathy and enlarged gastric rugae in childhood. Am J Dis Child 135:29, 1981.

8. Waldman, T. A. : Protein-losing enteropathy. Gastroenterology 50:422, 1966.

9. Schussheim, A. : Protein-losing enteropathies in children. Am J Gastroenterol 58:124, 1972.

10. Colon, A. R. , and D. H. Sandberg: Protein-losing enteropathies in children. South Med J 66:641, 1973.

11. Florent, C. , C. L'Hirondel, C. Desmazures, C. Aymes, and J. J. Bernier: Intestinal clearance of alpha1-antitrypsin. Gastroenterology 81:777, 1981.

12. Tift, W. L. , and J. K. Lloyd: Intestinal lymphangiectasia: Long term results with MCT diet. Arch Dis Child 50:269, 1975.

19

THE EXOCRINE PANCREAS

Arnold Schussheim, M. D.

INTRODUCTION

The exocrine pancreas consists of acinar cells arranged around a lumen and the centroacinar cells of the duct system. The function of the former is the secretion of the digestive enzymes, and the latter secretes fluid and bicarbonate. The intestinal polypeptide hormones are the major regulators of pancreatic function. Cholecystokinin-pancreozymin stimulates the secretion of enzymes from the acinar cells. The proteolytic enzymes are secreted as inactive (zymogen) forms under normal circumstances, and are only activated when they reach the duodenum, thus preventing "autodigestion." Along with pancreatic enzymes, the average healthy child secretes fluid (3ml/kg/50 min) containing large amounts of bicarbonate (15 mEq/L), when stimulated by secretin. The pancreas can alter both rate and type of secretion and is affected by many variables, including the type of diet, neural (vagal), and humoral factors (1). Duodenal factors affecting the activity of pancreatic enzymes include pH, bile salts, electrolytes, and enterokinase. These, as well as abnormal anatomical arrangements, may cause an apparent pancreatic insufficiency. Pancreatic enzymes bind with the substrate and are subsequently digested, thus accounting for a significant dietary protein requirement. Since pancreatic enzymes are secreted into the intestinal lumen and act there, deficiencies of these enzymes may be replaced orally.

Insufficiency of exocrine pancreatic function is responsible for what has been called maldigestion. Clinically, this is manifested by oily, malodorous stools and failure to thrive, often while maintaining a voracious appetite. In addition to these presentations, pancreatic disease should be thought of in children with acute or recurrent abdominal pain, abdominal masses, and a variety of systemic manifestations. Except for cystic fibrosis, the number of children with exocrine pancreatic insufficiency is not thought to be large (2).

METHODS OF STUDYING PANCREATIC DISEASE

Recent development of more sophisticated methods of studying pancreatic disease has led to further interest in these disorders in children despite their relative infrequency. Samples of urine, stool, serum, duodenal fluid, and effusions all have a place in diagnosis. Many factors in the patient's and family history should direct attention to the pancreas. These include pancreatic disease, chronic undiagnosed abdominal pain, oily stools, neutropenia, disturbances in serum calcium and lipid levels, or suspicion of cystic fibrosis. Gallbladder disease and alcohol ingestion as a cause of pancreatic disease are infrequent problems in pediatrics as is pancreatic cancer.

The volume of the pancreatic secretions and its bicarbonate neutralize gastric acidity and can be measured directly. Amylase activity may be measured in serum, urine, and duodenal juice, as can the lipases (technically much more difficult). Measurement of serum trypsin is of no clinical value because of the existence of serum trypsin inhibitors. Ascitic fluid and pleural effusions also may be studied for pancreatic enzyme activity in specific situations to clarify their etiologies. Fecal proteolytic enzymes can be determined to circumvent the difficulties of duodenal intubation. Here, most attention has been directed toward the study of trypsin and chymotrypsin in random or 24-hour stool collections. Stool chymotrypsin seems to have a place in screening for pancreatic disorders, perhaps because of its resistance to degradation by bacteria in the stool. The synthetic peptide N-benzoyl-L-tyrosyl-p-aminobenzoic acid which, when given by mouth, is cleaved by pancreatic peptidase, and the resultant para-aminobenzoic acid (PABA) excreted and measured in the urine, may be shown to be of use as another indicator of pancreatic function (3).

Generally, enzyme activity is measured by the rate of a chemical reaction on a specific substrate. Methodology and age of the child must be critically evaluated. Normal values for pancreatic enzymes in children have been given by various authors. Approximately 90% of pancreatic function must be destroyed before clinical symptomatology appears.

Pancreatic stimulation tests have been used and standardized in children (4). Intraluminal tubes that have been designed to obtain duodenal juice separate from gastric contents and in measurable quantitative amounts are available for this purpose. Secretin-pancreozymin stimulation is now more frequently employed than test meals. Volume, viscosity, pH, bicarbonate, microscopic examination, as well as enzyme analysis, should be done on the material obtained. Clinical response to pancreatic replacements by mouth is indicative of pancreatic malabsorption, but this as well as the variety of other stool and serum tests point to pancreatic disease only in a nonspecific manner.

Various other procedures have been used in studying pancreatic disease. Radiographic techniques include plain films of the abdomen, gastrointestinal series, retrograde duct pancreatography, and angiography. These studies may reveal pancreatic calcifications, segmental gaseous distention of jejunal loops (sentinal loops), fat necrosis, bone infarction, cholelithiasis, and duodenal displacement. Less frequently used techniques that may be of value in specific cases include cytology, radioimaging (selenomethionine), and most recently, computerized tomography and ultrasound. Increased size of the pancreas and an echodensity less than that of the liver suggests pancreatitis (5).

The causes of exocrine pancreatic insufficiency are listed in Table 1. It should be emphasized that cystic fibrosis accounts for the vast majority of cases seen.

CYSTIC FIBROSIS (CF) (See also Chap. 15)

INTRODUCTION AND PATHOGENESIS

Cystic fibrosis is a hereditary disorder with widespread manifestations due to dysfunction of the exocrine glands—mucous, salivary, and sweat. It is the purpose of this section to discuss the general diagnosis of CF, and to describe some of the gastrointestinal manifestations (6).

TABLE 1   Exocrine Pancreatic Insufficiency in Children

Cystic fibrosis
Shwachman syndrome
Protein-calorie malnutrition
Chronic pancreatitis
Isolated enzyme defects
    Lipase, amylase, trypsin, trypsinogen,
    physiologically delayed amylase
Apparent enzyme insufficiency
    Enterokinase deficiency
    Surgical rerouting
    Zollinger-Ellison syndrome
Anatomical
    Congenital hypoplasia of Bodian (?)
    Ductal obstruction
Miscellaneous
    Prenatal viral infections
    Postvaricella
Associated with other anomalies and syndromes

Cystic fibrosis of the pancreas was described in 1938 and became the first specific entity to be separated from the general group of the "celiac affections." It represents the major disorder of the pancreas in children, one of the most common chronic illnesses seen in pediatrics (with one of the highest mortalities in Caucasians), and in most areas of the United States, the most frequent cause of steatorrhea in children.

Cystic fibrosis is a genetic autosomal-recessive disorder and is estimated to occur in approximately 1:2000 live births in the United States. Its incidence in American blacks (1:17,000) is strikingly less than in Caucasions and it is rare in Orientals. There is an estimated 5% carrier rate with no reliable clinical or biochemical abnormalities detectable in the heterozygote.

Up to the present, no complete animal model has been available to study this disease. The pathogenesis is based mainly on the abnormal type of secretions from the exocrine glands, a process which may start in utero. The secretions become dry and inspissated with resulting ductular blockage. The current prolonged survival time of patients with cystic fibrosis has brought to light some new associations and complications of this disease. In view of the increasing number of patients surviving into adult life and significant number of patients initially diagnosed in late adolescence, there has been wider interest in CF outside the field of pediatrics. Many CF patients have married. Males seem to survive longer but are frequently infertile. Most patients can be expected to live to approximately 20 years of age. Though many biochemical and histological abnormalities have been reported, the basic defect still remains unknown. Various authors have focused attention on calcium, hyperpermeable mucus, abnormal mucus and glycoproteins, autonomic nervous system dysfunction, humoral factors, and ciliary dysfunction. Cell culture abnormalities indicate that CF may affect all somatic cells as well as exocrine glands. Since 1953, the elevation in the level of sweat electrolytes has formed the basis for diagnosis and screening along with signs of pancreatic insufficiency and pulmonary disease.

CLINICAL FEATURES OF CF

Extraintestinal Manifestations

Pulmonary disease often has an early onset. It is chronic and recurrent. This obstructive lung process starts in the peripheral airways with secretions that accumulate, lead to obstruction, air trapping, and ectasia. Bronchiolitis, pneumonia, and wheezing with subsequent clinical signs of overinflation of the lungs, high residual lung volume, and reduced expiratory flow rates ultimately are noted. Other pulmonary problems such as abscesses, atelectasis, hemoptysis, and pneumothorax occur frequently. Relentless pulmonary disease is usually the major factor in determining the ultimate outlook for CF.

A variety of nonpulmonary manifestations of CF have been reported. Nasal polyps, heat stroke, male sterility, diabetes, cor pulmonale, digital clubbing, failure to thrive, and salivary gland enlargement are some of the extraintestinal manifestations of CF.

Intestinal Manifestations

Table 2 lists the major intestinal manifestations of cystic fibrosis, some of which are discussed next (7, 8).

Malabsorption

Eighty-five percent of patients with CF eventually have clinically significant generalized exocrine pancreatic insufficiency. Pathological changes in the pancreas may be seen at birth, and advance to classical fibrosis with cystic dilatation of the ducts which contain hyaline material. When untreated this leads to malabsorption, steatorrhea, and failure to thrive, usually with a voracious appetite. The malabsorption is due to intraluminal maldigestion, as revealed by normal D-xylose absorption and normal histology of the small bowel. Oral pancreatic enzyme replace-

TABLE 2   Gastrointestinal Manifestations of Cystic Fibrosis

Malabsorption	Gallbladder disease
Vitamin A, E, K	Cholelithiasis-cholecystitis
Lactose	Atrophic gallbladder
Protein	
Bile acids	Meconium ileus equivalents
Fat	Abdominal pain
Calcium	Mass impaction
Meconium ileus	Rectal prolapse
Obstruction	
Peritonitis	Pneumatosis intestinalis
Small-bowel atresia	
	Duodenal ulcer
Liver disease	
Silent, focal	Intussusception
Fatty liver	
Biliary cirrhosis	Pancreatitis
Portal hypertension	
Neonatal jaundice	Complications of antibiotic therapy
Hemosiderosis	

ment controls pancreatic insufficiency in most children. The deficiency in pancreatic lipase seems to be clinically more important than amylase or protease deficiency. There have been some reports of absorptive defects and protein-losing enteropathy with CF (9). The mucous-secreting glands of the intestinal tract may be markedly affected in some patients, with mucous plugging. This may be responsible for abnormal intestinal x-rays with nodularity, coarsened folds, and segmentation, which in some cases is difficult to differentiate from Crohn or celiac disease. Hypoprothrombinemia, neuroaxonal dystrophy, or bulging fontanel may be seen as a result of malabsorption of the fat-soluble vitamins K, E, and A, respectively. Usually absorption of vitamin D is clinically not significantly affected. Intestinal lactase deficiency leading to impaired hydrolysis of lactose (10) as well as facilitated iron absorption from the small bowel has been reported. Malabsorption of calcium may lead to hypocalcemic tetany. The relationship of pancreatic proteases to intestinal lactase activity is under study.

Meconium ileus

Neonatal intestinal obstruction may be the earliest manifestation of CF, occurring in 10-15% of the patients. Vomiting and distention develop in the first few days of life, and usually no meconium stools are passed. Radiographic studies of the abdomen reveal distended loops of bowel in the right lower quadrant with a ground-glass appearance and no air-fluid levels.

Calcifications may be seen; these may be diffuse and extraintestinal when perforation has occurred. A barium enema, if done, reveals a microcolon. The diagnostic sweat test, although technically difficult to do in the newborn period, may be tried, but the operative intervention need not be delayed if one is unable to obtain this confirmation. Pancreatic trypsin is absent from the meconium. Volvulus, atresia, perforation, and meconium peritonitis may be found at surgery. The distal ileum is filled with tenacious meconium and mucus. The prognosis for these patients depends upon the associated pulmonary disease. It does, however, tend to recur in the same form in subsequently affected members of the same family. Meconium plug usually is not associated with a higher incidence of CF, but rather Hirschsprung disease, and trypsin levels are normal in this meconium.

Liver Disease

Liver disease in CF is frequently silent, focal, and only found at autopsy or surgery. Prolonged direct-reacting hyperbilirubinemia of the neonatal period may occur. CF accounts for a small number of patients involved in the differential diagnosis of "neonatal cholestasis"; bile duct plugging and pericholangitis may be seen on biopsy. Hemosiderosis and fatty liver may be found in older children. The liver appears enlarged at times due to the downward displacement by overinflated lungs; however, true hepatomegaly with minimal laboratory evidence of disease may occur. Portal hypertension and all its consequences is found in cases with multilobular biliary cirrhosis. Splenic infarction, hypoprothrombinemia, and hepatic failure may become additional problems. The clinical course of the liver and lung disease need not be parallel.

Hypoalbuminemia

Under most circumstances, pancreatic protease activity is sufficient to achieve adequate digestion of dietary proteins to maintain serum protein levels. The diet must, however, contain adequate amounts of quality protein. Breast milk has a relatively low protein content and CF patients fed exclusively on the breast have been reported to become hypoproteinemic. The development of loose bowel move-

ments in a young CF child with additional respiratory problems can easily be mis-
interpreted clinically as some form of "allergy." When a soy-based formula is instituted, significant hypoproteinemia and edema in CF patients may then result
either because of the peculiar quality of the soy protein or because of its inhibitory
effect on pancreatic enzymes.

Advanced liver disease with reduced synthesis of albumin and cor pulmonale
with expansion of plasma volume are additional contributory factors to be considered in the development of hypoalbuminemia.

Meconium Ileus Equivalents

Older children with CF may suffer episodes of acute, crampy abdominal pain together with signs of intestinal obstruction and palpable abdominal fecal masses in
the right lower quadrant. In essence this is a picture of acute right colonic constipation. Intussusception or volvulus may complicate the clinical picture. Abnormal mucus production and altered motility are thought to be responsible for
this situation. Additional causes of abdominal pain in CF patients also should be
considered. These include air swallowing during periods of respiratory distress,
swelling of the liver capsule due to fatty liver or heart failure, and coincidental
conditions.

Other Gastrointestinal Manifestations

Recurrent acute pancreatitis tends to occur in adolescent and young adult patients. The pancreatitis may predate the diagnosis of CF. The described acid-
peptic disease may be secondary to chronic pulmonary or liver disease or to reduced bicarbonate buffering. It is frequently difficult to decide if a condition such
as gallstones or atrophic gallbladder is only incidentally associated. There have
been suggestions that malabsorption of bile salts exists. The reason is unclear
but may be related to the degree of pancreatic insufficiency. The pathological implications of bile acid malabsorption may be far reaching. Rectal prolapse occurs
early in life and is related to frequent stooling and malnutrition.

DIAGNOSIS OF CF (Table 3)

Because of its frequency of occurrence in pediatrics CF should be considered in
the differential diagnosis of malabsorption, chronic diarrhea, chronic pulmonary
or liver disease, hypoproteinemia, and the full range of pulmonary, intestinal,
and extraintestinal disorders mentioned in this discussion. The onset of symptoms may be in the postnatal period with meconium ileus or neonatal jaundice; in
childhood with pulmonary disease; or in adolescence with growth failure, abnormal
stool patterns, or even with cirrhosis. Special differential diagnostic attention
should be directed toward celiac disease, asthma, allergy, immunoglobulin deficiency, and alpha$_1$-antitrypsin deficiency. Children born into families with siblings or parents having CF should be screened early. Early diagnosis and treatment may prolong the longevity of these children and certainly prevents many of
the disastrous complications. Antenatal and heterozygote testing are not reliable
at this time. Abnormal sodium transport in skin fibroblasts for detection of heter-
ozygotes is under study. The methylumbelliferylguanidinobenzoate (MUGB) reac-
tivity with amniotic fluid proteases has been suggested for prenatal detection (11).
Screening of all newborns in the general population has some merit for early identification of affected individuals and determination of incidence and natural course of
the disease. This screening has both cost-benefit and methodological limitations.
The quantitative sweat test following pilocarpine iontophoresis is the most reliable
test for CF and one of the most specific tests in all of medicine. However, it must
be meticulously performed and it is rather cumbersome and expensive. Both false-

TABLE 3   Available Diagnostic Tests for Cystic Fibrosis

Sweat test: quantitative pilocarpine iontophoresis; skin resistance; chloride electrode

Duodenal intubation: enzymes, viscosity, bicarbonate, volume

Stool enzymes: gelatin digestion; chymotrypsin/trypsin

Newborn stool screening: elevated meconium-albumin content (various techniques)

Fingernails and hair: neutron activation for Na^+ content

Rectal suction biopsy: "mucosis"

Palm print: chloride, silver nitrate

Chest x-ray

---

positive and false-negative results occur in inexperienced hands. Screening of newborns and young infants is made more complicated by the fact that it is difficult to collect sufficient sweat in the first few months of life. A minimum of approximately 50 mg (0.05 ml) of sweat is necessary for accurate quantitation. Testing of meconium for increased albumin content (B-M strip) has not been satisfactory. The 15% of CF infants with little or no pancreatic insufficiency will not be diagnosed and other causes of false results with this test also have been reported.

At the present time a properly executed abnormal sweat test (above 60 mEq chloride) repeated at least once, together with an appropriate clinical picture, is considered to be diagnostic of CF (12, 13). Sweat chloride determinations below a concentration of 40 mEq/L are considered to be normal. Persistent values between 40 and 60 mEq/L form a somewhat gray area but are also considered to be normal. Sweat electrolytes in normal adolescents and young adults are not infrequently in this gray range and must be more critically evaluated. Generally, the level of sweat electrolytes bears no relationship to the severity of the disease. Diagnosis by duodenal drainage studies is not common at present. As already noted 15% may have no exocrine pancreatic insufficiency. The duodenal aspirate findings may sometimes corroborate a diagnosis and consist of decreased fluid, bicarbonate, and enzyme production, with low pH and increased viscosity.

The old gelatin digestion test for semiquantitative stool trypsin may be used when other tests are unavailable. In children 6 years of age or older, the test is usually negative unless the stool sample is obtained by laxative action to preserve enzyme activity.

TREATMENT OF CF

The institution of early and vigorous treatment can both prolong the life of these patients as well as minimize complications and discomfort. As in any chronic illness, the physician must treat the entire patient and be aware of the emotional impact of the disease on both the child and the family. A comprehensive team approach is usually used. There is no known cure for this disease.

The cornerstones of treatment of pulmonary disease are appropriate systemic antibiotics, inhalation therapy, and physiotherapy. Treatment must be adjusted to the specific problem. It is important to relieve bronchial obstruction by liquifying secretions with humidification, concentrated mist, aerosols, and postural drainage. The organisms usually encountered are often resistant to many antibiotics, i. e., Staphylococcus pyogenes and Pseudomonas aeruginosa. There is some difference of opinion as to whether or not antibiotics should be prescribed continuously, rotated, or selected on the basis of sensitivity tests. In well-controlled pulmonary disease, patients are seen every 2-3 months, with the administration of appropriate antibiotics in therapeutic dosages for 2-3 weeks before each visit. These children should attend special centers where expert help with breathing exercises, postural drainage techniques, and appropriate equipment is available. Preoperative clearance should take into account detailed evaluation of cardiac and pulmonary function as well as coagulation studies. The therapy of other extraintestinal complications includes prophylactic salt replacement during hot weather to prevent heat prostration, and surgery for obstructing nasal polyps. The child should remain in as normal an environment as possible and attention should be paid to the full range of emotional and developmental aspects of childhood, including proper immunization schedules. Genetic counseling and screening of siblings is important.

The pancreatic insufficiency usually is treated satisfactorily with replacement therapy and diet. Pancreatic extracts are given with each meal and snacks, or more frequently in individualized trial and error doses. Supplemental water, fat-soluble vitamins, and reduction in fat and dietary lactose may be needed in some patients. Appetite is generally excellent and adequate caloric intake must be supplied. Caloric intake is usually above normal for age to replace excessive metabolic losses. In infants, medium-chain triglyceride-containing formulas increase caloric intake and decrease steatorrhea. The use of enteric coating, or oral bicarbonate, antacids, or cimetidine to raise intraduodenal pH to prevent lipase inactivation by gastric acidity, is helpful in otherwise intractable cases. Problems with pancreatic extracts may include allergies and a recently described renal damage due to the high purine load and subsequent hyperuricosuria.

Liver disease is frequently silent and progressive. In addition to maintaining good nutrition the treatment is ultimately that of cirrhosis and portal hypertension. Portosystemic shunting can be done, but these children are frequently poor operative risks.

In meconium ileus, oral mucolytic agents and enemas using hyperosmolar agents and detergents may be tried in some cases, to dislodge the tenacious mucus-meconium mixture (14). The newborn infant usually requires surgical intervention because of inability to dislodge the inspissated meconium, and the association of other surgical conditions such as atresia, gangrene, perforation, peritonitis, and volvulus. The amount of resected bowel may complicate matters by reducing specific absorptive capabilities in the future. Meconium ileus equivalents should be treated conservatively, if possible. Increased doses of oral pancreatic extracts, acetylcysteine, Tween 80, and arginine have been used. Such use frequently has avoided surgery. Avoidance of infrequent or hard stools, as prophylaxis is advised. Intravenous feedings may be needed in preparation for surgery or to treat pancreatitis. Elemental or other special diets need further study.

OTHER DISORDERS OF EXOCRINE PANCREATIC FUNCTION

SHWACHMAN SYNDROME (15, 16)

This hereditary syndrome described in 1964 may be the same as congenital hypoplasia of the pancreas with fatty replacement of the acinar tissue as previously described by Bodian. The Shwachman syndrome consists of neutropenia, which may be cyclic, bone marrow dysfunction, elevated fetal hemoglobin and several associated conditions such as metaphyseal dysostosis, dwarfism, and Hirschsprung disease. These children usually present in the first year of life with generalized pancreatic insufficiency and poor growth. The hematological manifestations may occur later. The patients do not fully respond to exocrine pancreatic replacement and the ultimate prognosis is still uncertain. The sweat test is normal.

Some authors have described an unusual susceptibility to infection. This disorder may represent the most common cause of pancreatic insufficiency in children after cystic fibrosis (15, 16).

DELAYED AMYLASE ACTIVITY

Full pancreatic amylase production may not be achieved until age 6 months to 1 year in some children. Inability to digest dietary starch may cause loose bowel movements, with starch granules seen on smear. Most authors would consider delay of amylase activity after 1 year of age as pathological. An oral starch tolerance test has generally had poor results in identifying these children. They respond to starch withdrawal and use of simple sugars in the diet. Starch granules alone in the stool are not diagnostic of this or any other abnormality. Rapid transit, antimicrobial agents, and premature evacuation of the stool from the rectum, artifically, with enemas, etc. , may result in significant amounts of starch granules, which would have been otherwise digested by bacterial fermentation, in the stool. Glucoamylase found in the intestinal brush border of infants may explain the satisfactory starch digestion observed clinically (17).

ISOLATED LIPASE DEFICIENCY

There have been several reports of isolated lipase deficiency leading to severe steatorrhea. The onset is shortly after birth.

PROTEOLYTIC ENZYME DEFICIENCY

There have been reports of isolated trypsin and trypsinogen deficiencies alone or with lipase deficiency. Diarrhea, hypoproteinemia, and edema result shortly after birth. The use of a protein-hydrolysate-based formula leads to rapid improvement. The proteolytic enzyme deficiency syndromes may, however, be a secondary phenomenon. Protease enzymes are secreted as inactive zymogens. The initial activation is probably by enterokinase, which is a measurable enzyme of the duodenal mucosa. Deficiency of enterokinase (18) results in symptoms and laboratory results similar to reported cases of isolated trypsinogen deficiency, and the two are difficult to separate (19).

PROTEIN-CALORIE MALNUTRITION

Diminished exocrine pancreatic function has been noted in a variety of conditions when protein and calorie quotas are not met. All of the pancreatic enzymes are affected; however, bicarbonate secretion and volume often remain normal. The deficiencies are generally reversible when the nutritional situation improves. At the time of the initial examination it is often difficult to differentiate this secondary condition from a genetic absence of one or more enzymes. One should be cautious about drawing conclusions regarding pancreatic enzyme insufficiency in the presence of caloric deficiency and especially with hypoproteinemia.

MISCELLANEOUS CAUSES OF PANCREATIC INSUFFICIENCY

In addition, pancreatic insufficiency has been noted after intrauterine and postnatal viral infections, and as a sequel to chronic pancreatitis. Recently, various reports have called attention to the possibility that pancreatic insufficiency can be associated with a wide variety of abnormalities. These include the XXY Klinefelter syndrome, chronic liver damage, asphyxiating thoracic dystrophy, diabetes, and IgA deficiency. A recently described syndrome with aplastic alae nasi, scalp and hair defects, oligodentia, deafness, and other deficits may help uncover other cases of pancreatic insufficiency (20). One previously described case of pancreatic insufficiency has been reclassified as part of this syndrome (21). A new syndrome of refractory sideroblastic anemia with vacuolization of marrow precursors together with pancreatic exocrine dysfunction further enlarges the conditions with which one must also consider pancreatic insufficiency (22).

PANCREATITIS

INTRODUCTION

Causes of pancreatitis in children are outlined in Table 4. The number of cases seen in the pediatric age group is not large, with trauma and mumps accounting for most of the cases seen in practice. Classification is not completely adequate. Acute pancreatitis is more common than the chronic form which has more hereditary than acquired causes. There is some doubt if acute pancreatitis, even with recurrent episodes, leads to chronic pancreatitis and insufficiency. Episodes may be acute, chronic, or acute relapsing and associated with a significant mortality. Acute pancreatitis returns to histological and functional normality between attacks (23).

PATHOLOGY

Hemorrhagic, interstitial, or suppurative forms of pancreatitis have been described. Autodigestion of the pancreas, necrosis, edema, hemorrhage, and calcification form a pathological spectrum depending on the etiological agent, severity, and duration. Autodigestion is due to activated proteolytic enzymes. The exact initiating factor is not clear but is probably related to trypsin or phospholipase activation. Lipase and amylase released into the blood and tissue account for some of the extrapancreatic pathology, and form part of the basis of laboratory diagnosis. Large amounts of fluid are lost from the circulation during acute attacks.

Chronic pancreatitis ultimately may lead to fibrosis and pancreatic insufficiency. Diabetes may result from the destruction of islet tissue. Other pathological

TABLE 4   Causes of Pancreatitis

Trauma: Mumps: ⎱ account for more than 50% of cases	
Unknown: accounts for more than 30% of cases	
Infectious: with various viral agents, hepatitis, bacterial infections	
Anatomic: obstruction to pancreatic ducts or sphincter of Oddi, gallbladder disease, penetrating ulcer	
Drugs: corticosteroids, sulfasalazine (salicylazosulfapyridine), alcohol, azathioprine, valproic acid, chlorthiazide	
Metabolic: cystic fibrosis, hyperparathyroidism, hyperlipemia, aminoaciduria, hereditary	
Miscellaneous: collagen-vascular, Reye syndrome, graft-vs-host reactions, postsurgical	

changes include pseudocyst formation or encapsulated peritonitis of the lesser sac, calcifications, fat necrosis, and bone necrosis.

CLINICAL FEATURES

A history of concurrent infections such as mumps, or of blunt abdominal trauma, such as a bicycle handlebar injury, may point to an etiology. One should take a careful history as to medication use (24), gallbladder disease, or a family history of pancreatitis.

Abdominal pain, vomiting, and signs of shock are noted in acute attacks. Tenderness can be elicited in the epigastrium but the physical findings may not parallel the serious systemic signs. Pleural effusions and ascites, both with elevated pancreatic enzymes, may be noted. Hemorrhagic pancreatitis is sometimes associated with bluish discoloration near the umbilicus (Cullen sign) or the flanks (Grey Turner spots). Painless forms of pancreatitis are seen in cystic fibrosis, hemochromatosis, and lipomatosis.

Hypocalcemia occurring during acute episodes is often associated with a poor prognosis. Clinical and laboratory evidence of hemoconcentration, shock, renal failure, and abnormal liver function tests are variably present.

Amylase determinations form an important part of the diagnosis of pancreatitis. Amylase may originate from many organs including salivary glands, small bowel, liver, and fallopian tubes. Pancreatic amylase isoenzyme may be specifically identified by a variety of research techniques. Increases up to three times normal of serum amylase generally are thought to be diagnostic, but pancreatitis may be present in the face of normal serum amylase. The degree of elevation does not parallel the severity of the pancreatitis. Serum amylase rises early and may return to normal by 12 hours. Urinary amylase increases later and may remain elevated for days. Increased urinary clearance of amylase has been used as the basis for the amylase-creatinine clearance ratio (ACCR):

$$ACCR = \frac{urinary\ amylase}{serum\ amylase} \times \frac{serum\ creatinine}{urine\ creatinine} \times 100\%$$

Values above 5% may be significant.

TREATMENT

Initial therapy is directed toward the treatment of the pain, shock, and placing the pancreas at rest. Large amounts of intravenous fluids and plasma are needed. The patient must be carefully monitored. Nasogastric suction and anticholinergics reduce pancreatic enzyme output and help to avoid vomiting if ileus is present. Hypocalcemia and hyperglycemia must be treated appropriately. Antibiotics may be needed. Surgery is reserved for acute gallbladder complications, pancreatic abscess, intestinal perforation, or rarely for diagnosis. Pseudocyst formation is the main late complication of pancreatitis and requires some form of surgical drainage. The patient's nutritional requirements may be met by total parenteral hyperalimentation, when needed. Refeeding by mouth should be cautious and a low fat, high carbohydrate diet is used. In severely affected patients, particularly in the presence of renal or hepatic insufficiency, the prognosis must be guarded.

Unproven therapeutic approaches include antitryptic agents, dialysis of kinins, and steroids. The treatment is a total organ support system in an intensive care unit.

Chronic fibrosing and chronic relapsing pancreatitis are rare forms of pancreatitis and are responsible for a small group of difficult-to-diagnose chronic recurrent episodes of abdominal pain (25). The hereditary pancreatitis variety has a well-defined familial clustering, and most kindred reveal an autosomal-dominant pattern of inheritance. Elevated serum amylase and signs of pancreatic insufficiency are not seen in early childhood. Episodes terminate in 4-7 days. Shock is unusual. There is intensive interstitial fibrosis at pathological examination. Calcific radiographic densities over the area of the pancreas are late signs and are seen in less than half of the cases. The originally reported association of aminoaciduria is extremely rare. Diagnosis is frequently made at exploratory laparotomy. Many of the complications are delayed until adult life.

REFERENCES

1. Wormsley, K. G. , and D. M. Goldberg: The interrelationships of the pancreatic enzymes. Gut 13:398, 1972.

2. Hadorn, B. : Diseases of the pancreas in children. Clin Gastroenterol 1:125, 1972.

3. Nousia-Arvanitakis, S. , C. Arvanitakis, N. Desai, et al. : Diagnosis of exocrine pancreatic insufficiency in cystic fibrosis by the synthetic peptide N-benzoyl-L-tyrosyl-p-aminobenzoic acid. J Pediatr 92:734, 1978.

4. Hadorn, B. , G. Zoppi, D. H. Shmerling, et al. : Quantitative assessment of exocrine pancreatic function in infants and children. J Pediatr 73:39, 1968.

5. Cox, K. L. , M. E. Ament, W. F. Sample, et al. : The ultrasonic and biochemical diagnosis of pancreatitis in children. J Pediatr 96:407, 1980.

6. Di Sant'Agnese, P. A. , and R. C. Talamo: Pathogenesis and pathophysiology of cystic fibrosis of the pancreas. N Engl J Med 177:1287, 1967.

7. Kopel, F. B. : Gastrointestinal manifestations of cystic fibrosis. Gastroenterology 62:483, 1972.

8. Chase, H. P. , M. A. Long, and M. H. Lavin: Cystic fibrosis and malnutrition. J Pediatr 95:337, 1979.

9. Weber, A. M. , C. C. Roy, C. L. Morin, et al. : Malabsorption of bile acids in children with cystic fibrosis. N Engl J Med 289:1001, 1973.

10. Seetharam, B. , R. Perrillo, and D. H. Alpers: Effect of pancreatic proteases on intestinal lactase activity. Gastroenterology 79:827, 1980.

11. Nadler, H. L. , and M. M. J. Walsh: Intrauterine detection of cystic fibrosis. Pediatrics 66:690, 1980.

12. Shwachman, H. , and A. Mahmoodian: Pilocarpine iontophoresis sweat testing. Results in seven years' experience. Mod Probl Pediatr 10:158, 1967.

13. Goldbloom, R. B. , and P. Sekel: Cystic fibrosis of the pancreas. Diagnosis by application of a sodium electrode to the skin. N Engl J Med 269:1349, 1963.

14.   Meeker, I. A. , and W. N. Kincannon: Acetylcysteine used to liquify inspissat-
       ed meconium causing intestinal obstruction in the newborn. Surgery 56:419,
       1964.

15.   Shwachman, H. , L. K. Diamond, F. A. Oski, et al. : The syndrome of pan-
       creatic insufficiency and bone marrow dysfunction. J Pediatr 65:645, 1964.

16.   Shmerling, D. H. , A. Prader, W. H. Hitzig, et al. : The syndrome of exo-
       crine pancreatic insufficiency: Neutropenia, metaphyseal dysostosis and
       dwarfism. Hel Paediatr Acta 24:547, 1969.

17.   Lebenthal, E. , and P. C. Lee: Glucoamylase and disaccharidase activities
       in normal subjects and in patients with mucosal injury of the small intestine.
       J Pediatr 97:389, 1980.

18.   Hadorn, B. , J. B. Tarlow, J. K. Lloyd, and O. N. Wolff: Intestinal enteroki-
       nase deficiency. Lancet 1:812, 1969.

19.   Lebenthal, E. , A. Antonowicz, and H. Shwachman: Enterokinase and trypsin
       activities in pancreatic insufficiency of the small intestine. Gastroenterology
       70:508, 1976.

20.   Schussheim, A. , S. J. Choi, and M. Silverberg: Exocrine pancreatic insuf-
       ficiency with congenital anomalies. J Pediatr 89:782, 1976.

21.   Townes, P. L. , and M. R. White: Identity of two syndromes. Am J Dis
       Child 135:248, 1981.

22.   Stoddard, R. A. , D. C. McCurnin, S. J. Shultenover, et al. : Syndrome of re-
       fractory sideroblastic anemia with vacuolization of marrow precursors and
       exocrine pancreatic dysfunction presenting in the neonate. J Pediatr 99:259,
       1981.

23.   Jordan, S. C. , and M. E. Ament: Pancreatitis in children and adolescents.
       J Pediatr 91:211, 1977.

24.   Mallory, A. , and F. Kern: Drug-induced pancreatitis: A critical review.
       Gastroenterology 78:813, 1980.

25.   Warwick, W. J. , and S. R. Leavitt: Chronic relapsing pancreatitis in child-
       hood. Am J Dis Child 99:648, 1960.

20

LABORATORY METHODS

Raul A. Wapnir, Ph. D. , M. P. H. and Hyacinth Spencer, M. S.

TESTS FOR CARBOHYDRATE DIGESTION AND ABSORPTION

EXAMINATION OF STOOLS

Specimens

Freshness of the stools is essential to avoid alterations in sugar composition, pH, or lactic acid content. The rapidity of these changes has been documented (1) as shown in Table 1.

A device patterned on an electronic timing aid for alerting personnel for urine collections (2) has been applied to warn of every bowel movement of infants and to allow immediate removal of diapers and testing of stools.

Several **preservatives** have been tested for effectiveness in maintaining fecal glucose and retarding bacterial fermentation as an alternative to immediate freezing (3).

The most effective appears to be 0. 04% sodium fluoride in 1 N hydrochloric acid, in sufficient amounts to saturate the stools (approximately equal volumes). Table 2 (1) exemplifies the effectiveness of various potential **preservatives** in terms of the loss of glucose after 24 hours of standing at room temperature and the coincident increase in lactic acid concentration.

Reducing Carbohydrates in Stools

Normally, the amount of reducing substances in feces is very low, since the small intestine is extremely effective in absorbing monosaccharides. When dietary disaccharides are poorly hydrolyzed by small-intestinal mucosal disaccharidases, they pass into the large bowel and are excreted in the stools. This usually is associated with osmotic diarrhea. Common tests for reducing substances would exclude sucrose. Specimens investigated for this sugar require examination before and after acid hydrolysis with boiling 1 N hydrochloric acid for 20 minutes. The analysis of the monosaccharides may be carried out by paper chromatography (4), thin-layer chromatography (5), or high-voltage paper electrophoresis (6).

TABLE 1   Change in Fecal Glucose and Lactic Acid Concentrations in a Specimen Maintained at Room Temperature

Time After Excretion (min)	pH	Glucose (mg/dl)	Lactic Acid (mg/dl)
0	7. 18	167. 2	22. 4
30	6. 67	147. 2	41. 3
60	6. 45	136. 0	51. 0
90	6. 19	122. 0	62. 4
120	5. 85	112. 3	82. 7
24 hr	5. 17	1. 24	103. 4

TABLE 2   Effectiveness of Preservatives

Preservatives	Glucose (mg/dl)		Lactic Acid (mg/dl)	
	Initial	24 Hours	Initial	Final
0. 04% sodium fluoride in 1 N hydrochloric acid	173. 4	167. 2	22. 4	27. 5
Toluene	151. 8	160. 9	26. 9	68. 9
1 N NaOH	151. 0	118. 5	24. 1	48. 2
Chloroform	169. 2	173. 4	15. 5	25. 8
10% formaldehyde	180. 9	92. 7	244. 8	537. 9

Clinitest* for Reducing Sugars (7)

These sugars include glucose, galactose, fructose, maltose, and lactose.

1. A small amount of stool is shaken in twice its volume of deionized water. If the suspension is very turbid, it should be cleared by centrifugation for 10 minutes at 3000 rpm in a clinical centrifuge, preferably in a refrigerated apparatus (2-4°C).
2. Transfer 15 drops of the clear supernatant into a test tube. Add 1 tablet of Clinitest without shaking. After exactly 15 seconds, shake the tube gently and compare with the color chart. The scale of + to ++++ approximately corresponds to the range 0. 25-2% glucose.
3. If the specimen reads ++++, the test should be repeated by diluting the original stool suspension 1:3 (5 drops of clear suspension plus 10 drops of water) in a test tube before taking a new aliquot and repeating the test with a fresh Clinitest tablet.

*Trademark: Ames Co. , Elkhart, IN 46514

Specific Test for Glucose

A suspension prepared as in (1) can be rapidly tested for glucose by dipping reagent strips of Clinistix[a] or Diastix[a].

Determination of pH

This may be done in the same original suspension described previously (1) using a pH meter, or with narrow-range pH paper, either Nitrazinc[b] paper for a range 4. 5-7. 5, or Alkacid[c] pH 6. 0-8. 5. Most normal stools, negative for reducing substances, will have a pH between 6-8 (3). Feces with elevated sugar content and short-chain, volatile, organic acids have a pH of 5. 5 or less.

Determination of Organic Acids (8)

Excess short-chain organic acids are produced by bacterial fermentation when unabsorbed disaccharides reach the terminal ileum and colon.

For this determination, interfering carbonates and phosphates are precipitated as calcium salts and the resulting solution is titrated back to the isoelectric pH range of commonly found organic acids.

A 5-ml aliquot of a stool homogenate (1:3) prepared in water with fresh or quickly frozen stools is treated with 0. 2 g of calcium hydroxide, or more if necessary, to ensure alkalinity. After waiting for 15 minutes, the sample is centrifuged; 1 ml of the supernatant is transferred to a titrating vessel, diluted with deionized water, and adjusted to pH 8. 0-8. 3 (phenolphtalein turning point). The titration is continued with 0. 1 N hydrochloric acid to pH 2. 7 (by pH meter, or end point with tropeolin 00, orange IV, or thymol blue as indicators). The number of milliequivalents of organic acids is calculated from the volume of acid used per gram of stools.

Determination of Lactic Acid

The presence of excess lactic acid is indicative of proliferating anaerobic bacteria thriving on unabsorbed carbohydrate. Enzymatic methods used for its determination in plasma and other physiological tissues are not appropriate for stools, since lactic acid originated from bacterial fermentation is the D(-) form, as opposed to the L(+) optical isomer present in animal tissues. The classical Barker and Summerson procedure (9) determines both isomers.

A 0. 050-ml aliquot of a 1:3 stool suspension in the hydrochloric acid-sodium fluoride preservative (see previous text) is added to 1. 0 ml of water and 1. 0 ml of tungstic acid (prepared by mixing, just before use, equal volumes of 2. 2% sodium tungstate and 0. 15 N sulfuric acid), mixed and centrifuged. Reducing substances are eliminated by taking 1. 5 ml of the supernatant into a test tube and adding 0. 2 ml of 20% (w/v) cupric sulfate pentahydrate, and a small amount of calcium hydroxide powder, mixing and centrifuging. The assay of lactic acid is carried out on 0. 5 ml of the supernatant from that treatment. While keeping the tubes on ice, 1 drop of 1% (w/v) cupric sulfate solution and 3 ml of concentrated sulfuric acid are carefully added and the contents well mixed before immersing them in boiling water for 4 min. After removal of the tubes from the bath, they are cooled and 0. 1 ml of p-hydroxydiphenyl (0. 8% in 0. 25% sodium hydroxide) is added and allowed to react

---

[a]Trademark: Ames Co. , Elkhart, IN 46514
[b]Trademark: E. R. Squibb & Sons, Inc. , Princeton, NJ 08540, #52620
[c]Trademark: Fisher Scientific Co. , Fairlawn, NJ ,07410, #A-983

for 30 minutes. The tubes are then immersed in boiling water again for 90 seconds, cooled at room temperature, and the absorbancy read at 570 nm against a reagent blank. Standards are carried through the same procedure and the calculation of lactic acid concentration is computed, taking into account the dilution of the samples.

No lactic acid should be detectable in stools, by this method, in healthy individuals.

XYLOSE ABSORPTION TEST (10-12)

This five-carbon sugar is absorbed and excreted essentially unchanged in the urine. It has served as a test for the integrity of the duodenal and jejunal mucosa. Xylose is absorbed mostly by passive diffusion and its rate of absorption is considered to be proportional to the surface of intact absorptive membrane. The xylose absorption test is useful in the differential diagnosis of malabsorption due to upper intestinal mucosal disease.

Children are given 0.5 g/kg, to a maximum of 25 g, as a 5 or 10% solution. The patient is urged to drink more water at 1 and 2 hours. Sometimes the reliability of the test can be improved by infusing the solution via nasogastric tube directly into the duodenum. Determination of the rate of absorption can be assessed either by determination of serum xylose after 30, 60, and 120 minutes, or in the urine during the 5 hours following administration. Falsely low results will be obtained with delayed gastric emptying and in the presence of renal insufficiency. A minimum excretion of 15-20% of the dose given in children under 3 years of age and over 25% in older patients is considered to be normal. A level of at least 20 mg/dl in the serum of any of the postabsorptive specimens is an indicator of normal absorption. A 0.20 ml sample of serum is deproteinized by the standard Somogyi procedure to a 1:10 dilution. Urines are adjusted to a uniform volume of 1 L. A second 1:25 dilution is then carried out. Two 0.50 ml aliquots are mixed with 2.50 ml of p-bromoaniline reagent (2% w/v solution in glacial acetic acid saturated with thiourea) in small test tubes. Standards containing 0.1 and 0.2 mg/ml xylose are treated identically. The tubes are incubated in a water bath at 70°C for 10 minutes. After cooling, the reaction is allowed to proceed in the dark for 1 hour. The absorbance is read at 520 nm in a spectrophotometer using a nonincubated tube as a blank.

INTESTINAL DISACCHARIDASES (13-23)

The presence or absence of hydrolytic enzymes in the brush border of the intestinal mucosa will indicate whether the individual is physiologically capable of breaking down the three nutritionally most important disaccharides, i.e., lactose, sucrose, and maltose. It has been shown that all lactase, sucrase, and maltase activity is associated with the jejunal mucosa and is not present in cell-free debris in the intestinal lumen.

Specimens for the assay of disaccharidases are generally obtained by a peroral intestinal biopsy, or during endoscopy. For the former, either a Crosby capsule, or a Rubin multipurpose suction device with a double-port capsule is preferred. Some investigators have advocated the recovery of duodenal washings as the means to obtain mucosal cells, via a double-lumen tube (19). An appropriate attachment of the endoscope is also effective for the securing of biopsies.

Red blood cell contamination is eliminated by washing the biopsy with 10 mM EDTA buffered at pH 7.4 and spinning down the epithelial cells at 500 x g. The cells so harvested can be weighed on a polyethylene film and stored in the refrigerator at 4°C for up to 1 week. Freezing and thawing the material three times will disrupt cells and liberate surface-attached disaccharidase enzymatic activity. A final suspension in a small volume of saline is used for the assays.

The determination is carried out on 50 μl aliquots, added to 50 μl of the appropriate substrate dissolved in 0.1 M maleate buffer, pH 6.0. Sucrose and lactose are used in 56 mM concentrations; maltose in 28 mM concentration. The specimens are incubated for 60 minutes at 37°C.

The hydrolysis of the disaccharides is stopped with 1.50 ml of TRIS glucose oxidase reagent (PGO)* rapidly added to all tubes. After an additional 30 minutes at 37°C the enzymatic reaction is stopped by the addition of 1 drop of 6 N hydrochloric acid to each tube. All tubes are mixed well and read in a spectrophotometer at 420 nm 15 minutes later. Glucose standards are carried through a simultaneous reaction procedure. The color is stable for several hours.

The activity can be expressed in IU/g wet mucosa or in IU/mg protein. One international unit (IU) is equivalent to 1 μmol of substrate hydrolyzed per minute under the conditions of the assay. The normal ranges listed in Table 3 apply to children over 3 months of age.

However, it should be noted that in certain patients disaccharide intolerance, as expressed by its clinical symptomatology, fails to correlate with biochemically defined disaccharidase deficiency (13, 15-18, 21, 23).

CARBOHYDRATE TOLERANCE TESTS

These tests are based on the increase of blood glucose levels following an oral load of a specific carbohydrate. Clinically, determination of tolerance to lactose is the most often investigated problem in gastrointestinal pediatric practice. Occasionally, fructose, galactose, or glucose are administered for diagnostic purposes of monosaccharide intolerance or a congenital defect in carbohydrate metabolism (galactosemia, fructose intolerance, fructosuria, etc.). Since disaccharides are absorbed following hydrolysis at the intestinal mucosa brush border, the absence or diminution of disaccharidases often is cause for apparent malabsorption. However, since blood levels are an indirect measurement of events at the intestinal mucosal site, other factors such as congenital enzymatic deficiencies, temporary or permanent damage to the intestinal mucosa and its transport mechanisms can also be responsible for the observed alterations.

Load Test Performance (24)

In overnight-fasted patients, or for infants, at least 4 hours after the last feeding, a zero time blood specimen is obtained by finger or heel prick in a heparinized capillary tube. Only 20 μl are necessary to prepare a Somogyi 1:100 filtrate.

TABLE 3   Intestinal Disaccharidases in the Small Intestinal Mucosa of Children 3 Months of Age or Older

Enzyme	U/g Mucosa	U/g Protein
Lactase	1-11	3-83
Sucrase	1-15	4-120
Maltase	6-45	27-445

Adapted from refs. 16-18

*Trademark: PGO Enzymes. Sigma Chemical Co., St. Louis, MO 63178. #510-6

Glucose standards are prepared the same way. The carbohydrate is given orally at a dose of 40 g/m^2 with a maximum dose of 50 g, as a 20% (w/v) solution. In uncooperative patients, the disaccharide may be given via a nasogastric tube. Blood samples are taken at 15, 30, 45, 60, and 90 minutes. Capillary blood sugar levels are usually higher and are more accurate than peripheral venous blood samples (25).

The glucose assay is carried out on 0.50 ml of filtrates placed in 10 x 75 mm tubes. An equal volume of PGO reagent is added and the tubes are incubated in a water bath at 37°C for 30 minutes. The reaction is stopped with 1 drop of 6 N HCl. After 15 minutes the absorbancy is measured at 420 nm. A minimum rise of 20 mg/dl glucose over baseline levels at any time after ingestion of a disaccharide would be a normal response. A smaller rise may occur in normal individuals, usually due to delayed gastric emptying or unusual peripheral utilization. Patients are monitored for clinical complaints of diarrhea, abdominal pain, and borborygmi. Stools are examined over the 24 hours following the load for a drop in pH or/and the appearance of reducing substances (see previous text). Tolerant individuals have stools with pH greater than 5.5 and only trace or no reducing substances.

BREATH HYDROGEN TEST (26, 27)

Performance of the Procedure

The analysis of breath hydrogen after a carbohydrate load is performed with increasing frequency as a noninvasive means of detecting malabsorption and/or bacterial overgrowth in the small intestine. The carbohydrate that reaches the colon unchanged is fermented by bacteria with the production of hydrogen. Approximately 14% of the hydrogen produced is absorbed into the bloodstream and excreted via the lungs. This hydrogen can be measured quantitatively by means of a thermal conductivity gas chromatograph. Expired air is collected in a syringe by using a face mask. The syringe is fitted with a three-way valve that assures against loss of air. The patient is instructed to take a deep breath and expire into the mask. During the latter half of expiration about 5 ml of air is collected in the syringe, by actively withdrawing the plunger. This procedure is repeated until a total of 25 ml of air is collected. The sample is then introduced into the chromatograph and the hydrogen concentration determined by comparison of the height of the hydrogen peak of the subject's breath to that of a standard (Fig. 1).

Lactose Tolerance Test

The patient is given a standard dose of lactose (40 g/m^2 to a maximum of 50 g, as a 20% solution). Breath samples are collected, as previously described, at 0, 60, 90, and 120 minutes after ingestion of the challenge. An increase in hydrogen concentration greater than 10 ppm above the fasting (baseline) level is indicative of lactose malabsorption.

Lactulose Hydrogen Breath Test

This substance is administered as a 50% solution. Breath sampling is carried out at 0, 5, 10, 15, 20, and 30 minutes, and thereafter every 15 minutes for at least 3 hours. Evidence of small bowel bacterial overgrowth is indicated by the appearance of two peaks, the former occurring at least 15 minutes before the colon peak and greater than 10 ppm above the baseline.

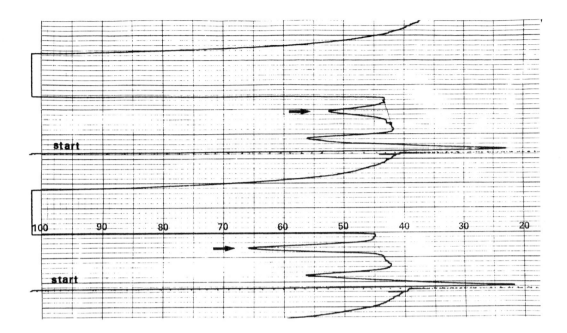

FIGURE 1   Two consecutive tracings of a breath hydrogen gas chromatographic recording. The arrows indicate the hydrogen peaks. The lower peak represents a hydrogen concentration of 55 ppm. The upper peak corresponds to 25 ppm. The equipment used was a model S gas chromatograph, QuinTron Instruments, Milwaukee, WI. Attenuation = 1.

TESTS FOR FAT DIGESTION AND ABSORPTION

STOOL FAT DETERMINATION

The assessment of stool fat in a 72-hour collection is the most accurate method of estimating steatorrhea. The original Van de Kamer method (28), or its variations, are still the most widely used.   Additional modifications are needed when medium-chain fatty acids are a substantial part of the diet (29).

The patient is usually given a high-fat diet (i. e. , in excess of 35% of total diet), for at least 2 days before the test. This diet is continued for the subsequent 3 days while stools are collected. Food intake over the entire period should be recorded and made available to the laboratory for estimation of fat intake. A charcoal marker may be used, in which case it is ingested at the beginning of the high-fat diet intake and 72 hours later. Stools are then collected from the appearance of the first marker until appearance of the second marker. In most situations, a timed 72-hour collection is adequate. All stools are collected in a mason jar and are kept refrigerated until assayed. No medication or gastrointestinal radiocontrast studies should be prescribed during the test.

The 72-hour stool collection is weighed, an equal volume of water is added and the entire specimen homogenized in a mechanical blender. A 5 g portion is then transferred to a 250 ml round bottom flask; 10 ml of 33% potassium hydroxide and 40 ml of 95% ethanol containing a 0. 4% amyl alcohol are added. The mixture is boiled under reflux for 20 minutes and then cooled at room temperature. Next, 17 ml of 25% hydrochloric acid solution is added and the mixture cooled again, after which 50 ml of petroleum ether is added to extract lipids and the two phases are vortex-mixed for 5 minutes. The layers are allowed to separate. The upper, petroleum ether layer is removed to a separatory funnel, dehydrated with a few grams of anhydrous sodium sulfate and a 25 ml aliquot transferred to a weighed Erlenmeyer flask. The petroleum ether is then evaporated at 60°C and the flask reweighed. The difference in weights is the amount present in 2.5 g of sample. The total fat excreted is calculated. Fatty acids also can be assayed by adding 10 ml of neutral ethanol to the flask and titrating with 0.1 N sodium hydroxide from a microburette, using thymol blue as indicator. The titration is complete when the yellow color begins shifting to green.

A daily excretion of up to 5 g of fat per day is normal in adults and older children. When the fat intake is known, results are usually reported as a percentage coefficient of fat absorption, i.e. (fat ingested - fat in stool) x 100/fat ingested. Normal values are no less than 95% fat absorption for children and adults, and no less than 85% for infants. To obtain technically reliable results, patients should ingest no less than 30 g of fat per day, for children under 12.

VITAMIN A ABSORPTION TEST (30)

This also is referred to as vitamin A tolerance test, and provides an indication of fat absorption. Regular food intake need not be altered, provided that no extra vitamin preparations are given during the preceding 24 hours. A zero time blood specimen is obtained before the oral administration of a test dose of 7500 IU/kg body weight, to a maximum of 350,000 IU, as vitamin A alcohol or palmitate in arachis oil. Another blood sample is taken after 4 hours, and vitamin A and carotene are assayed in both specimens.

The serum is extracted in alcohol-petroleum ether and estimated colorimetrically at 450 nm against a beta-carotene standard. The ether extract is evaporated to dryness and the residue, redissolved in chloroform, is reacted with acetic anhydride and antimony trichloride reagent for determination of vitamin A colorimetrically at 620 nm. The absorbency is compared to a stable standard.

Normal individuals will reach serum vitamin A levels of 500 IU/dl or higher, 4 hours after ingestion of the test dose. A lower level often correlates with steatorrhea.

TOTAL BILE SALTS IN DUODENAL FLUID

Bile salts activate pancreatic lipase and they aid in solubilization of fats by forming micelles. Therefore, they have a key role in the absorption of fats (31). The enzyme beta-hydroxy steroid dehydrogenase reversibly oxidizes or reduces the 3-OH or 3-0 portion of most steroid mixtures. The reaction is nicotinamide adenine dinucleotide (NAD) dependent. Such a reaction can be used for the determination of total bile salt content in duodenal fluid. The assay can also be performed in stools (32).

To an aliquot of 0.01-0.03 ml of aspirated duodenal fluid, or 0.01 ml of a 30 mM standard (61.3 mg cholic acid in 5 ml methanol), add 2 ml buffer (0.1 M potassium phosphate, pH 9.5), 0.25 ml of the enzyme preparation (1 mg/ml in cold water), 0.5 ml of 1 M hydrazine hydrate pH 9.5, and 0.25 ml of NAD (40 mg/ml), neutralized just before use). After mixing and leaving at room temperature for 1 hour, the absorbancy is measured at 340 nm. A bile-containing blank is made up with all reagents, except the NAD, and a reagent blank is also read, using all the reagents, minus the sample.

Thin layer chromatography (33) also can be used to identify the bile acids present. Precoated silica plates (0.25 mm thick, F 254, Brinkman, Westbury, NY) are used with an eluting solvent made up with isooctane:isopropyl alcohol:ethyl acetate:acetic acid (40:20:10:10). The bile acids are visualized with a cupromolybdate spray. This procedure separates most individual glycine-conjugates and individual taurine conjugates from unconjugated bile acids. Free acids are usually absent in the upper gastrointestinal tract except in cases of bowel flora overgrowth. Gas chromatography (34) will identify and quantitate the individual bile acids. The bile acids are extracted, hydrolyzed, methylated, and purified using thin-layer chromatography (hexane: ethyl acetate 10:4). The purified product is extracted, from the silica gel, acetylated and injected in the gas chromatograph apparatus (Hewlett-Packard 7610A, or comparable), at a column temperature of 260°C.

ORAL FAT-LOADING TEST (35)

Recently it has been proposed that the measurement of the increase of serum triglycerides following a fat-loading test is a reliable and rapid screening approach to determine fat malabsorption in children.

After either 6 or 12 hours of fasting, according to the age, the patient ingests 2 g/kg of a flavored margarine preparation. In the case of small babies or young children, the load can be given via a nasogastric tube after melting the mixture at 60°C. Fasting and 2-hour postingestion levels of triglycerides are determined by semiautomated procedures (Technicon), or enzymatically (Sigma, kit 320-UV).

Patients with steatorrhea fail to show an increase of 55 mg/dl (0. 6 mM), or more, in serum triglycerides. This cutoff point discriminates well between affected individuals and normal controls or children with functional disturbances. The test also correlates well with the coefficient of fat absorption in normal individuals. Children with other types of biopsy proven mucosal pathology showed abnormal correlation between gravimetric fat absorption and postingestive triglyceride levels.

TESTS FOR PROTEIN ASSIMILATION

The ability to absorb proteins, provided an adequate diet is available, cannot be directly assessed by short-term tests. Plasma levels of protein and amino acids can be altered in liver and kidney diseases, malnutrition, starvation, and specific conditions of the small bowel, such as celiac sprue and granulomatous ileitis (36).

In infantile diarrhea, protein loss in the stools can entail an important source of nutritional imbalance. Its origin may include the proteins exuded from the serum and the turnover of intestinal mucosa, as well as protein of bacterial origin.

CHROMIUM-TAGGED ALBUMIN (37)

Specific information can be obtained from the determination of excretion of albumin tagged with chromium 51 (^{51}Cr) from the bloodstream into the gastrointestinal tract. This test can reveal excessive breakdown, loss, or exudation of albumin, as in protein-losing enteropathy. The normal turnover of body albumin is estimated at 0. 2 g/kg body weight per day, of which less than one-tenth is lost in the stools.

Either ^{51}CrCl$_3$ or ^{51}Cr-labeled albumin is administered intravenously, using a 25-30 μ Ci dose. All stools, free of urine contamination, are collected for 96 hours, homogenized, and an aliquot is assayed in a scintillation counter.

^{51}Cr is excreted into the intestine, albumin bound. The free ion is not secreted or absorbed in the gastrointestinal tract. Normal persons excrete less than 1% of the administered dose. In protein-losing enteropathy, up to 40% can be recovered in the stool. ^{51}Cr has a short half-life (27. 8 days) and is a weak beta and gamma emitter. Since the commercial availability of ^{51}Cr-tagged albumin is severely limited, this test may not be accessible to the practitioner, in spite of its usefulness.

Gastrointestinal protein loss also has been estimated with radiolabeled copper ceruloplasmin (38). This compound is very expensive and the half-life of ^{67}Cu is inconveniently brief.

PROTEIN IN STOOLS (39)

Extraction

A 24-hour collection of feces is carried out directly in 1-qt mason jars (cf. fat in stools). The weight is recorded and an equal amount of deionized water is added. The jar is attached to a Waring-type blender and the contents are homogenized for 60 seconds. A 2-ml aliquot is transferred to a centrifuge tube and the proteins precipitated with an equal volume of 20% (w/v) trichloroacetic acid. After a 10-minute wait, the tube is spun down. The supernatant is removed and the precipitate is washed twice with 5% (w/v) trichloroacetic acid, discarding the washings. The proteins in the residue are dissolved in approximately 5 ml of 0.3 N sodium hydroxide with the help of a glass rod and a vortex mixer. Undissolved residues are separated by centrifugation. A small amount of Hyflo Supercel (Fisher H-333) added before centrifugation can help in clarifying the solution. The supernatant is transferred to a 10-ml volumetric flask and made up to volume with 0.2 N sodium hydroxide.

Protein Assay (40)

This is carried out on 0.40-ml aliquots transferred to 10 x 75 mm test tubes. One milliliter of 2% (w/v) sodium carbonate is added and mixed. After 10 minutes, 0.1 ml of Folin-Ciocalteu reagent (Sigma F 9252, previously diluted with an equal volume of water) is added and mixed immediately in a vortex buzzer. A protein standard containing 0.1 mg/ml of bovine serum albumin is carried through the same procedure with the exception that the sodium carbonate reagent used for the study also must contain sodium hydroxide (0.1 N). After 30 minutes the absorbancy is measured at 540 nm in a spectrophotometer. The protein concentration in the sample is calculated taking into account dilutions.

TESTS FOR PANCREATIC EXOCRINE FUNCTION

A deficiency in pancreatic exocrine function can be reflected in malabsorption resulting essentially from a partial breakdown of proteins into peptides and amino acids and an insufficient hydrolysis of fats into absorbable glycerides and fatty acids.

A definitive diagnosis of pancreatic insufficiency should be directly assessed by enzymatic assay of pancreatic enzymes present in the duodenal fluid.

Duodenal fluid is obtained by intubation after an overnight fast. A double- or triple-lumen tube, providing for separate aspiration of gastric and duodenal contents, is passed into the duodenum. Fluoroscopy is used as a guide and the gastric fluid is constantly aspirated. Contamination with gastric secretions, and consequent pH drop will destroy the enzymes and negate the test. This requires constant check of the pH of the fluid, which should be alkaline.

More definitive information can be obtained by stimulation of the pancreas with hormones after the fasting specimen is obtained.

HORMONAL STIMULATION (CHOLECYSTOKININ-PANCREOZYMIN (CCK-PZ))-SECRETIN TEST (41)

Preceding this test, sensitivity to these hormones should be checked by injecting intradermally 0. 1 ml (0. 1 unit each) of CCK-PZ and secretin in separate sites of one forearm. As a control, 0. 1 ml of saline is injected in the other forearm. A positive test is when hyperemia greater than 1 cm diameter or pseudopodia appear in the hormone-injected sites. Patients with a positive skin test should not be given the CCK-PZ or secretin challenges. Once the tube described previously is located in the duodenum of the patient, a fasting specimen is collected for 10-20 minutes. The CCK-PZ (Boots, 2 units/kg) is then administered intramuscularly. Specimens are collected for two 10-minute periods. Secretin (Boots, 2 units/kg) is subsequently administered and the fluid collected for three 10-minute periods. The determination of volume, pH, bicarbonate concentration, and lipase activity are done immediately. Trypsin, chymotrypsin, and amylase can be assayed on frozen samples. All specimens must be collected in ice-cold containers.

The normal ranges for this test are, for duodenal fluid volume: 1. 6-4. 9 ml/kg body weight; bicarbonate concentration: ≥ 70 mEq/L, and total amylase output: $\geq 98,000$ units. In serum, amylase values are expected to be between 80-200 units/dl, and lipase between 0. 08-0. 3 units/dl. Patients with pancreatic insufficiency may have all or most of the preceding values lower than those indicated.

TRYPSIN AND CHYMOTRYPSIN ASSAYS

Trypsin and chymotrypsin can also be assayed in stool. Some of the enzymes are destroyed by bacterial proteolytic activity in the gut, but generally simultaneous determinations of enzymes from stool and duodenal fluid show good correlation (42). Since duodenal intubation is a difficult procedure and poorly tolerated by patients, particularly in the pediatric age group, stool enzymes are usually assayed, and, if abnormal, it may be followed by duodenal intubation, if indicated.

Stool specimens may be either a single random sample or a 24-hour or 72-hour collection (43, 44). Specimens should be refrigerated, not frozen, and the test done as soon as possible. Chymotrypsin is more stable than trypsin and gives fewer false-positive results.

Both enzymes are measured spectrophotometrically (45), or by titrimetry (46). Certain amino acid esters, such as p-toluene-sulfonyl-L-arginine methyl ester (TAME), show substrate specificity for trypsin, in the presence of chymotrypsin. Similarly, benzoyl-L-tyrosine ethyl ester (BTEE) or acetyl-L-tyrosine ethyl ester (ATEE) are specific for chymotrypsin, in the presence of trypsin. Both methods are suitable for the assay of these enzymes in duodenal fluid. The spectrophotometric method is not recommended for stool analysis.

Spectrophotometric Method

A 0. 01-ml aliquot of duodenal fluid, or 0. 01 ml of standard (0. 03 mg/ml trypsin, or 0. 3 mg/ml chymotrypsin in 0. 005 N HCl)is added to 3. 00 ml of buffered substrate (TAME, 0. 87 mM dissolved in 0. 05 M phosphate buffer, pH 8. 0 for trypsin assay, or 0. 5 mM BTEE dissolved in 25% methyl alcohol with 0.08 M TRIS and 0.1 M $CaCl_2$ at pH 7.8 for chymotrypsin). After mixing rapidly, the change in absorbence with time is measured on a recording spectrophotometer for approximately 5 minutes, and the initial rate of reaction is calculated. Trypsin is read at 247 nm; chymotrypsin is read at 253 nm.

Titrimetric Assay of Trypsin and Chymotrypsin

Stool is homogenized with normal saline to give a 1:10 dilution and the pH is adjusted to 9.0.

A volume between 0.025 ml and 2 ml of stool homogenate is mixed with 0.005 M TRIS buffer containing 0.04 M sodium chloride and 0.2 M calcium chloride, adjusted to pH 7.8 with hydrochloric acid and made up to a total volume of 7.5 ml for trypsin determination. TAME 2.5 ml of a 0.1 M solution in TRIS buffer is added and the mixture is adjusted to pH 8.2. Titrations are made at 25°C maintaining the solution at pH 8.2 with sodium hydroxide in concentrations from 0.01 N-0.0025 N depending on the degree of enzymatic activity. The volume of sodium hydroxide delivered is recorded, and tryptic activity is measured as microequivalents of titrant delivered per unit time to maintain a constant pH. This is converted to micrograms of crystalline trypsin, by comparison with a standard curve.

For the assay of chymotrypsin, between 0.025-2 ml of stool homogenate is added to TRIS buffer (0.005 M TRIS containing 0.5 M of sodium chloride and 0.005 M of calcium chloride, adjusted to pH 7.8 with hydrochloric acid) to a total volume of 5 ml of ATEE substrate (0.036 M prepared in 50% methanol and 50% 0.01 M TRIS buffer). Titration is carried out as for trypsin and quantitated from a standard curve (100 mg pure chymotrypsin in 100 ml of 0.005 N hydrochloric acid, and appropriate dilutions).

AMYLASE ASSAY (47)

An aqueous suspension of amylase in phosphate buffer is treated with Cibachron Blue F3GA*, left in contact with the dye at 50°C, and air dried. This mixture is commercially available as Amylochrome (Roche Diagnostics, Div. of Hoffman-La Roche Inc., Nutley, N.J.). The amylase destroys the bond releasing the dye which is quantitated.

A standard curve to estimate dye release is prepared with 0.5, 1.0, 2.0, and 3.0 ml of 0.2 g/L Cibachron Blue F3GA and diluted to 10 ml with an acid buffer (1 M sodium phosphate, pH 4.3). The absorbance is read at 625 nm and a graph is plotted.

For the assay, 200 mg of substrate and 0.8 ml of neutral buffer (0.04 M phosphate buffer pH 7.0 containing 0.02 M of sodium chloride) is added to a test tube. The tube is warmed to 37°C and 0.1 ml of fluid is added with mixing. After 15 minutes incubation at 37°C, 9.1 ml of acid buffer is added. The tube is mixed well, centrifuged and the supernatant's absorbance is measured against a control at 625 nm. The control is identical to the test except that the fluid is added after incubation and addition of the acid buffer. This method is unaffected by bilirubin, and is comparable to other methods frequently used.

Amylase activity, expressed as the quantity of colored product formed in terms of free dye, is obtained by reference to the calibration curve. Normal values for duodenal fluid are 63-500 mg dye/ml.

LIPASE ASSAY (48)

Pancreatic lipase is highly specific for triglycerides and is activated by bile salts at pH 9.0. Pancreatic lipase acts on ester linkages of triglycerides and is activated by bile salts at pH 9.0. The enzyme is measured by the decrease in turbidity of a dilute olive oil emulsion as a result of progressive hydrolysis. The substrate is

---

*Trademark: Ciba Chemical & Drug Co., Fairlawn, NJ

a 7. 5 ml olive oil solution (1% purified olive oil in absolute ethanol) diluted to 500 ml with TRIS buffer (3 g TRIS, 6 g sodium deoxycholic acid in 1 L of water adjusted to pH 8. 8). A 3-ml aliquot of the olive oil emulsion is pipetted into a cuvette and placed in a water bath at 37°C. The solution is warmed to this temperature (approximately 5 minutes), then 0. 05 ml of the duodenal fluid is added. The contents are mixed by inversion. The change in absorbance at 340 nm is recorded for two 1-minute intervals. The absorbance is converted to IU (micromoles per liter per minute) using a standard curve of buffered olive oil emulsion. Normal values for duodenal fluid are 5-267 IU.

DETERMINATION OF BICARBONATE IN DUODENAL FLUID

The acidity of gastric contents is neutralized beyond the pylorus mostly by duodenal and jejunal secretion of bicarbonate. Its concentration is assayed using the Natelson gasometer which measures carbon dioxide content. A 0. 3-ml aliquot of fluid is treated with lactic acid. The carbon dioxide released is measured manometrically (P_1). Sodium hydroxide is used to absorb the carbon dioxide and a second pressure reading is taken (P_2). The difference between the two pressure readings (P_1-P_1) is the carbon dioxide released which is converted to milliequivalents per liter. The lower limit of normal results for maximum bicarbonate (hormonal stimulation) is 70 mEq/L (49).

DETERMINATION OF SWEAT CHLORIDE BY
PILOCARPINE IONTOPHORESIS

In the pediatric age group, the most common cause of malabsorption of pancreatic origin is cystic fibrosis. It is characterized by a reduction in proteolytic and lipolytic enzymes of the pancreas, and an increased salt content of sweat. Both these parameters are employed in the diagnosis of the disease. The "sweat test" is the most widely used indicator for the diagnosis of cystic fibrosis since it is noninvasive and the material easily collectible. A minimum of 100 mg of sweat is required for the test. Lesser amounts tend to give erratic values because of increased procedural error.

An electric current is used to introduce the pilocarpine into the skin (50). The inside of the forearm is usually the area of choice. A 2 x 2 in. gauze saturated with 0.5% pilocarpine nitrate is attached to the positive electrode. A similar gauze dipped in 1% sodium nitrate is the conductor for the negative electrode. The current is slowly increased to 1. 5 mA and maintained for 5-7 minutes. Following iontophoretic stimulation and careful rinsing of the area, a preweighed gauze or filter paper patch is placed on this area, and covered with a polyethylene (Parafilm) layer. This area is sealed with adhesive tape to make it airtight and the patch left in place for about 1 hour. It is then removed and reweighed. As indicated previously, a minimum amount of sweat is required for reliability. A known, accurate volume of deionized water is used as an eluent and an aliquot analyzed for chloride and sodium.

Chloride is most accurately determined with a chloridometer (Buchler Instruments, Fort Lee, NJ) with microsetting and an automatic titrator. Standards in the 0. 5 mEq/L range should be used. In determining sodium, a flame photometer is used and standards in the 10-30 mEq/L range are required. Direct application on the skin of a sodium electrode allows direct estimation of sweat electrolyte content. However, many laboratories still consider this procedure unreliable and lacking consistency of results.

In children, sweat chloride concentrations over 60 mEq/L are diagnostic for cystic fibrosis. Levels between 50-60 mEq/L in the absence of adrenal insufficiency require repeated confirmatory determinations. Most normal children have sweat chloride levels below 30 mEq/L (Fig. 2). Sodium values run up to 20 mEq/L higher than chloride. Newborn infants tend to sweat very little, even with stimula-

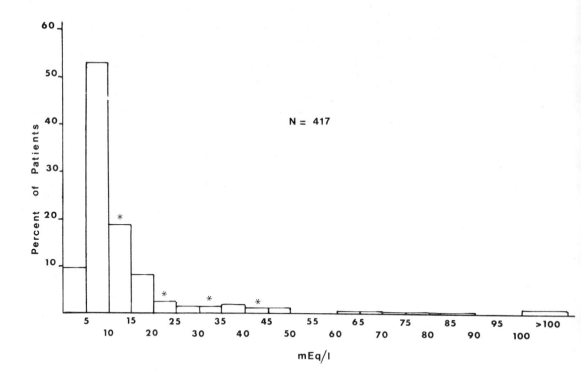

FIGURE 2   Percentage distribution of sweat chloride concentrations in 417 consecutive tests. Sweating was induced by iontophoresis and the samples collected in
gauze pieces. In the groups marked *, one specimen each from parents of patients
with cystic fibrosis is included.

tion. Serial testings at monthly intervals should be carried out on infants suspected
of the disease, or who may have siblings with the disease.

The overnight collection of sweat in patients admitted into hospitals is often
fraught with additional problems. The estimation of sodium in hair and nail clip-
pings for diagnostic value has only marginal utility.

More important is the estimation of albumin in the soluble proteins of meconium.
It is known that about 10% of infants who develop cystic fibrosis have meconium
ileum requiring surgical intervention. The composition of their meconium is abnormal, containing large concentrations of serum proteins, albumin in particular
(51). By immunological complement-fixation techniques (52) it has been shown
that, in normal infants, the proportion of albumin in the soluble proteins of meconium is less than 1%, while in infants with cystic fibrosis the mean concentration
of albumin in meconium is ten times higher.

The desirability of mass screening of newborns by determination of meconium
albumin, or meconium lactase, has been recently advised by some investigators
(53). However, the present state of the art entails an unacceptable proportion of
false-positive results. Since all the previously mentioned determinations do not
reflect directly the yet undetermined basic metabolic defect, early screening by
this procedure has been discouraged (54).

REFERENCES

1. Lifshitz, F.: Clinical studies in diarrheal disease and malnutrition associated with carbohydrate intolerance. Proc. 9th Int. Cong Nutr., Mexico, 1972, S. Karger, Basel, 1975, p. 173.

2. Kallen, R. J., and F. Burg: An electronic aid for timing urine collection periods in non-catheterized infants. Pediatrics 34:703, 1964.

3. Lindquist, B. L., and L. Wranne: Problems in analysis of faecal sugar. Arch Dis Child 51:319, 1976.

4. Smith, I. (ed.): Chromatographic and Electrophoretic Techniques, Vol. 1. Chromatography, 2nd ed. Interscience Publishers, New York, 1960, p. 246.

5. Randerath, K.: Thin Layer Chromatography, 2nd ed. Academic Press, New York, 1966, p. 235.

6. Mabry, C. C., J. D. Gryboski, and E. A. Karam: Rapid identification and measurement of mono- and oligosaccharides: An adaptation of high-voltage paper electrophoresis for sugars and its application to biologic materials. J Lab Clin Med 62:817, 1963.

7. Kerry, K. R., and C. M. Anderson: A ward test for sugar in feces. Lancet 1:981, 1964.

8. Oser, B. L., (ed): Hawk's Physiological Chemistry, 14th ed. McGraw-Hill Book Co., New York, 1965, p. 1210.

9. Barker, S. B., and W. H. Summerson. Colorimetric determination of lactic acid in biological material. J Biol Chem 138:535, 1941.

10. Sammons, H. G., D. B. Morgan, A. C. Frazer, R. D. Montgomery, W. M. Philip, and M. J. Phillips: Modification in the xylose absorption test as an index of intestinal function. Gut 8:348, 1967.

11. Hawkins, K. I.: Pediatric xylose absorption test: Measurements in blood preferable to measurements in urine. Clin Chem 16:749, 1970.

12. Hindmarsh, J. T.: Xylose absorption and its clinical significance. Clin Biochem 9:141, 1976.

13. Dahlqvist, A.: The intestinal disaccharidases and disaccharide intolerance. Gastroenterology 43:694, 1962.

14. Dahlqvist, A.: Method for assay of intestinal disaccharidases. Anal Biochem 7:18, 1964.

15. Sunshine, P., and N. Kretchmer: Studies of small intestine during development. Infantile diarrhea associated with intolerance to disaccharides. Pediatrics 34:38, 1964.

16. Townley, R. R. W.: Disaccharidase deficiency in infancy and childhood. Pediatrics 38:127, 1966.

17. Huang, S. , and T. M. Bayless: Lactose intolerance in healthy children. N Engl J Med 276:1283, 1967.

18. Newcomer, A. D. , and D. B. McGill: Disaccharidase activity in the small intestine: Prevalence of lactase deficiency in 100 healthy subjects. Gastroenterology 53:881, 1967.

19. Torres-Pinedo, R. , C. Rivera, and S. Garcia-Castiñeiras: Intestinal exfoliated cells in infants: A system for study of microvillus particles. Gastroenterology 66:1154, 1974.

20. Kidder, D. E. , and M. J. Manners: A method for automatic measurement of lactase and sucrase. Clin. Chim. Acta 61:233, 1975.

21. Newcomer, A. D. , D. B. McGill, P. J. Thomas, and A. F. Hofman: Prospective comparison of indirect methods for detecting lactase deficiency. N Engl J Med 293:1232, 1975.

22. Peters, T. J. , R. M. Batt, J. R. Heath, and J. Tilleray: The microassay of intestinal disaccharidases. Biochem Med 15:145, 1976.

23. Gray, G. M. , K. A. Conklin and R. R. W. Townley: Sucrase-isomaltase deficiency. N Engl J Med 294:750, 1976.

24. Basford, R. L. , and J. B. Henry: Lactose intolerance in the adult. Postgrad Med 41A:70, 1971.

25. McGill, D. B. , and A. D. Newcomer: Comparison of venous and capillary blood samples in lactose tolerance testing. Gastroenterology 53:371, 1967.

26. Solomons, N. W. , F. E. Viteri, and L. H. Hamilton: Application of a simple gas chromatographic technique for measuring breath hydrogen. J Lab Clin Med 90:856, 1977.

27. Rhodes, J. M. , P. Middleton, and D. P. Jewell: The lactulose hydrogen test as a diagnostic test for small-bowel bacterial overgrowth. Scand J Gastroenterol 14:336, 1979.

28. Van de Kamer, J. H. , H. ten Bokkel Huinink, and H. A. Weijers: A rapid method for the determination of fat in faeces. J Biol Chem 177:347, 1949.

29. Massion, C. G. , and M. S. McNeely: Accurate micromethod for estimation of both medium and long-chain fatty acids and triglycerides in fecal fat. Clin Chem 19:499, 1973.

30. Patterson, J. C. S. , and H. S. Wiggins: Estimation of plasma vitamin A and vitamin A absorption. J Clin Pathol 7:56, 1954.

31. Iwata, T. , and K. Yamasaki: Enzymatic determination and thin layer chromatography of bile acids in blood. J Biochem 56:424, 1964.

32. Weber, A. M. , L. Chartland, G. Doyan, S. Gordon, and C. C. Roy: The quantitative determination of fecal bile acids in children by the enzymatic method. Clin Chim Acta 39:524, 1972.

33. Goswami, S. K. , and C. F. Frey: A novel method for the separation and iden-
     tification of bile acids and phospholipids of bile on thin layer chromato-
     grams. J Chromatog 89:87, 1974.

34. Ali, S. S. , and N. B. Javitt: Quantitative estimation of bile salts in serum.
     Can J Biochem 48:1054, 1970.

35. Jonas, A. , S. Weiser, P. Segal, and D. Katznelson: Oral fat loading test.
     A reliable procedure for the study of fat malabsorption in children. Arch
     Dis Child 54:770, 1979.

36. Waldmann, T. A. : Protein-losing enteropathy. Gastroenterology 50:422,
     1966.

37. Waldmann, T. A. : Gastrointestinal protein loss demonstrated by ^{51}Cr label-
     led albumin. Lancet 2:121, 1961.

38. Waldmann, T. A. , A. G. Morell, R. D. Wochner, and I. Sternlieb: Quanti-
     tation of gastrointestinal protein loss with copper 67-labelled ceruloplas-
     min. J Clin Invest 44:1107, 1965.

39. Ghadimi, H. , S. Kumar, and F. Abaci. Endogenous amino acid loss and
     its significance in infantile diarrhea. Pediatr Res 7:161, 1973.

40. Lowry, O. H. , N. J. Rosebrough, A. L. Farr, and R. J. Randall: Protein
     measurement with the Folin phenol reagent. J Biol Chem 193:265, 1951.

41. Hadorn, B. , G. Zoppi, D. Shmerling, A. Prader, I. McIntire, and C. M.
     Anderson: Quantitative assessment of exocrine pancreatic function in infants
     and children. J Pediatr 73:39, 1968.

42. Sacks, H. , S. Bank, I. Kramer, B. Novis, and I. N. Marks: A comparison
     between spectrophotometric and titrimetric methods of estimating trypsin.
     Gut 12:727, 1971.

43. Ammann, R. W. , E. Tagwercher, H. Kashiwagi, and H. Rosenmund: Di-
     agnostic value of fecal chymotrypsin and trypsin assessment for detection
     of pancreatic disease. Am J Dig Dis 13:123, 1968.

44. Bonin, A. , C. C. Roy, R. Lasalle, A. Weber, and C. L. Morin: Fecal
     chymotrypsin. A reliable index of exocrine pancreatic function in children.
     J Pediatr 83:594, 1973.

45. Schwert, G. W. , and Y. Takenaka: A spectrophotometric determination of
     trypsin and chymotrypsin. Biochim Biophys Acta 16:570, 1955.

46. Haverback, B. J. , B. J. Dyce, P. J. Gutentag, and D. W. Montgomery:
     Measurement of chymotrypsin in stool. Gastroenterology 44:588, 1963.

47. Klein, B. , J. A. Foreman, and R. L. Searcy: New chromogenic substrate
     for determination of serum amylase activity. Clin Chem 16:32, 1970.

48. Shihabi, Z. K. , and C. Bishop: Simplified turbidimetric assay for lipase
     activity. Clin Chem 17:1150, 1971,

49. Natelson, S.: Techniques of Clinical Chemistry, 3rd ed. Charles C Thomas, Springfield, IL, 1971, p. 220.

50. Gibson, L. E., and R. E. Cooke: Test for concentration of electrolytes in sweat in cystic fibrosis of pancreas utilizing pilocarpine by iontophoresis. Pediatrics 23:545, 1959.

51. Green, M. N., J. T. Clarke, and H. Shwachman: Studies in cystic fibrosis of the pancreas: Protein pattern in meconium ileus. Pediatrics 21:635, 1958.

52. Rule, A. H., D. T. Baran, and H. Shwachman. Quantitative determination of water-soluble proteins in meconium. Pediatrics 45:847, 1970.

53. Berry, H. K., F. W. Kellogg, S. R. Lichstein, and R. L. Ingberg: Elevated meconium lactase activity. Its use as a screening test for cystic fibrosis. Am J Dis Child 134:930, 1980.

54. Gibson, L. E.: Screening of newborns for cystic fibrosis. Am J Dis Child 134:925, 1980.

BOOKS OF RELATED INTEREST:

HANDBOOK OF GASTROINTESTINAL EMERGENCIES
 edited by Gary Gitnick, M.D.
  $27.50--paperbound 1982 #057
PEDIATRIC GASTROENTEROLOGY CASE STUDIES
 by William Liebman, M.D.
  $23.00--paperbound 1980 #084
PEDIATRIC HEPATOLOGY--Medical Outline Series
 by A.R. Colón, M.D.
  About $30.00--paperbound 1982 #407
GASTROENTEROLOGY--Specialty Board Review, Second Edition
 by William A. Sodeman, Jr., M.D., and Thomas A. Saladin, M.D.
  $27.50--paperbound 1981 #316
Medical Examination Review--Volume 34:GASTROENTEROLOGY,
Fourth Edition
 by Lawrence D. Wruble, M.D., Myron Lewis, M.D., and
 Michael Levinson, M.D.
  $23.50--paperbound 1982 #141

MEDICAL EXAMINATION PUBLISHING CO., INC.
an Excerpta Medica company
3003 New Hyde Park Road
New Hyde Park, New York 11040

IBP

ORDER ON APPROVAL

If not completely satisfied, I may return the book(s) within 30 days for a credit
or refund.

Please print your selection(s):

quantity	code #	author	title		price
				@	
				@	
				@	

ALL PRICES SUBJECT TO CHANGE

☐ To save shipping and handling charges, my check is enclosed. (New York
 residents, please add sales tax.)
☐ Bill me. I will remit payment within the 30-day approval period, including
 mailing charges.

NAME _____

ADDRESS _____

CITY _____ STATE _____ ZIP _____

SIGNATURE _____

AVAILABLE AT BOOKSTORES OR BY USING THIS COUPON

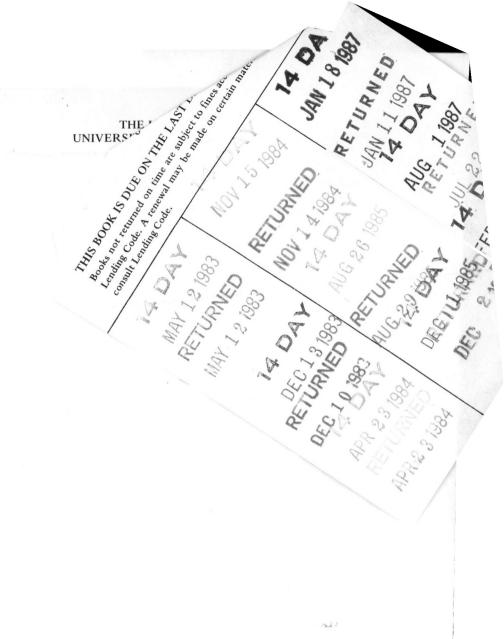